to Accompany Nelson Textbook of Pediatrics, 16th Ed.

Pediatric Decision-Making Strategies to Accompany Nelson Textbook of Pediatrics, 16th Ed.

Albert J. Pomeranz, MD
Associate Professor of Pediatrics
Medical College of Wisconsin
Department of Pediatrics
Children's Hospital of Wisconsin
Milwaukee, Wisconsin

Sharon L. Busey, MD
Assistant Professor of Pediatrics
Medical College of Wisconsin
Department of Pediatrics
Children's Hospital of Wisconsin
Milwaukee, Wisconsin

Svapna Sabnis, MD
Assistant Professor of Pediatrics
Medical College of Wisconsin
Department of Pediatrics
Children's Hospital of Wisconsin
Milwaukee, Wisconsin

Richard E. Behrman, MD
Clinical Professor of Pediatrics
Stanford University School of Medicine and
University of California, San Francisco,
School of Medicine
Senior Vice-President for Medical Affairs
The Lucile Packard Foundation
for Children's Health
Palo Alto, California

Robert M. Kliegman, MD
Professor and Chair
Department of Pediatrics
Medical College of Wisconsin
Pediatrician-in-Chief
Children's Hospital of Wisconsin
Milwaukee, Wisconsin

An Imprint of Elsevier
SAUNDERS

The Curtis Center
Independence Square West
Philadelphia, Pennsylvania 19106

Library of Congress Cataloging-in-Publication Data

Pediatric decision-making strategies to accompany Nelson textbook of pediatrics, 16th ed. / Albert Pomeranz . . . [et al.].

p.   cm.

ISBN 0–7216–8246–4

1. Pediatrics—Decision making.   2. Pediatrics.   I. Title: Pediatric decision making strategies.   II. Pomeranz, Albert.
   [DNLM: 1. Pediatrics.   2. Diagnosis.   WS 200 N432 2002]

RJ47.N45 2002

618.92—dc21   2001032080

Editor-in-Chief: Richard Zorab
Acquisitions Editor: Judith Fletcher
Production Manager: Frank Morales
Illustration Specialist: Peg Shaw

PEDIATRIC DECISION-MAKING STRATEGIES
TO ACCOMPANY NELSON TEXTBOOK OF PEDIATRICS, 16th Ed.   ISBN 0–7216–8246–4

Permissions may be sought directly from Elsevier's Health Sciences Rights Department in Philadelphia, USA: phone: (+1)215-238-7869, fax: (+1)215-238-2239, email: healthpermissions@elsevier.com. You may also complete your request on-line via the Elsevier Science homepage (http://www.elsevier.com), by selecting 'Customer Support' and then 'Obtaining Permissions'.
Printed in the United States of America.

Last digit is the print number: 9   8   7   6   5   4   3

To Emily and Kate
AP

To Craig
SB

To Nishant and Samir
SS

To Steve Koeff, MD, a kind and loving person—the greatest role model a student of medicine could have
AP

PREFACE

Pediatric Decision-Making Strategies to Accompany Nelson Textbook of Pediatrics was written with the purpose of assisting the student, house officer, and clinician in the evaluation of common pediatric signs and symptoms and abnormal laboratory findings. The algorithmic format allows for a rapid and concise, step-wise approach to a diagnosis. The text accompanying each algorithm helps to clarify certain approaches and to supply additional useful information regarding the steps leading to a differential diagnosis and eventually a diagnosis. For more detailed information about the manifestations of the diseases discussed, each algorithm is cross-referenced to the corresponding chapters in *Nelson Textbook of Pediatrics* and *Practical Strategies in Pediatric Diagnosis and Therapy*.

The information in this book is the most up-to-date information available. The literature has been extensively reviewed, and most of the algorithms have been discussed with the appropriate specialists. We believe that we have created algorithms that are easy to follow, yet complete and accurate. We realize that not all diagnoses fit neatly into algorithms, nor can any one algorithm be all-inclusive or demonstrate the only approach to a problem. However, we hope that our logical step-wise approach promotes consideration, in a time efficient manner, of reasonable differential diagnoses for the common clinical problems discussed. This task could not have been completed without the generous help of many of the faculty members at the Medical College of Wisconsin and Children's Hospital of Wisconsin.

ACKNOWLEDGMENTS

We wish to thank the many physicians and staff at the Medical College of Wisconsin and Children's Hospital of Wisconsin who were subjected to the multitude of questions we asked to ensure the accuracy and completeness of this text. They have all been extremely helpful and patient. In particular, we would like to extend special thanks to the following faculty members for their help on chapters related to their specialties: Laurence Greenbaum for Fluids and Electrolytes and Genitourinary System; Arnold Slyper for Endocrine System; Jay Nocton for Musculoskeletal System; Lee Rusakow for Respiratory System; Cheryl Hillery and John Paul Scott for Hematology; David Walsh for Neurology; Michael J. Chusid for Infectious Disease; Mark Ruttum for Ophthalmology; and Steven Matson for Genitourinary System.

We also wish to thank Carolyn Redman for editorial assistance at the Medical College of Wisconsin and Lisette Bralow and Judith Fletcher at the W.B. Saunders Company for all of their support and encouragement. We are thankful for the opportunity to create a text we hope will be useful to health-care workers in promoting the health of our children.

ABBREVIATIONS

ABG	arterial blood gases	EMG	electromyogram	PCR	polymerase chain reaction
ALT	alanine aminotransferase	ENT	ear, nose, and throat	PPD	purified protein derivative (of tuber-culin)
ALTE	apparent life-threatening event	ESR	erythrocyte sedimentation rate		
ANA	antinuclear antibody	FSH	follicle-stimulating hormone	PT	prothombin time
AP	anteroposterior	GER	gastroesophageal reflux	PTT	partial thromboplastin time
ARF	acute rheumatic fever	GGT	γ-glutamyl transferase	RBC	red blood cell
AST	aspartate aminotransferase	GI	gastrointestinal	RF	rheumatoid factor
AVN	avascular necrosis	GU	genitourinary	RSV	respiratory syncytial virus
BP	blood pressure	H and P	history and physical	RTA	renal tubular acidosis
BUN	blood urea nitrogen	HEENT	head, eyes, ears, nose, and throat	SCIWORA	spinal cord injury in the absence of radiographic abnormalities
CBC	complete blood count	Hgb	hemoglobin		
CMV	cytomegalovirus	HIV	human immunodeficiency virus	SI	sacroiliac
CNS	central nervous system	I and D	incision and drainage	Sp gr	specific gravity
Cr	creatinine	ICP	intracranial pressure	s/p	status/post
CRP	C-reactive protein	IV	intravenous	T_4	thyroxine
CSF	cerebrospinal fluid	JRA	juvenile rheumatoid arthritis	Td	tetanus-diphtheria toxid
CT	computed tomography	KUB	kidney, ureter, bladder (X-ray study)	TSH	thyroid-stimulating hormone
CXR	chest X-ray	LFT	liver function test	UA	urinalysis
DTP	diphtheria-tetanus-pertussis	LH	luteinizing hormone	UGI	upper gastrointestinal series
EBV	Epstein-Barr virus	LP	lumbar puncture	URI	upper respiratoy infection
ECF	extracellular fluid	MRI	magnetic resonance imaging	US	ultrasound
EEG	electroencephalogram	O&P	ova and parasites	UTI	urinary tract infection
EKG	electrocardiogram	OM	otitis media	WBC	white blood cell

CONTENTS

HEAD, NECK, AND EYES

Chapter 1 **Ear Pain**

Ear pain is common, particularly in the first few years of life. Acute otitis media (AOM) accounts for most cases. Eighty-five percent of children have at least one episode of AOM by the age of 3 years.

(1) Signs of AOM may be nonspecific in the child less than 2 years (e.g., fever, irritability, vomiting). Ear tugging is not a specific sign. It is unusual to have AOM without preceding or concomitant upper respiratory symptoms. The presence of a middle ear effusion is most accurately predicted by determining altered mobility of the tympanic membrane (TM) with an insufflator.

(2) AOM is the diagnosis when the examination reveals an inflammatory drum or a yellow or white effusion behind the TM. About two thirds of AOM episodes are a result of bacterial infection. The major pathogens are *Streptococcus pneumoniae*, nontypable *Haemophilus influenzae,* and *Moraxella catarrhalis.* Inappropriate diagnosis of AOM contributes to the overuse of antibiotics and the serious problem of antimicrobial resistance.

(3) With periostitis, infection within the mastoid air cells has spread to the periosteum that covers the mastoid process. Further spread of infection results in osteitis, which involves destruction of mastoid air cells and abscess formation. Resultant swelling is often severe enough to cause outward displacement of the pinna.

(4) Otitis media with effusion (OME) is the presence of fluid in the middle ear space without signs of inflammation or infection. It is commonly associated with upper respiratory infection or a successfully treated AOM. OME should, in general, not be treated with antibiotics. Mild discomfort or a feeling of "fullness" is not unusual. Diagnosis can be aided by the use of tympanometry and acoustic reflectometry. These diagnostic tools determine the presence or absence of effusion but not infection.

(5) Cholesteatoma is related to negative middle ear pressure, retraction pockets, and AOM. The increasing size of the tumor results in destruction of the middle ear and temporal bone in addition to intracranial spread.

(6) The main clue to the diagnosis of a furuncle in the canal, although uncommon, is the severe pain elicited when the otoscope tip is placed in the canal. The canal appears generally normal except for the erythematous papule or pustule.

(7) The canal is protected by the waxy, water-repellent coating (cerumen). Excessive wetness or trauma or various skin dermatoses (e.g., eczema) can disrupt this cerumen. Frequent water exposure (e.g., swimming), hearing aids, eczematous skin lesions, and aggressive use of cotton-tipped swabs or other devices in the canal are risks for development of otitis externa. Edema, erythema, and discharge are common. Occasionally, the disease is due to drainage from a perforated tympanic membrane or to infection in the presence of tympanostomy tubes. The moist, irritant nature of the purulent drainage results in superinfection from bacterial colonization. Pathogens include *Pseudomonas aeruginosa, Staphylococcus aureus,* other gram-negative organisms, and occasionally fungi.

BIBLIOGRAPHY

Bluestone CD, Stool SE, Kenna MA: Pediatric Otolaryngology, 3rd ed, pp 388–582. Philadelphia, WB Saunders Company, 1996.

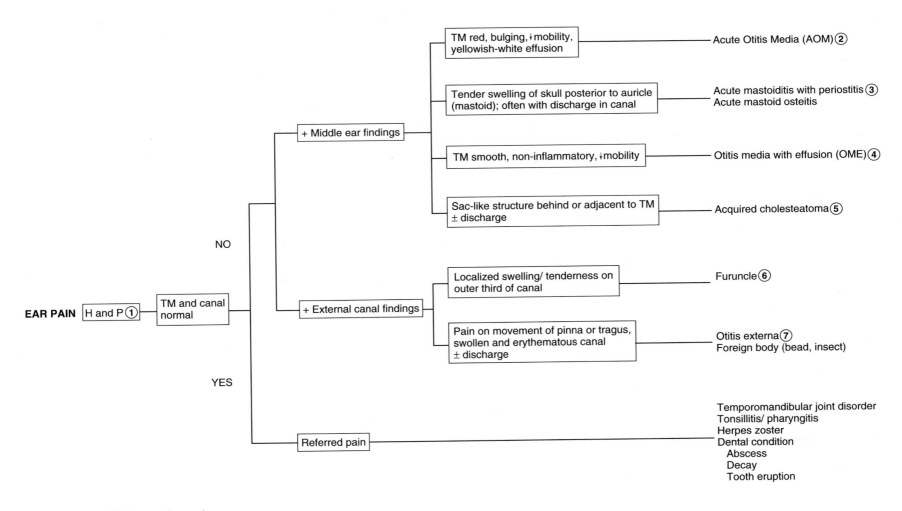

EAR PAIN | H and P ① | → TM and canal normal

NO

+ Middle ear findings
- TM red, bulging, ↓mobility, yellowish-white effusion —— Acute Otitis Media (AOM) ②
- Tender swelling of skull posterior to auricle (mastoid); often with discharge in canal —— Acute mastoiditis with periostitis ③ / Acute mastoid osteitis
- TM smooth, non-inflammatory, ↓mobility —— Otitis media with effusion (OME) ④
- Sac-like structure behind or adjacent to TM ± discharge —— Acquired cholesteatoma ⑤

+ External canal findings
- Localized swelling/ tenderness on outer third of canal —— Furuncle ⑥
- Pain on movement of pinna or tragus, swollen and erythematous canal ± discharge —— Otitis externa ⑦ / Foreign body (bead, insect)

YES

Referred pain —— Temporomandibular joint disorder / Tonsillitis/ pharyngitis / Herpes zoster / Dental condition /   Abscess /   Decay /   Tooth eruption

TM= tympanic membrane

Nelson chapters 645, 646
Practical Strategies chapter 9

Rhinorrhea is a common complaint in childhood. It is most frequently due to a viral upper respiratory infection but must be distinguished from allergies and other less common etiologies.

(1) A careful head, eyes, ears, nose, and throat (HEENT) examination is essential. Stigmata suggestive of genetic syndromes should be noted because congenital nasal anomalies (e.g., atresia, stenosis, hypoplasia) are frequently associated with other anomalies. Examination of the nose should include the appearance of the mucosa (e.g., swelling, pallor, erythema, degree of patency), character of the secretions, and presence of any obvious obstructing lesions (e.g., polyps, foreign bodies).

(2) Viral nasopharyngitis or the "common cold" is the most common cause of rhinorrhea. The nasal mucosa is usually inflamed and erythematous. Secretions are normally thin and watery initially and gradually become thicker and purulent.

(3) Rarely, an acute form of sinusitis can occur with a short duration of severe symptoms (e.g., high fever, purulent rhinorrhea, headache, and swelling of the eyes).

(4) The vasomotor responses of increased secretion and mucosal swelling are the normal responses of the nasal mucosa to a variety of stimuli. External stimuli (e.g., cold temperature, change in humidity, cigarette smoke, spicy food) are the most common. The autonomic system response, hormones, and stress are other triggers.

(5) Bronchiolitis, roseola infantum, measles, mononucleosis, hepatitis, pertussis, and erythema infectiosum may appear with a prodromal, acute watery rhinorrhea.

(6) Cerebrospinal fluid (CSF) of rhinorrhea is clear and usually unilateral, and it may vary noticeably with a change in head position, Valsalva maneuver, or jugular compression. Detection of glucose (50 mg/100 ml or higher) in the fluid is highly suggestive. The condition may occur acutely with head trauma or chronically with congenital conditions (e.g., fistulas, encephaloceles) or tumors.

(7) Allergic rhinitis is an IgE-mediated condition that may be seasonal (e.g., hay fever) or perennial. The nasal mucosa is typically boggy and pale or bluish. The rhinorrhea is clear and watery. Other allergic signs and symptoms, such as upward rubbing of the nose (allergic salute, allergic shiners, sneezing, eye symptoms) are common. Atopic disorders may be present (e.g., asthma, eczema). Fever suggests an alternative (infectious) diagnosis.

(8) Foreign bodies usually have a unilateral foul-smelling, purulent or bloody discharge.

(9) When the clinical course and examination are not specific for a diagnosis, especially when considering sinusitis versus allergic rhinitis, a microscopic examination of the nasal secretions may be helpful. An eosin-methylene blue stain of these secretions can help to identify eosinophils, white blood cells (WBCs), and bacteria. A predominance of WBCs and bacteria suggests sinusitis, and at least 5% eosinophils suggests allergic rhinitis. The two diseases may occur together.

(10) Clinical diagnosis of sinusitis is made by findings of prolonged symptoms of rhinorrhea and cough without improvement for more than 10 to 14 days. Other suggestive symptoms include halitosis, fever, nocturnal cough, and postnasal drip. Older children may have headache, facial pain, tooth pain, and periorbital swelling. A limited CT scan of the sinuses is the preferred imaging test when the diagnosis is unclear.

(11) Rhinitis medicamentosa results from overuse of vasoconstrictor nose drops or sprays. A rapid toxic reaction of the nasal mucosa causes the rebound swelling and obstruction.

(12) Cocaine, marijuana, and inhaled solvents may result in mucoid or purulent rhinorrhea. Medications causing rhinorrhea include hormones, aspirin, iodide, and bromides. The syndrome of nasal polyps, asthma, and aspirin intolerance is called **triad asthma**.

(13) Symptoms of nasal obstruction with increasing frequency of episodes of epistaxis, particularly unilateral, in boys are suggestive of juvenile nasopharyngeal angiofibroma.

(14) Infants with congenital syphilis may present between the second week and third month of life with a watery nasal discharge that progresses to a mucopurulent or bloody discharge. Significant obstruction results in noisy breathing ("snuffles"). Chronic mucopurulent rhinorrhea, septal perforation, and saddle nose deformity are late complications. Serologic tests for treponemal antibodies and specimens for dark field microscopy examination should be obtained whenever this diagnosis is suspected.

(15) Bilateral choanal atresia occurs early in the newborn period with respiratory distress. Unilateral choanal atresia appears later with chronic unilateral rhinorrhea that can be clear or purulent. Feeding difficulties are also common since most newborns are nose breathers. Inability to pass a nasal catheter suggests this diagnosis. An ENT consultation should be obtained whenever choanal atresia is suspected.

BIBLIOGRAPHY

Belenky WM, Madgy DN: Nasal obstruction and rhinorrhea. In Bluestone CD, Stool SE, Kenna MA (eds): Pediatric Otolaryngology, 3rd ed, p 765. Philadelphia, WB Saunders Company, 1996.

RHINORRHEA

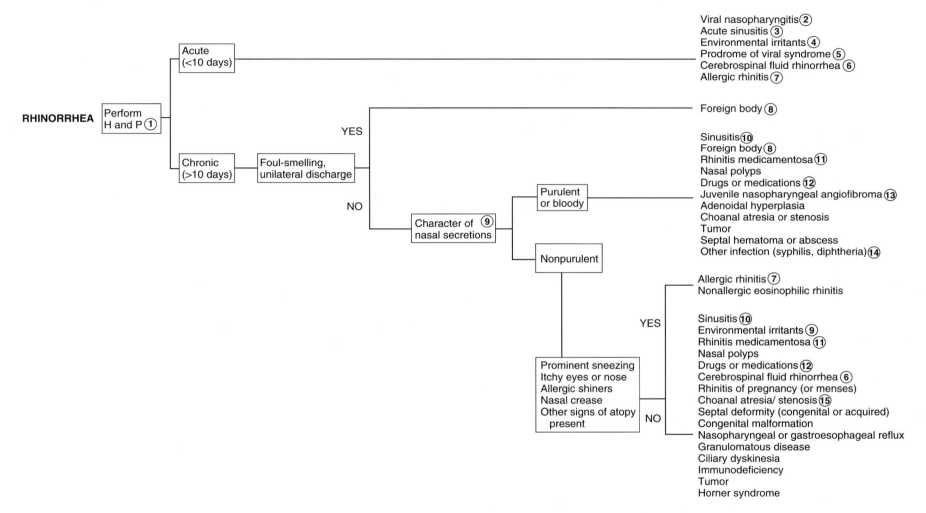

Perform H and P ①

Acute (<10 days)

Viral nasopharyngitis ②
Acute sinusitis ③
Environmental irritants ④
Prodrome of viral syndrome ⑤
Cerebrospinal fluid rhinorrhea ⑥
Allergic rhinitis ⑦

Chronic (>10 days)

Foul-smelling, unilateral discharge

YES

Foreign body ⑧

NO

Character of nasal secretions ⑨

Purulent or bloody

Sinusitis ⑩
Foreign body ⑧
Rhinitis medicamentosa ⑪
Nasal polyps
Drugs or medications ⑫
Juvenile nasopharyngeal angiofibroma ⑬
Adenoidal hyperplasia
Choanal atresia or stenosis
Tumor
Septal hematoma or abscess
Other infection (syphilis, diphtheria) ⑭

Nonpurulent

Prominent sneezing
Itchy eyes or nose
Allergic shiners
Nasal crease
Other signs of atopy present

YES

Allergic rhinitis ⑦
Nonallergic eosinophilic rhinitis

NO

Sinusitis ⑩
Environmental irritants ⑨
Rhinitis medicamentosa ⑪
Nasal polyps
Drugs or medications ⑫
Cerebrospinal fluid rhinorrhea ⑥
Rhinitis of pregnancy (or menses)
Choanal atresia/ stenosis ⑮
Septal deformity (congenital or acquired)
Congenital malformation
Nasopharyngeal or gastroesophageal reflux
Granulomatous disease
Ciliary dyskinesia
Immunodeficiency
Tumor
Horner syndrome

Nelson chapters 144, 381
Practical Strategies chapter 7

Most sore throats are benign, self-limiting viral illnesses. The practitioner should always consider the likelihood of group A β-hemolytic streptococcus *(S. pyogenes)*, which is important to identify and treat because of its potentially serious complications. Other less common causes should be considered when symptoms are worrisome or prolonged.

(1) A history of exposure to a family member or classmate with a cold or documented group A streptococcal infection is helpful. A history of sexual activity or abuse should raise the suspicion for pharyngeal gonococcal infection.

The degree of pharyngeal inflammation is not always consistent with the severity of the complaint. Tonsillar exudates are suggestive of streptococcus but also of mononucleosis and adenovirus. Many patients with streptococcal pharyngitis have only mild erythema without tonsillar enlargement or exudates. Small ulcers or vesicles on the soft palate suggest a viral etiology.

Associated symptoms of stridor, drooling, and air hunger or an unwillingness to recline suggests impending airway obstruction. The patient warrants emergent management for airway stabilization and treatment for potentially life-threatening conditions such as epiglottitis and retropharyngeal abscess. (See also Ch. 12.)

(2) Group A streptococcal pharyngitis is most common between 5 and 11 years of age and unlikely under 2 years of age. The occurrence of conjunctivitis, rhinitis, cough, and hoarseness is more indicative of a virus than group A streptococcus. Significant diarrhea also makes streptococcal disease unlikely.

(3) Even when the clinical picture is highly suggestive of streptococcal pharyngitis, laboratory confirmation is strongly recommended. Rapid antigen detection tests (RST) are highly specific with sensitivities from 85% to 95%. Throat cultures are the standard for diagnosis whenever the RST results are negative. The RST and the most commonly used culture methods do not identify organisms other than group A streptococcus. In cases in which another family member has a positive culture finding, or in which a typical scarlatina rash is present, group A streptococcus should still be considered despite negative test results.

(4) Scarlet fever is the occurrence of group A streptococcal pharyngitis with a characteristic sandpaper-like blanching erythematous rash. The rash begins on the face, affecting primarily the cheeks (resulting in circumoral pallor) then generalizes. The erythema is accentuated in flexor creases (Pastia signs). Desquamation typically begins within a week of onset and progresses in a cephalad to caudad direction. This is a normal sequela even in treated patients. The desquamation may be especially noticeable around the fingernails. Treatment of group A streptococcal disease is indicated to relieve symptoms and to prevent rheumatic fever.

(5) Viral pharyngitis is most commonly accompanied by "common cold" symptoms such as rhinitis and cough. The most common etiologies are rhinovirus, coronavirus, adenovirus, and enterovirus. Viral pharyngitis is usually gradual in onset with early signs of fever, malaise, and anorexia generally preceding the sore throat.

(6) Adenovirus may cause an exudative pharyngitis. Diarrhea and conjunctivitis are also common.

(7) Coxsackie A16 is responsible for hand-foot-mouth disease, a characteristic outbreak of vesicles on the palms and soles with accompanying ulcerating vesicles throughout the oropharynx. Herpangina is a disorder characterized by discrete painful vesicular lesions of the posterior pharynx and fever. It is caused by Coxsackie virus A and B, echovirus, and occasionally herpes simplex virus.

(8) Primary herpes simplex virus infection can cause gingivostomatitis characterized by painful ulcerating vesicles in the anterior portion of the oral cavity, including the lips. An exudative tonsillitis may occur. Fevers and impaired fluid intake are common. Herpetic gingivostomatitis may last up to 2 weeks.

(9) Pharyngitis characterized by intense erythema but absent tonsillar enlargement or exudate is an early finding in measles. Fever, cough, coryza, conjunctivitis, and Koplik spots (i.e., blue-white enanthem on the buccal mucosa) suggest the diagnosis.

(10) Although non-group A streptococci have been implicated in pharyngitis, they cause a self-limiting illness, are not associated with complications, and require no treatment.

(11) Other bacteria have occasionally been implicated in pharyngitis: *Staphylococcus aureus, Streptococcus pneumoniae, Haemophilus influenzae, Moraxella catarrhalis,* and *Arcanobacterium haemolyticum.* The etiologic role of *Chlamydia* (both *C. trachomatis* and *C. pneumoniae*) and *Mycoplasma pneumoniae* in pharyngitis is controversial.

(12) A severe exudative pharyngitis is often a manifestation of infectious mononucleosis. Patients experience an abrupt onset of fatigue, malaise, fever, and headache preceding the pharyngitis. Hepatosplenomegaly and generalized lymphadenopathy are common. Preadolescents tend to have milder symptoms than adolescents and young adults. Atypical lymphocytosis is suggestive of the disorder, and a positive "monospot" (heterophile antibody test) finding confirms EBV mononucleosis. The test is not considered reliable in children younger than 5 years of age because of a low titer of heterophile antibody. EBV serology should be used in young patients or in patients with heterophile negative cases. CMV serology should also be considered as CMV causes approximately 5% to 10% of cases.

(13) *Corynebacterium diphtheriae* is a rare but serious cause of pharyngitis. The disease is suggested by a systemic illness and grayish membrane over the tonsils and pharyngeal walls. It should be suspected in unimmunized persons or in persons from underdeveloped countries. Culture of the organism and confirmation of its toxin are necessary to confirm the diagnosis.

14 *Arcanobacterium haemolyticum* causes a scarlet fever–like illness but requires special

culture methods. It is not routinely sought in the evaluation of pharyngitis.

15 Immunocompromised patients are at risk for fungal oropharyngeal infections. *Candida* is the most common pathogen. Diagnosis is made by examination of a specimen treated with potassium hydroxide or by culture.

16 Agranulocytosis may manifest as a pharyngitis with a white or yellow exudate with underlying necrosis and ulceration.

BIBLIOGRAPHY

Kenna MA: Sore throat in children. In Bluestone CD, Stool SE, Kenna MA (eds): Pediatric Otolaryngology, 3rd ed, p 958. Philadelphia, WB Saunders Company, 1996.

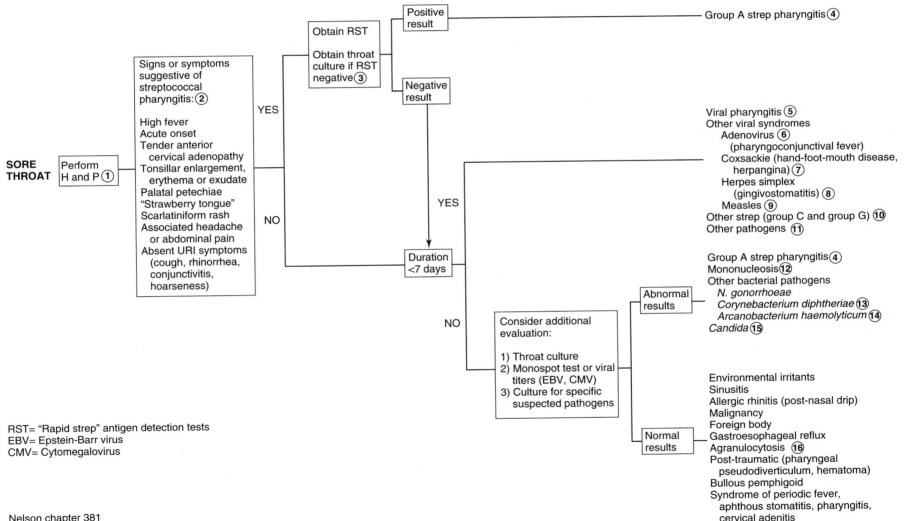

RST= "Rapid strep" antigen detection tests
EBV= Epstein-Barr virus
CMV= Cytomegalovirus

Nelson chapter 381
Practical Strategies chapter 6

Most neck masses are benign, but it is important not to miss rare malignant masses. A directed history and physical examination allows for successful diagnosis and, if necessary, referral for further evaluation and treatment.

1 Neck masses may be distinguished broadly into two categories: congenital and acquired. Masses present since birth, or with chronic drainage or recurrent episodes of swelling, are usually congenital. History of fever may indicate inflammation or infection. Constitutional symptoms, such as fever, night sweats, and weight loss, may indicate a malignancy or a granulomatous process. Rapidly enlarging, painless masses may be malignant. Those due to infection are often painful. Symptoms indicating compression of the trachea, esophagus, or recurrent laryngeal nerve should be elicited because rapid progression of the mass may be life-threatening. A history of recurrent infections such as thrush, sinopulmonary infections, or cellulitis may indicate an immunodeficiency syndrome. A mass associated with dry mouth or with pain when eating may involve a salivary gland.

The location of the mass is very important in making the diagnosis. The neck is divided into two triangles: the anterior triangle is bounded by the mandible, the sternocleidomastoid, and the anterior midline; the posterior triangle is bounded by the posterior border of the sternocleidomastoid, the distal two thirds of the clavicle, and the posterior midline. It is also important to determine the consistency of the lesion. Cystic lesions may show fluctuance and transilluminate. A bruit may be heard with vascular lesions.

2 Thyroglossal duct cysts are usually painless and may move with tongue protrusion. They may occur with recurrent inflammation associated with upper respiratory tract infection. Their location can be anywhere from the base of the tongue to behind the sternum, but are usually near or below the hyoid bone. Ultrasound may be done to confirm the diagnosis. A thyroid scan is important to identify ectopic gland tissue in the cyst.

3 In newborn infants, a goiter may be associated with hypothyroidism. This may occur with defects in thyroid hormone synthesis, administration of goitrogenic substances to the mother (e.g., antithyroid drug, iodide, amiodarone, radioiodine), or iodide deficiency, causing endemic goiter, which is rare in the United States. Congenital hyperthyroidism in infants born to mothers with Graves disease may cause a goiter that usually resolves in 6 to 12 weeks.

4 Dermoid cysts are benign congenital neoplasms located in the midline. They are nontender, smooth, and doughy or rubbery in consistency. They may be difficult to distinguish from thyroglossal duct cysts. In cases in which the diagnosis is difficult to make, aspiration of the cyst may be considered.

5 Teratomas are usually midline but may be paramedian. They are firm and irregular and do not transilluminate. Teratomas have classic radiologic findings of calcifications.

6 Laryngoceles are cystic dilations of the laryngeal ventricle located between the true and false vocal cords. They appear as soft compressible masses just lateral to the midline. Laryngoceles may enlarge with Valsalva maneuver. They may cause hoarseness or stridor. Air fluid levels may be seen radiographically.

7 Branchial cleft anomalies include cysts, sinuses, and fistulas. They are located in the lateral aspect of the anterior triangle. Most anomalies arise from the second branchial arch along the anterior border of the sternocleidomastoid. Some may arise from the first branchial arch at the angle of the mandible or in the postauricular region. These may not be present at birth but may manifest when older as drainage or a mass, if infected. Diagnosis may be confirmed by CT, MRI, or fistulography.

8 Cystic hygromas (lymphangiomas) are cystic masses formed by dilated, anomalous lymphatic channels. These are most common in the posterior triangle but may occur in the submandibular or submental region. They are soft, nontender, diffuse, and compressible masses that may increase in size with straining or crying. Most transilluminate. Diagnosis may be confirmed by ultrasound. A chest X-ray may be considered to look for mediastinal extension in patients with stridor or respiratory compromise.

9 Congenital torticollis is usually noted within the first few weeks of life. There is a firm, nontender, fibrous mass within the body of the sternocleidomastoid. It results in tilting of the head towards the mass with the chin in the opposite direction. It is believed to be caused by trauma or abnormal positioning *in utero*. Prolonged, severe, untreated torticollis may result in a deformed face and skull.

10 Hemangiomas are vascular anomalies, which appear at birth, often enlarging in the first year of life. They are soft, compressible, red or purple colored masses. They may increase in size with crying or Valsalva maneuver. They do not transilluminate. Bruits may be heard, particularly over large hemangiomas. The diagnosis can usually be made on physical findings, but an ultrasound may be used to confirm the diagnosis.

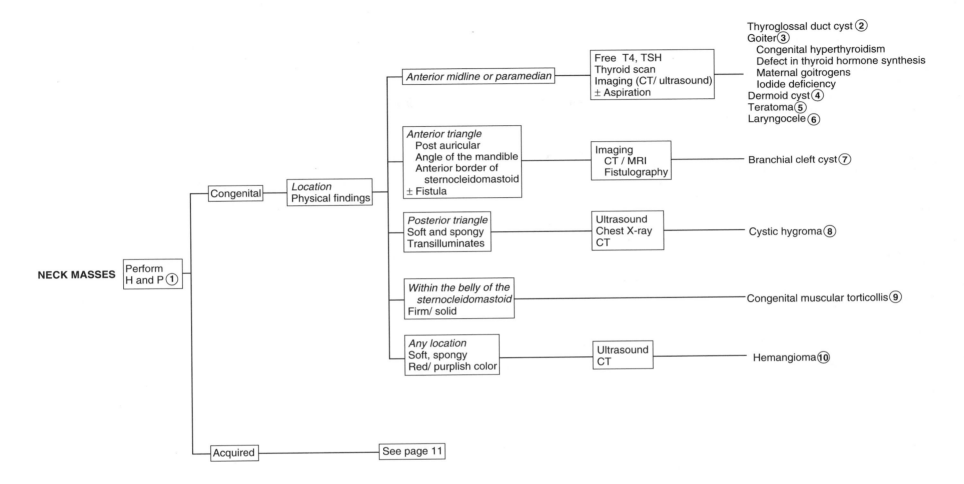

NECK MASSES — Perform H and P ①

Congenital — Location / Physical findings

Anterior midline or paramedian → Free T4, TSH / Thyroid scan / Imaging (CT/ ultrasound) / ± Aspiration →
- Thyroglossal duct cyst ②
- Goiter ③
  - Congenital hyperthyroidism
  - Defect in thyroid hormone synthesis
  - Maternal goitrogens
  - Iodide deficiency
- Dermoid cyst ④
- Teratoma ⑤
- Laryngocele ⑥

Anterior triangle
Post auricular
Angle of the mandible
Anterior border of
 sternocleidomastoid
± Fistula
→ Imaging / CT / MRI / Fistulography → Branchial cleft cyst ⑦

Posterior triangle
Soft and spongy
Transilluminates
→ Ultrasound / Chest X-ray / CT → Cystic hygroma ⑧

**Within the belly of the
 sternocleidomastoid**
Firm/ solid
→ Congenital muscular torticollis ⑨

Any location
Soft, spongy
Red/ purplish color
→ Ultrasound / CT → Hemangioma ⑩

Acquired → See page 11

Nelson chapters 242, 316, 504, 506, 575-579, 686
Practical Strategies chapters 48, 50

(11) Salivary gland enlargement most commonly involves the parotid that obscures the angle of the mandible but may involve the submandibular or minor glands. Parotitis occurs with tender swollen parotid glands classically caused by mumps but also associated with Coxsackie A and HIV. In suppurative parotitis caused by *Staphylococcus aureus,* pus can be expressed from the gland's duct.

(12) Bilateral enlargement of submaxillary glands may occur in AIDS, cystic fibrosis, and malnutrition. Parotid enlargement occurs with chronic emesis as in bulimia. Salivary calculus formation may be associated with anticholinergic-antihistamine drugs. Recurrent idiopathic parotitis occurs at times lasting 2 to 3 weeks. It is usually unilateral with little pain. The condition is believed to be allergic in etiology. Tumors of the salivary gland are rare, and they are usually benign (e.g., hemangiomas, hamartomas, pleomorphic adenoma).

(13) A goiter is an enlargement of the thyroid. It is a midline mass that moves with swallowing. A hard, rapidly growing nodule in the thyroid area should be assessed using a thyroid scan. "Cold" nodules may indicate malignancy. Ultrasound or CT may also be done. Histologic examination of specimens obtained by fine needle aspiration or open biopsy are diagnostic indicators of carcinoma of the thyroid, including papillary, follicular, mixed differentiated, and medullary. Benign adenomas may also appear as solitary nodules.

(14) Thyroid function tests should be obtained with all cases of thyroid enlargement. These enable classification into euthyroid, hyperthyroid, or hypothyroid goiters. Antithyroid antibodies (i.e., antiperoxidase antibodies and antithyroglobulin antibodies) may indicate an autoimmune etiology. Radiographic studies may be useful in defining the nature of the mass. Ultrasound helps to differentiate cystic from solid lesions. Thyroid scan demonstrates "hot" or "cold" areas, which indicate increased or decreased activity. If the etiology cannot be determined fine-needle aspiration or biopsy should be done to exclude malignancy.

(15) Lymphocytic thyroiditis (Hashimoto thyroiditis) is the most common cause of thyroid disease in children. It occurs most commonly during adolescence. Most children are asymptomatic and euthyroid. Although a significant proportion of patients eventually becomes hypothyroid, an occasional patient has hyperthyroidism. Thyroid antibodies are usually present. Endemic goiter due to iodine deficiency is rare in the United States, with iodized salt availability. Goitrogenic drugs include lithium, amiodarone, and iodides in cough medicines. Defects in thyroid hormone synthesis may also cause hypothyroid goiters.

(16) Children with Pendred syndrome (i.e., goiter and congenital deafness) are often euthyroid but may be hypothyroid. It is believed to be caused by a defect in hormone synthesis. Simple colloid goiters are of unknown etiology. The thyroid scans are normal, and thyroid antibodies are absent.

(17) Hyperthyroidism is most commonly due to Graves disease. In addition to the thyroid, there is increase in size of the thymus, spleen, and retro-orbital tissue (exophthalmos). Patients exhibit classic signs and symptoms of hyperthyroidism, such as heat intolerance, weight loss, palpitations, and tremor. TSH level is decreased, T3 and T4 are increased, and antimicrosomal antibodies are present. Thyroid scan is not usually needed but shows rapid and diffuse concentration of radioiodine in the thyroid. Hyperthyroidism may rarely be seen with McCune-Albright syndrome and hyperfunctioning thyroid carcinoma.

(18) Rhabdomyosarcoma may occur with cervical node enlargement with or without pain. The diagnosis should be considered in patients with chronic ear or nose drainage, which is refractory to therapy. Neuroblastoma should be suspected in patients with a cervical mass and Horner syndrome, which consists of homolateral miosis, mild ptosis, and apparent enophthalmos with slight elevation of the lower lid. Horner syndrome is due to oculosympathetic paresis. If it occurs before age two, there may be hypopigmentation of the iris on the affected side (i.e., heterochromia of the iris).

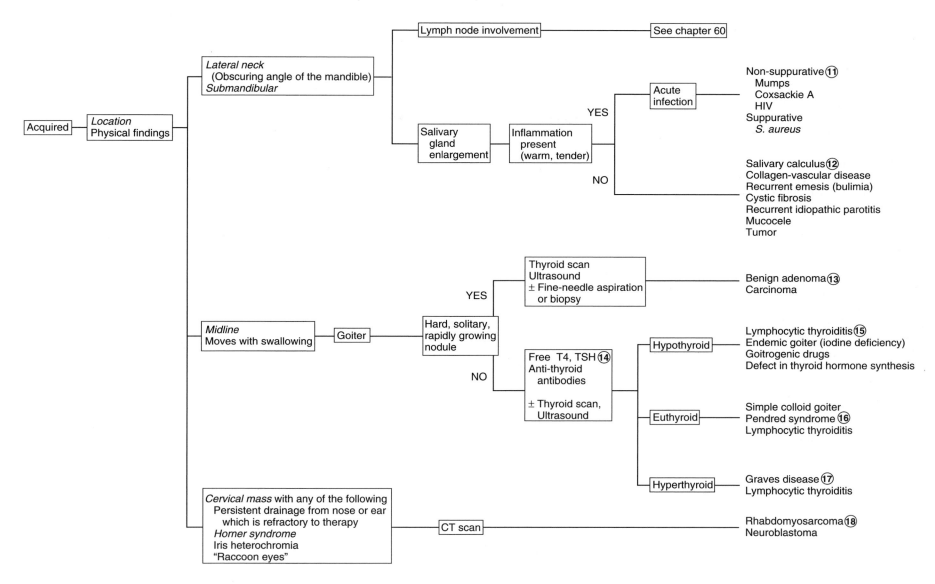

Acquired — *Location* Physical findings

Lateral neck (Obscuring angle of the mandible) *Submandibular*

Lymph node involvement — See chapter 60

Salivary gland enlargement — Inflammation present (warm, tender)

YES — Acute infection

Non-suppurative ⑪
  Mumps
  Coxsackie A
  HIV
Suppurative
  S. aureus

NO

Salivary calculus ⑫
Collagen-vascular disease
Recurrent emesis (bulimia)
Cystic fibrosis
Recurrent idiopathic parotitis
Mucocele
Tumor

Midline Moves with swallowing — Goiter — Hard, solitary, rapidly growing nodule

YES — Thyroid scan Ultrasound ± Fine-needle aspiration or biopsy

Benign adenoma ⑬
Carcinoma

NO — Free T4, TSH ⑭ Anti-thyroid antibodies

± Thyroid scan, Ultrasound

Hypothyroid — Lymphocytic thyroiditis ⑮
Endemic goiter (iodine deficiency)
Goitrogenic drugs
Defect in thyroid hormone synthesis

Euthyroid — Simple colloid goiter
Pendred syndrome ⑯
Lymphocytic thyroiditis

Hyperthyroid — Graves disease ⑰
Lymphocytic thyroiditis

Cervical mass with any of the following
  Persistent drainage from nose or ear which is refractory to therapy
  Horner syndrome
  Iris heterochromia
  "Raccoon eyes"

CT scan — Rhabdomyosarcoma ⑱
Neuroblastoma

Nelson chapters 242, 316, 504, 506, 575-579, 686
Practical Strategies chapters 48, 50

Macrocephaly is defined as a head circumference greater than 2 standard deviations above the mean. Microcephaly is a head circumference 2 standard deviations below the mean. An acceleration in growth rate with crossing of percentiles is of more concern than the case of a child with a large head growing at a normal rate.

(1) A birth history and a developmental history are important components of the initial evaluation. For macrocephaly, inquire about familial head sizes (e.g., ask about hat sizes).

(2) Imaging is usually recommended to help rule out the treatable causes of macrocephaly. Ultrasound can be done if the anterior fontanel (AF) is open. Otherwise, a head CT without contrast is usually adequate. Radiologic evaluation may not be necessary if development is normal, a parent is macrocephalic, and the child's head is growing at a normal rate.

(3) Megalencephaly means a large brain. In the case of a child with normal development and other family members with macrocephaly, the brain is large but normal. In other cases, the megalencephaly represents an underlying problem (e.g., storage disease, neurofibromatosis).

(4) Occasionally, premature infants or infants suffering from deprivation dwarfism (e.g., malnutrition, congenital heart disease) demonstrate a rapid period of percentile crossing ("catch-up") head growth. Growth rate normalizes as the expected size is approached.

(5) Occasionally, benign fluid collections (e.g., subarachnoid, subdural) cause macrocephaly without other clinical significance. A pediatric neurosurgeon should be consulted for recommendations.

(6) Familial microcephaly is usually associated with some degree of mental retardation.

(7) Exposure to noxious agents during periods of rapid brain growth in utero or during the first 2 years of life can cause microcephaly. Examples include congenital infection (rubella, CMV), maternal radiation, drugs (alcohol, hydantoin), CNS infection, hypoxic-ischemic events, and metabolic disorders (maternal PKU).

(8) Intracerebral calcifications on CT or MRI are suggestive of congenital infection. Toxoplasmosis, rubella, cytomegalovirus, and herpes simplex virus (TORCH) titers of both mother and child may help to confirm the diagnosis. A urine culture for cytomegalovirus (CMV) is also helpful.

(9) Cleidocranial dysostosis is a hereditary condition characterized by incomplete ossification of membranous bones, including the cranium, clavicle, and pelvis. Cranial sutures are often wide and contain wormian bones.

(10) Skull deformational malformations occur as the result of an alteration of the normal forces (in utero, perinatal, or postnatal) acting upon the growing cranium. Positional "flat head" or plagiocephaly (skull asymmetry) is the most common type of deformational malformation. Its incidence has increased because of the recommendations to place infants on their back while sleeping. Plagiocephaly is a benign condition that must be distinguished from true cranial suture synostosis. In plagiocephaly, sutures are open, and a frontal and temporal prominence occurs on the same side as the flat occiput. Frontal flattening occurs on the side opposite the flat occiput. In true synostosis of a lambdoidal suture, frontal and parietal bossing would occur on the opposite side because of compensatory growth. Symmetric occipital flattening that is believed to be positional does not require imaging. Rarely, cases of plagiocephaly progress to secondary synostosis. Ventriculoperitoneal shunting, prematurity, microcephaly, hypotonia, and developmental delay are risk factors.

(11) In craniosynostosis there is often palpable ridging over the fused sutures. The condition may occur as a primary isolated disorder, which is most common, or as part of a syndrome. Common associated disorders include Crouzon, Apert, and Pfeiffer syndromes; congenital hyperthyroidism; and adrenal hyperplasia.

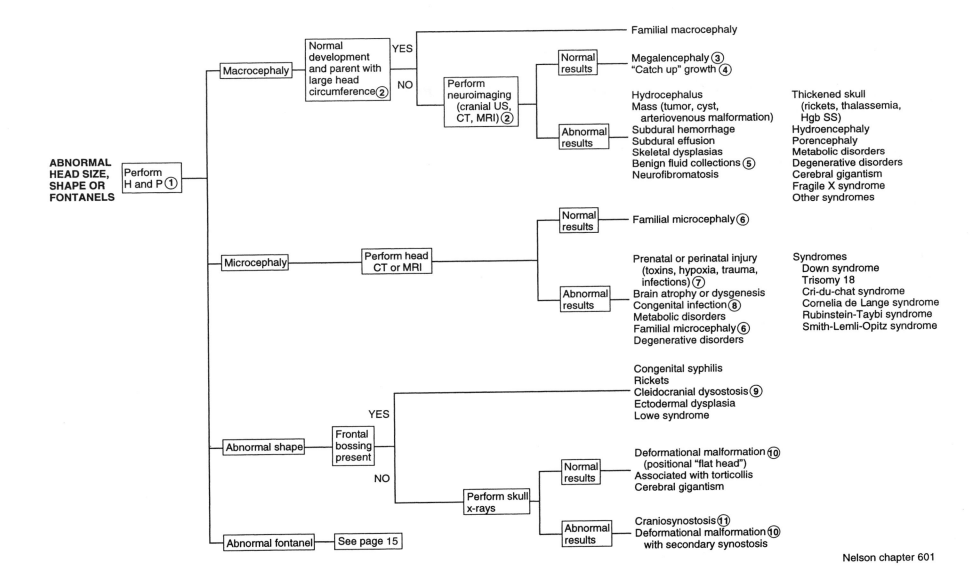

ABNORMAL HEAD SIZE, SHAPE OR FONTANELS — Perform H and P ①

Macrocephaly

Normal development and parent with large head circumference ②
- YES → Familial macrocephaly
- NO → Perform neuroimaging (cranial US, CT, MRI) ②
  - **Normal results** → Megalencephaly ③ / "Catch up" growth ④
  - **Abnormal results**:
    - Hydrocephalus
    - Mass (tumor, cyst, arteriovenous malformation)
    - Subdural hemorrhage
    - Subdural effusion
    - Skeletal dysplasias
    - Benign fluid collections ⑤
    - Neurofibromatosis
    - Thickened skull (rickets, thalassemia, Hgb SS)
    - Hydroencephaly
    - Porencephaly
    - Metabolic disorders
    - Degenerative disorders
    - Cerebral gigantism
    - Fragile X syndrome
    - Other syndromes

Microcephaly — Perform head CT or MRI
- **Normal results** → Familial microcephaly ⑥
- **Abnormal results**:
  - Prenatal or perinatal injury (toxins, hypoxia, trauma, infections) ⑦
  - Brain atrophy or dysgenesis
  - Congenital infection ⑧
  - Metabolic disorders
  - Familial microcephaly ⑥
  - Degenerative disorders
  - Syndromes
    - Down syndrome
    - Trisomy 18
    - Cri-du-chat syndrome
    - Cornelia de Lange syndrome
    - Rubinstein-Taybi syndrome
    - Smith-Lemli-Opitz syndrome

Abnormal shape — Frontal bossing present
- YES →
  - Congenital syphilis
  - Rickets
  - Cleidocranial dysostosis ⑨
  - Ectodermal dysplasia
  - Lowe syndrome
- NO → Perform skull x-rays
  - **Normal results**:
    - Deformational malformation ⑩ (positional "flat head")
    - Associated with torticollis
    - Cerebral gigantism
  - **Abnormal results**:
    - Craniosynostosis ⑪
    - Deformational malformation ⑩ with secondary synostosis

Abnormal fontanel — See page 15

Nelson chapter 601

(12) The anterior fontanel averages 2.5 cm in diameter. Average age of closure is between 7 and 19 months. As long as head growth is normal and sutural ridging is absent, early closure is not a concern.

(13) Imaging is recommended except in the case of a crying infant in whom the bulging resolves spontaneously or in an infant with a clinical picture of meningitis. A lumbar puncture should be performed if meningitis is suspected.

(14) Normal fullness occurs with crying in an infant with a normal fontanel. It should be distinguished from true bulging, such as occurs in hydrocephalic infants. Normally, the fontanel is pulsatile even when full due to crying. In hydrocephalus, the anterior fontanel is usually not visibly pulsatile. Examination of the fontanel should be performed while the infant is in a sitting position.

(15) Transient, unexplained benign bulging of the fontanel may occur in normal infants. This, however, should be a diagnosis of exclusion.

BIBLIOGRAPHY

Ellison PH: Abnormal head: Size and shape. In Berman S: Pediatric Decision Making, 3rd ed, p 425. St. Louis, Mosby, 1996.

Green M: Pediatric Diagnosis: Interpretation of Signs and Symptoms in Children and Adolescents, 6th ed. Philadelphia, W.B. Saunders Company, 1998.

Moe PG, Seay AR: Neurologic and muscular disorders. In Hay WW, Hayward AR, Levin MJ, Sondheimer JM (eds): Current Pediatric Diagnosis and Treatment, 14th ed, p 622. Stanford, CT, Appleton & Lange, 1999.

Rohan AJ, Golombek SG, Rosenthal AD: Infants with misshapen skulls. Contemp Pediatr 16:47,1999.

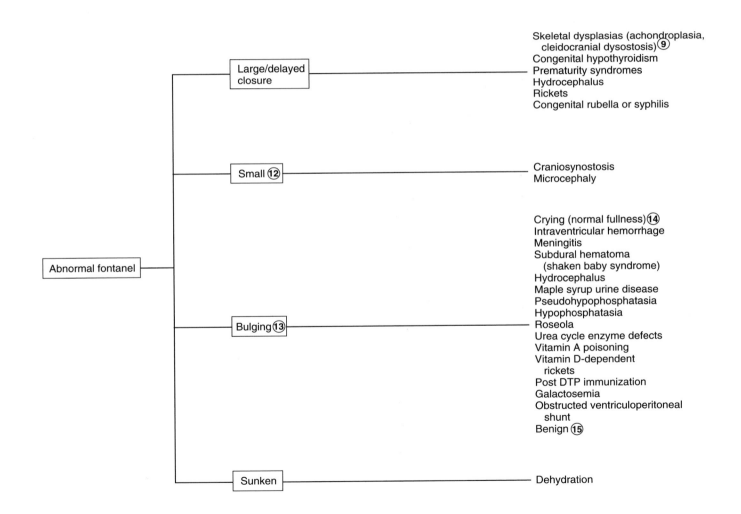

Large/delayed closure
- Skeletal dysplasias (achondroplasia, cleidocranial dysostosis) ⑨
- Congenital hypothyroidism
- Prematurity syndromes
- Hydrocephalus
- Rickets
- Congenital rubella or syphilis

Small ⑫
- Craniosynostosis
- Microcephaly

Abnormal fontanel

Bulging ⑬
- Crying (normal fullness) ⑭
- Intraventricular hemorrhage
- Meningitis
- Subdural hematoma (shaken baby syndrome)
- Hydrocephalus
- Maple syrup urine disease
- Pseudohypophosphatasia
- Hypophosphatasia
- Roseola
- Urea cycle enzyme defects
- Vitamin A poisoning
- Vitamin D-dependent rickets
- Post DTP immunization
- Galactosemia
- Obstructed ventriculoperitoneal shunt
- Benign ⑮

Sunken
- Dehydration

Red eye is a common pediatric complaint. It can occur secondary to a wide range of etiologies.

1 The age of onset of the red eye, the nature of any discharge, and the associated signs and symptoms are the most important components of the history. History of exposure to irritants (e.g., allergens, particulate matter, chemicals) and of trauma or infectious contacts (e.g., "pinkeye" in school or daycare settings) may also be helpful. For infants, inquire about the possibility of any maternal infections.

2 Gonococcal conjunctivitis typically appears as a fulminant, purulent conjunctivitis in the first two to six days of life. Chlamydial conjunctivitis is more likely beyond the first six days of life. Conjunctivitis caused by herpes simplex virus characteristically occurs as a unilateral bright red eye with thin watery discharge. Vesicles or erosions are present on the lid or surrounding skin. These clinical findings are not specific, however, and prompt evaluation and treatment are always indicated to avoid serious sequelae. A Gram stain will aid in the diagnosis of the gonococcus. Rapid antigen tests are available for the chlamydial infections. Herpes simplex is usually cultured but PCR may be helpful. Ophthalmologic consultation is indicated when herpes is suspected.

3 Conjunctivitis in the first 24 hours of life is probably a chemical conjunctivitis unless membranes were ruptured prematurely. Silver nitrate is more likely to produce this condition than other agents used for prophylaxis (e.g., erythromycin, tetracycline).

4 Tearing, photophobia, and blepharospasm make up the classic triad of presenting symptoms of infantile glaucoma. Conjunctival injection, corneal enlargement (>12 mm), and corneal clouding (edema) are the other findings.

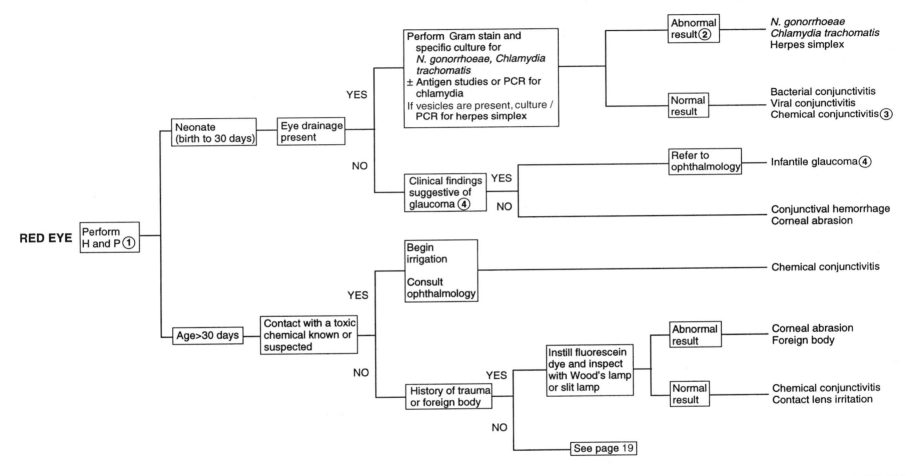

RED EYE — Perform H and P ①

Perform H and P ① → Neonate (birth to 30 days) → Eye drainage present

YES → Perform Gram stain and specific culture for *N. gonorrhoeae, Chlamydia trachomatis* ± Antigen studies or PCR for chlamydia. If vesicles are present, culture / PCR for herpes simplex

- Abnormal result ② → *N. gonorrhoeae*, *Chlamydia trachomatis*, Herpes simplex
- Normal result → Bacterial conjunctivitis, Viral conjunctivitis, Chemical conjunctivitis ③

NO → Clinical findings suggestive of glaucoma ④
- **YES** → Refer to ophthalmology → Infantile glaucoma ④
- **NO** → Conjunctival hemorrhage, Corneal abrasion

Perform H and P ① → Age>30 days → Contact with a toxic chemical known or suspected

YES → Begin irrigation / Consult ophthalmology → Chemical conjunctivitis

NO → History of trauma or foreign body
- **YES** → Instill fluorescein dye and inspect with Wood's lamp or slit lamp
  - Abnormal result → Corneal abrasion, Foreign body
  - Normal result → Chemical conjunctivitis, Contact lens irritation
- **NO** → See page 19

Nelson chapters 632, 633, 639
Practical Strategies chapter 44

Red Eye (continued)

(5) Dacryostenosis (i.e., congenital lacrimal duct stenosis) is a common disorder that occurs within two to four months of age but sometimes not until tear production with crying becomes evident. An excessive tear lake and overflow with crusting are evident on examination. Children so affected are at risk for inflammation and infection (i.e., dacryocystitis) of the obstructed nasolacrimal sac. Some systemic disorders, such as sarcoid, tuberculosis, and syphilis, may cause chronic dacryocystitis.

(6) The lacrimal gland (i.e., the site of tear production) is located in the lateral aspect of the upper eyelid. Rarely, inflammation of the lacrimal gland (i.e., dacryoadenitis) can occur as a result of infections (e.g., *Staphylococcus aureus,* infectious mononucleosis, and mumps).

(7) Pain with extraocular *eye* movements may accompany orbital cellulitis. Proptosis and impaired extraocular movement and vision are other signs. Orbital cellulitis must be distinguished from preseptal (periorbital) cellulitis. Minimal conjunctival redness usually occurs in orbital cellulitis, and extraocular muscle movements are intact in preseptal cellulitis.

(8) Iritis and iridocyclitis may occur secondary to localized infection or trauma, or they may be manifestations of a rheumatic disorder (e.g., juvenile rheumatoid arthritis, Reiter syndrome, Behçet disease). Inflammatory bowel disease and Kawasaki disease are other associated conditions. Photophobia is typically a significant finding with iritis and iridocyclitis.

(9) Scleritis or episcleritis may accompany certain autoimmune disorders including systemic lupus erythematosus and Henoch-Schönlein purpura. Pain is present, eye discharge is absent, and dilated blood vessels are larger than in conjunctivitis.

(10) Bacterial conjunctivitis may be unilateral or bilateral, but viral conjunctivitis is more commonly bilateral. Bacterial conjunctivitis is more likely to have purulent discharge than viral conjunctivitis, although significant overlap in the clinical presentation of the two etiologies does occur. A history of a recent upper respiratory tract infection, preauricular adenopathy, and scant eye discharge that is more mucoid than purulent suggests a viral etiology. Allergic conjunctivitis is characterized by itching, chemosis, papillae of the tarsal conjunctivae, and white stringy discharge.

BIBLIOGRAPHY

King RA: Common ocular signs and symptoms in childhood. Pediatr Clin North Am 40:753–765, 1993.

Lavrich JB, Nelson LB: Disorders of the lacrimal system apparatus. Pediatr Clin North Am 40:767–776, 1993.

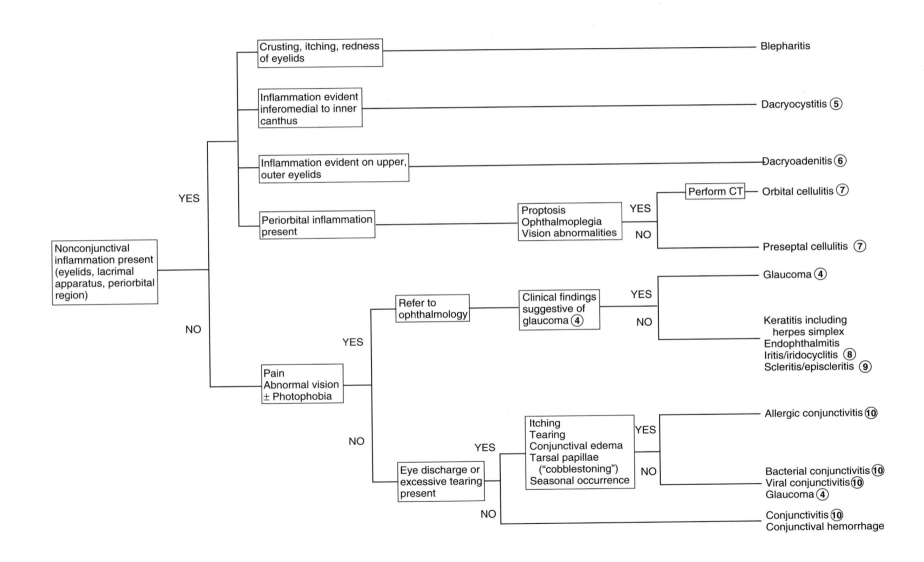

Strabismus ("crossed eyes" or "straying eyes") is a term used to describe any misalignment of the eyes. The condition is usually an isolated problem in children but can occasionally indicate an underlying pathology. Early diagnosis and treatment are essential to prevent the development of amblyopia (i.e., visual loss), which occurs in 30% to 50% of children with strabismus.

(1) The history should include age of onset, circumstances eliciting the deviation, and associated visual complaints. Prematurity, perinatal problems, and developmental delay are risk factors for early onset strabismus. A family history may also be helpful.

Evaluation of ocular motility and binocular alignment, using the cover tests and corneal light reflex test, is particularly important. Careful examination should result in being able to classify the problem as a heterophoria (latent) or heterotropia (manifest), paralytic or nonparalytic, and inward turning **(eso-)** or outward turning **(exo-)**. Based on the nature of the defect and the child's age at the time the problem develops, many cases can be identified as a specific clinical entity.

(2) Intermittent transient eye crossing is normal in infants up to 4 to 6 months of age. It frequently occurs when infants are tired.

(3) A wide flat nasal bridge or prominent epicanthal folds may create an optical illusion of inturning eyes (i.e., pseudostrabismus). Careful assessment of the corneal light reflexes confirms that the alignment is normal.

(4) In nonparalytic strabismus, the extraocular muscles and the nerves innervating them are normal. The degree of deviation is constant or relatively constant in all directions of gaze.

(5) Infantile (congenital) esotropia appears before 6 months of age, most by 2 to 3 months.

(6) In nystagmus blockage syndrome, early onset esotropia is accompanied by nystagmus.

(7) In dissociated vertical deviation (DVD), an upward movement of the eye occurs when a normal binocular gaze is interrupted.

(8) Cyclic esotropia is the rare occurrence of alternating periods of large angle esotropia with normal alignment or small angle esotropia.

(9) Acquired comitant esotropia is the acute onset of a large degree esotropia. It often follows a period of occlusion of one eye.

(10) Convergence insufficiency is an exodeviation that occurs or is exaggerated on near gaze.

(11) In accommodative esotropia, the inward turning of the eyes is linked to convergence. A high degree of hyperopia (i.e., farsightedness) necessitates a high degree of convergence, which results in esotropia that worsens when the child attempts to near focus. Onset is typically between two and three years of age.

(12) Intermittent exotropia typically develops between two and three years of age.

(13) Paralytic strabismus is suggested by an eye misalignment that varies according to the direction of the gaze. The condition is produced by an underlying nerve palsy, muscle weakness, or mechanical restriction of eye movement. Compensatory head tilting often occurs.

(14) Excessive fibrosis and anomalous insertion of extraocular muscles result in ptosis and external ophthalmoplegia. Convergence on attempted upward gaze, divergence on attempted downward gaze, and compensatory chin-up posturing are also characteristic of congenital fibrosis syndrome.

(15) In Duane syndrome, lateral movement of the affected eye is limited. Medial movement produces sharp upshoots or downshoots of the affected eye. These motions are also accompanied by globe retraction.

(16) A defect of the sixth and seventh cranial nerve nuclei results in congenital facial diplegia and defective abduction in the Möbius syndrome.

(17) In Brown syndrome, an abnormality of the superior oblique tendon results in an inability to elevate the eye in the medial position.

(18) Careful assessment of ocular motility and associated lid and pupillary functions should help identify cranial nerve palsies. Acquired cranial nerve palsies warrant careful evaluation to rule out CNS lesions.

(19) Palsies of the third cranial nerves with resultant pupillary dilation and ptosis are characteristic of most ophthalmoplegic migraines. The eye muscle paralysis may last for a few weeks following a headache.

(20) In Gradenigo syndrome, inflammation results in a sixth nerve palsy due to nerve entrapment along the petrosphenoidal ligament. Etiologies include otitis media, mastoiditis, and tumor.

BIBLIOGRAPHY

Lavrich JB, Nelson LB: Diagnosis and treatment of strabismus disorders. Pediatr Clin North Am 40:737–752,1993.

Rubin SE, Nelson LB: Amblyopia: Diagnosis and management. Pediatr Clin North Am 40:727–735, 1993.

STRABISMUS

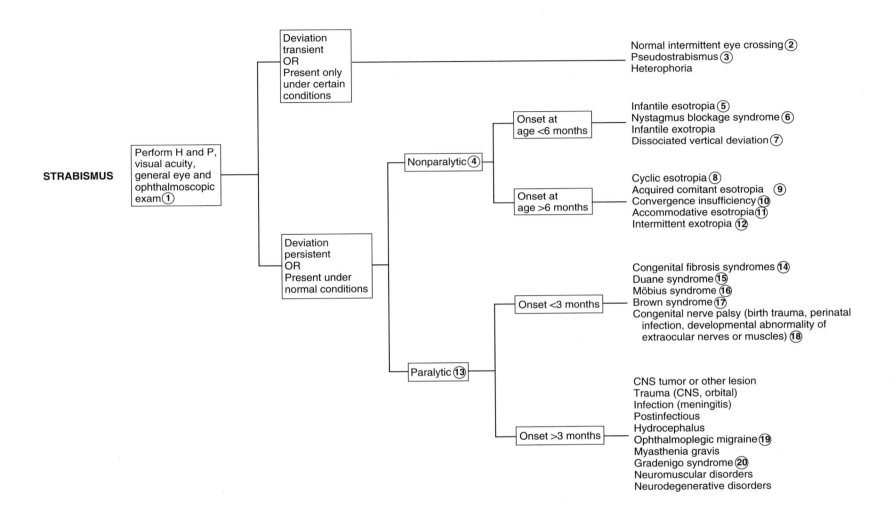

Perform H and P, visual acuity, general eye and ophthalmoscopic exam ①

Deviation transient OR Present only under certain conditions

Normal intermittent eye crossing ②
Pseudostrabismus ③
Heterophoria

Deviation persistent OR Present under normal conditions

Nonparalytic ④

Onset at age <6 months

Infantile esotropia ⑤
Nystagmus blockage syndrome ⑥
Infantile exotropia
Dissociated vertical deviation ⑦

Onset at age >6 months

Cyclic esotropia ⑧
Acquired comitant esotropia ⑨
Convergence insufficiency ⑩
Accommodative esotropia ⑪
Intermittent exotropia ⑫

Paralytic ⑬

Onset <3 months

Congenital fibrosis syndromes ⑭
Duane syndrome ⑮
Möbius syndrome ⑯
Brown syndrome ⑰
Congenital nerve palsy (birth trauma, perinatal infection, developmental abnormality of extraocular nerves or muscles) ⑱

Onset >3 months

CNS tumor or other lesion
Trauma (CNS, orbital)
Infection (meningitis)
Postinfectious
Hydrocephalus
Ophthalmoplegic migraine ⑲
Myasthenia gravis
Gradenigo syndrome ⑳
Neuromuscular disorders
Neurodegenerative disorders

Nelson chapter 630
Practical Strategies chapters 38, 44

When treating a child in whom there are visual concerns, consultation with a pediatric ophthalmologist or optometrist is frequently required, especially for a very young infant.

(1) A detailed description of the visual complaint is helpful, but in infants and young children the history tends to be based primarily on the observations of family and caretakers. For older children, inquire about focal versus general blurring, double images, night vision, and abnormal sensations (e.g., spots, lines). The birth history is an important component of the medical history as asphyxia or trauma (i.e., forceps injury) may be contributory. Recent illness may aid in the diagnosis of sudden visual loss caused by acute optic neuritis. A family history of neurocutaneous disorders, metabolic disorders, cataracts, or other visual problems may also be helpful.

The examination should include an assessment for visual acuity using a Snellen chart or one designed for preliterate children (e.g., tumbling E and picture tests). For infants and toddlers, referral for visual assessment using behavioral responses may be necessary.

Visual fields should also be assessed. Examination of the pupils, ocular motility, and eye alignment is necessary. A thorough ophthalmologic examination should be done. Common findings that may be helpful in diagnosis include strabismus, corneal opacity, leukocoria, and nystagmus.

(2) Leukocoria (i.e., white pupillary reflex) occurs secondary to a number of causes in children. Leukocoria is most common in the young infant, although it may occur with problems that develop at a later age. Referral to an ophthalmologist for a thorough diagnostic evaluation is always indicated.

(3) Cataracts are a common cause of leukocoria. Common etiologies of cataracts include infections (e.g., rubella, toxoplasmosis, cytomegalovirus); hereditary or metabolic disorders; chromosomal disorders (e.g., trisomy 18, trisomy 13, Turner syndrome), and other systemic disorders (Conradi, Marinesco-Sjögren, myotonic dystrophy).

(4) Premature infants less than 33 weeks' gestation, or less than 2000 grams birth weight, who received supplemental oxygen are at highest risk for retinopathy of prematurity (ROP). Guidelines exist for ROP classification. Recommended guidelines for examinations of infants at risk are also available.

(5) Infantile glaucoma occurs during the first 3 years of life; juvenile glaucoma occurs between 3 and 30 years of age. Glaucoma may be primary or secondary to structural, hamartomatous, inflammatory, metabolic, or congenital disorders. The classic triad of presenting symptoms is tearing, photophobia, and blepharospasm (i.e., eyelid squeezing). Signs include corneal haziness, corneal and ocular enlargement, and conjunctival injection as well as visual impairment. Corneal diameter greater than one centimeter is abnormal and should be evaluated. For young infants an examination under light anesthesia is frequently necessary to accurately measure intraocular pressure and make the diagnosis.

(6) Acute vision loss with or without pain on movement of the globe characterizes optic neuritis. Funduscopy may reveal hemorrhages and exudates of the optic disc (i.e., papillitis). Usually the findings are normal if the neuritis is retrobulbar. There is frequently a history of a preceding viral illness. Neuroimaging and electrophysiologic studies are often required to make the diagnosis. Multiple sclerosis is a possible etiology.

(7) Psychogenic vision loss is more likely to occur in older school-aged children. Complaints of visual loss or blurring may be accompanied by numerous other complaints (e.g., abnormal visual sensations, diplopia, polyopia, painful eyes, headaches). Diagnosis is suggested by normal examination findings and behavioral "red flags," such as inconsistent complaints in different situations, positive responses to examiner's suggestions of maneuvers to improve vision, and inappropriate affect (e.g., indifferent, belligerent, overdramatic) during the examination.

(8) Amblyopia is poor visual acuity despite correction of any refractive errors. Diagnosis is made when visual impairment occurs despite normal ophthalmoscopic examination findings. Obstruction of the light axis (cataracts) or creation of a double image (strabismus) extinguishes the cortical perception permanently.

(9) Optic gliomas are most commonly located in the optic chiasm but may occur anywhere along the optic pathway. They can occur with a variety of symptoms including unilateral vision loss, proptosis, bitemporal hemianopsia, and eye deviation. Craniopharyngiomas may occur with visual loss, pituitary dysfunction (e.g., diabetes insipidus, short stature, hypothyroidism), and increased intracranial pressure. Neuroimaging is indicated whenever a tumor is suspected.

(10) Degenerative disorders originating in the retina are Coats disease, retinoschisis, familial exudative vitreoretinopathy, and retinitis pigmentosa.

BIBLIOGRAPHY

Potter WS: Pediatric cataracts. Pediatr Clin North Am 40:841–853, 1993.
Repka MX: Common pediatric neuro-ophthalmologic conditions. Pediatr Clin North Am 40:777–788, 1993.
Rubin SE, Nelson LB: Amblyopia: Diagnosis and management. Pediatr Clin North Am 40:727–735, 1993.

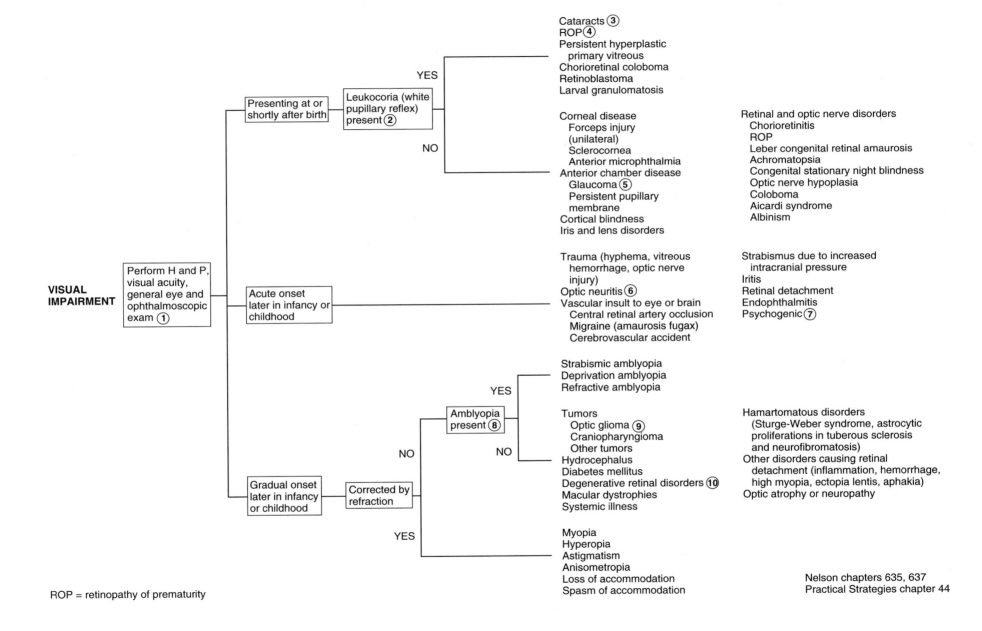

VISUAL IMPAIRMENT

Perform H and P, visual acuity, general eye and ophthalmoscopic exam ①

Presenting at or shortly after birth

Leukocoria (white pupillary reflex) present ②

YES:
Cataracts ③
ROP④
Persistent hyperplastic primary vitreous
Chorioretinal coloboma
Retinoblastoma
Larval granulomatosis

NO:
Corneal disease
  Forceps injury (unilateral)
  Sclerocornea
  Anterior microphthalmia
Anterior chamber disease
  Glaucoma ⑤
  Persistent pupillary membrane
Cortical blindness
Iris and lens disorders

Retinal and optic nerve disorders
  Chorioretinitis
  ROP
  Leber congenital retinal amaurosis
  Achromatopsia
  Congenital stationary night blindness
  Optic nerve hypoplasia
  Coloboma
  Aicardi syndrome
  Albinism

Acute onset later in infancy or childhood

Trauma (hyphema, vitreous hemorrhage, optic nerve injury)
Optic neuritis ⑥
Vascular insult to eye or brain
  Central retinal artery occlusion
  Migraine (amaurosis fugax)
  Cerebrovascular accident

Strabismus due to increased intracranial pressure
Iritis
Retinal detachment
Endophthalmitis
Psychogenic ⑦

Gradual onset later in infancy or childhood

Corrected by refraction

NO → Amblyopia present ⑧

YES:
Strabismic amblyopia
Deprivation amblyopia
Refractive amblyopia

NO:
Tumors
  Optic glioma ⑨
  Craniopharyngioma
  Other tumors
Hydrocephalus
Diabetes mellitus
Degenerative retinal disorders ⑩
Macular dystrophies
Systemic illness

Hamartomatous disorders (Sturge-Weber syndrome, astrocytic proliferations in tuberous sclerosis and neurofibromatosis)
Other disorders causing retinal detachment (inflammation, hemorrhage, high myopia, ectopia lentis, aphakia)
Optic atrophy or neuropathy

YES:
Myopia
Hyperopia
Astigmatism
Anisometropia
Loss of accommodation
Spasm of accommodation

ROP = retinopathy of prematurity

Nelson chapters 635, 637
Practical Strategies chapter 44

Chapter 9 *Abnormal Eye Movements*

Abnormal eye movements may occur as a benign finding or in association with other visual or ocular problems. They may indicate, however, an acquired, more severe underlying neurologic problem.

1 The history needs to include an accurate description of the eye movements, age of onset, and associated signs and symptoms. Specifically inquire about visual acuity, color vision, night vision, photophobia, abnormal head movements, tinnitus, and oscillopsia. Oscillopsia is a sensation of movement or swinging of the visual field.

Careful examination should yield an accurate description of the eye movements and other associated signs and symptoms. Eye movements should be initially classified as rhythmic (swinging, pendulum-like) or nonrhythmic. The association of any nonocular muscle movements should be discerned. Nystagmus is defined as the repetitive rhythmic oscillations of one or both eyes. The waveform, direction, amplitude, frequency, and velocity of oscillations further help to classify the pattern of nystagmus. It should be noted whether the movements are symmetric or asymmetric between the two eyes. Some patterns have diagnostic implications. For example, vertical nystagmus is associated with posterior fossa lesions. Some drug-induced nystagmus may occasionally be vertical.

Frequently, neuroimaging and sometimes more specialized studies (e.g., electroretinogram, visual evoked potential test) are necessary to rule out underlying etiologies.

2 In opsoclonus the eyes appear to dart around quickly in short unpredictable bursts. It may be associated with hydrocephalus and brainstem or cerebellar disorders. Opsoclonus may be the presenting symptom of neuroblastoma.

3 Ocular dysmetria describes a pathologic overshoot (hypermetria) of the eye followed by oscillation of decreasing amplitude during gaze refixation.

4 Ocular flutter describes brief intermittent horizontal oscillations of the eyes on forward gaze or occasionally on blinking. It may occur with hydrocephalus, cerebellar disease, or tumor.

5 Ocular bobbing is repeated downward jerking of the eyes followed by a slow drifting back to the primary position. It occurs in seriously ill patients (stuporous or comatose) with significant disease of the pons. The bobbing may be associated with pontine tumors.

6 Ocular myoclonus describes rhythmic oscillating eye movements accompanied by nonocular movements of the soft palate, tongue, face, pharynx, larynx, and diaphragm. It usually indicates cerebellar damage.

7 Sensory nystagmus is associated with impaired vision due to an abnormality of the eye or visual pathway. It is the most common type of nystagmus in infants. It generally occurs in children in the first 3 to 4 months of life and in children with congenital or perinatal vision defects. It may also be observed in children who develop blindness later in the first few years of life. The cause (microphthalmia, glaucoma, cataracts) is frequently evident on general or ophthalmoscopic examination. Electrophysiologic imaging may be necessary to rule out certain causes (achromatopsia, congenital stationary night blindness, Leber congenital retinal amaurosis), which are not evident on fundoscopic examination. (See Ch. 8.) Neuroimaging to rule out tumors is always recommended when the cause is not evident.

8 Congenital idiopathic nystagmus typically appears in the first 3 months of life and is associated with compensatory head tilting. A thorough examination including neuroimaging and electrophysiologic studies is usually necessary to rule out underlying ocular or neurologic disorders.

9 Both congenital and acquired disorders of the nervous system may be responsible for neurologic nystagmus. Examples include CNS infections, trauma, encephalopathy, demyelination, metabolic disorders, and neurodevelopmental syndromes. In some cases, both neurologic and sensory etiologies may contribute to the nystagmus.

10 Labyrinthitis is an infrequent complication of otitis media. Manifestations can include vertigo, ear pain, nausea, vomiting, hearing loss, and nystagmus.

11 Spasmus nutans is usually a benign condition that occurs as a combination of bilateral asymmetric nystagmus, head nodding, and torticollis in the first years of life. The etiology is unknown. It generally resolves by age 3 years without sequelae. Despite the benign nature of the condition, neuroimaging is recommended to rule out the possibility of a CNS neoplasm.

12 Both children and adults can exhibit an occasional one to two beats of lateral nystagmus on side gaze that is not considered significant.

BIBLIOGRAPHY

Repka MX: Common pediatric neuro-ophthalmologic conditions. Pediatr Clin North Am 40:777–788, 1993.

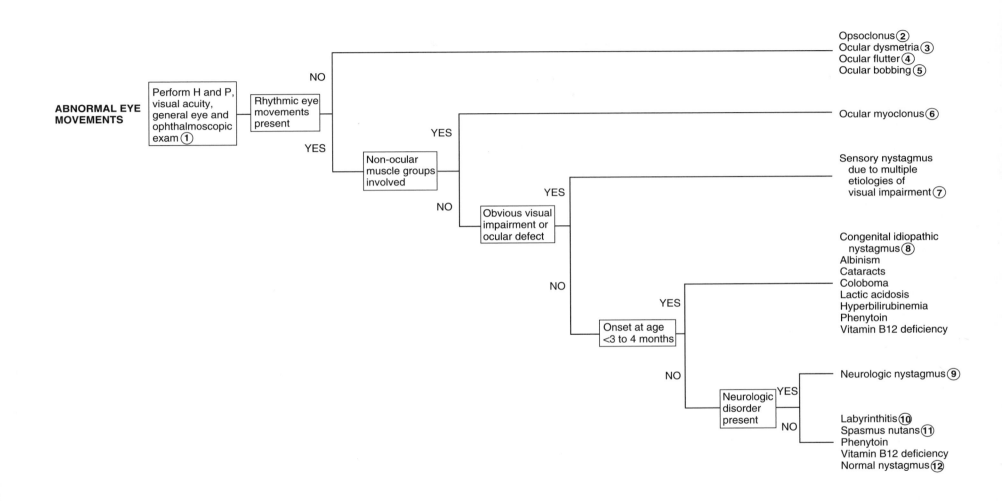

ABNORMAL EYE MOVEMENTS

Perform H and P, visual acuity, general eye and ophthalmoscopic exam ①

Rhythmic eye movements present

NO

Opsoclonus ②
Ocular dysmetria ③
Ocular flutter ④
Ocular bobbing ⑤

YES

Non-ocular muscle groups involved

YES

Ocular myoclonus ⑥

NO

Obvious visual impairment or ocular defect

YES

Sensory nystagmus due to multiple etiologies of visual impairment ⑦

NO

Onset at age <3 to 4 months

YES

Congenital idiopathic nystagmus ⑧
Albinism
Cataracts
Coloboma
Lactic acidosis
Hyperbilirubinemia
Phenytoin
Vitamin B12 deficiency

NO

Neurologic disorder present

YES

Neurologic nystagmus ⑨

NO

Labyrinthitis ⑩
Spasmus nutans ⑪
Phenytoin
Vitamin B12 deficiency
Normal nystagmus ⑫

RESPIRATORY SYSTEM

(1) The medical history should include a neonatal history and an assessment for immunodeficiency. An environmental history should include inquiries about potential irritants (e.g., wood burning stove, smoke, perfume, scented candle, incense). The review of systems should include respiratory and nonrespiratory symptoms (e.g., poor growth, malodorous stools, halitosis). Inquire specifically about any recent choking episodes. A family history for asthma and cystic fibrosis and current illnesses may be helpful.

(2) Clinical diagnosis of sinusitis is made by prolonged, nonspecific upper respiratory signs and symptoms (e.g., rhinorrhea, cough) without improvement at 10 to 14 days or more severe upper respiratory tract signs or symptoms. Older children may complain of facial pain and have sinus tenderness on examination.

(3) Croup (laryngotracheobronchitis) occurs most commonly in children younger than 2 years. It typically follows the onset of a cold by a few days and is characterized by a "barky" cough and inspiratory stridor. Fever is typically low grade. An anteroposterior neck film is more helpful than a chest X-ray in helping to make this diagnosis. A lateral neck film is more helpful if epiglottitis or retropharyngeal abscess is suspected. Spasmodic croup refers to a clinically similar condition but without evidence of infection. Possible etiologies include allergic, psychologic, viral, and gastroesophageal reflux.

(4) Children with pertussis generally appear well between paroxysmal coughing spells. The "whoop" may not occur in infants younger than 3 months of age. Diagnosis can often be difficult to make because nasopharyngeal culture and fluorescent antibody test results are most likely to be positive during the early (catarrhal) stage of illness and before the diagnosis is suspected. Polymerase chain reaction testing may improve the diagnostic yield. An elevated white blood cell count (as high as 20,000 to 25,000) with lymphocytosis supports the diagnosis. This finding may not occur in the very young infant. The chest X-ray and physical examination are typically noncontributory, although the chest X-ray may show atelectasis or perihilar infiltrates. Most cases of pertussis in infants and children can be traced to contact with a mildly symptomatic adult, presenting primarily with a prolonged nonspecific cough.

(5) Although "bronchitis" is a frequently used term in pediatrics, it probably does not typically occur as an isolated entity. Tracheobronchitis is probably a better descriptor of the common clinical scenario of a viral upper respiratory infection complicated by a prolonged cough, which may be productive, and malaise. Prolonged symptoms or late onset fever may be caused by secondary bacterial infections with the usual respiratory pathogens, such as *Streptococcus pneumoniae* and *Haemophilus influenzae*. *Mycoplasma pneumoniae* or *Chlamydia pneumoniae* may also be a cause.

(6) Foreign body aspiration is usually obvious immediately but occasionally a delay of weeks to months may occur before symptoms develop. Even when inspiratory and expiratory views are obtained, X-ray findings are still reported negative in 15% of children with aspirated foreign bodies. Fluoroscopy can also yield false-negative results. Computed tomography may be necessary for diagnosis. Rigid bronchoscopy confirms the diagnosis and removes the foreign body.

(7) Aspiration of food or secretions in neurologically abnormal children may cause cough of varying frequency or severity. Cough due to aspiration may be produced by airway inflammation, bronchospasm, or pneumonia. Aspiration pneumonia may or may not be superinfected. If infection does occur, it is usually due to anaerobes or gram-negative organisms when chronic or nosocomial. Radionuclide scans or barium contrast studies may help to diagnose swallowing abnormalities. The intermittent nature of aspiration, however, frequently makes diagnosis difficult.

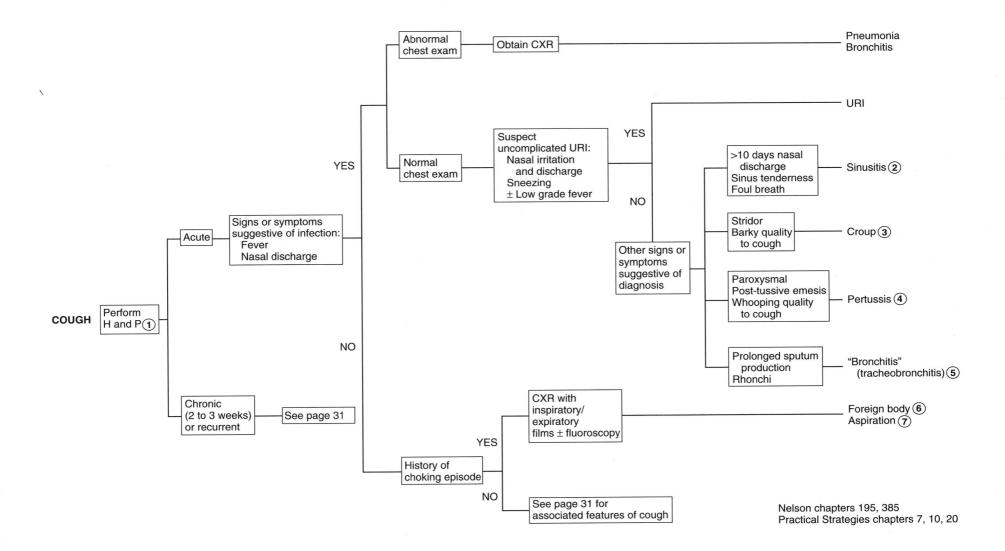

COUGH

Perform H and P ①

Acute

Signs or symptoms suggestive of infection:
Fever
Nasal discharge

YES

Abnormal chest exam — Obtain CXR —————————————— Pneumonia
Bronchitis

Normal chest exam — Suspect uncomplicated URI:
Nasal irritation and discharge
Sneezing
± Low grade fever

YES — URI

NO

Other signs or symptoms suggestive of diagnosis

>10 days nasal discharge
Sinus tenderness
Foul breath — Sinusitis ②

Stridor
Barky quality to cough — Croup ③

Paroxysmal
Post-tussive emesis
Whooping quality to cough — Pertussis ④

Prolonged sputum production
Rhonchi — "Bronchitis" (tracheobronchitis) ⑤

Chronic (2 to 3 weeks) or recurrent — See page 31

NO

History of choking episode

YES

CXR with inspiratory/ expiratory films ± fluoroscopy —————————— Foreign body ⑥
Aspiration ⑦

NO

See page 31 for associated features of cough

Nelson chapters 195, 385
Practical Strategies chapters 7, 10, 20

(8) Pulmonary contusions can occur as a result of chest trauma. The onset of symptoms may be acute or delayed. Contusions may be visible on a chest X-ray. Initial film findings are often negative.

(9) Gastroesophageal reflux (GER) is most common in infants but may occasionally cause a chronic cough of an unclear mechanism in older children. A history of coughing after meals or when lying down and of belching or substernal pain before or after meals are suggestive. Children with difficult to control asthma should also be evaluated for GER. Diagnostic choices include an upper GI series or endoscopy or a trial of antireflux therapy.

(10) Asthma (i.e., reactive airway disease) is the most common cause of chronic and recurrent cough in children. Wheezing may not be evident (i.e., cough variant). A history of an acute, significant cough with colds, exercise, hard laughter, crying, cold air, or smoke exposure or significant improvement with bronchodilators leads to the diagnosis. The chest X-ray may reveal hyperinflation and atelectasis.

(11) Cough due to certain viral pathogens (e.g., adenovirus, influenza) may last 8 to 12 weeks.

(12) Habit cough (i.e., psychogenic cough tic) is an infrequent cause of a prolonged cough in school-aged children that is often refractory to treatment. The harsh, barky cough occurs only during waking hours. The child appears well and is typically not bothered by the coughing. Attention seeking or underlying psychologic factors are commonly thought to be associated.

(13) Mediastinal disorders include tumor; lymphadenopathy due to sarcoidosis, tuberculosis, histoplasmosis, and coccidioidomycosis; pericardial cyst; and diaphragmatic hernia.

(14) A large number of rare conditions can occur with cough including interstitial lung disease, graft-versus-host disease, α_1-antitrypsin deficiency, pulmonary hemosiderosis, alveolar proteinosis, heart failure, pulmonary edema, sarcoidosis, obliterative bronchiolitis, and follicular bronchiolitis.

(15) Many types of medications can cause or aggravate a cough by a number of mechanisms (e.g., direct irritation, aggravation of reactive airways, GER), but this is rare.

BIBLIOGRAPHY

Guilbert TW, Taussig LM: Doctor, he's been coughing for a month. Is it serious? Contemp Pediatr 15:155, 1998.

Schidlow D: Cough. In Schidlow D, Smith D (eds): A Practical Guide to Pediatric Respiratory Diseases, p 49. Philadelphia, Hanley & Belfus, Inc, 1994.

COUGH continued

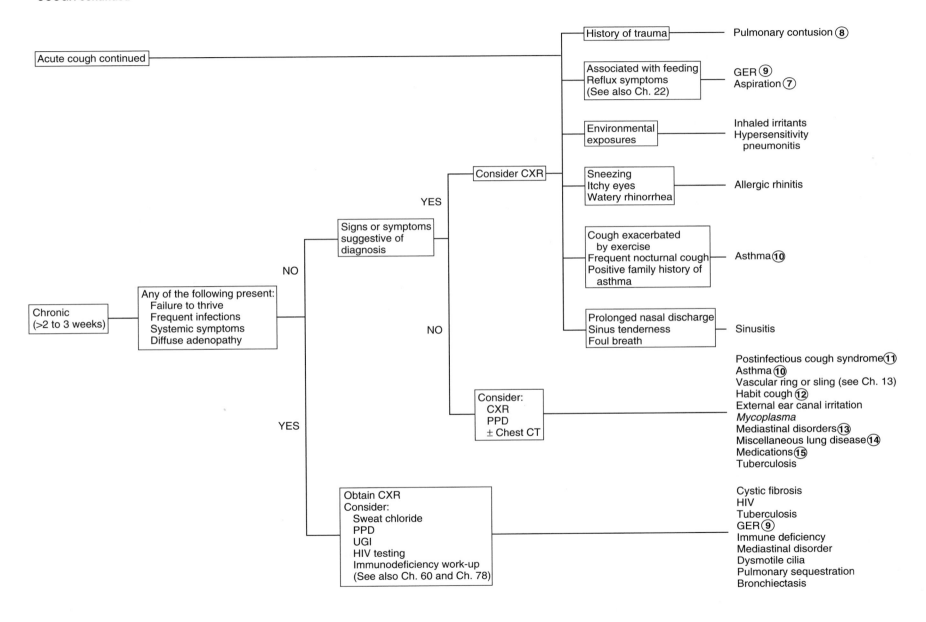

Chapter 11 Hoarseness

Hoarseness is a common, usually benign, pediatric symptom caused by alteration of the size, shape, or tension of the vocal cords. Evaluation is indicated for congenital hoarseness or acquired hoarseness that is associated with trauma or that persists longer than one to two weeks.

(1) Congenital anomalies of the larynx appearing as hoarseness include laryngoceles and webs. Laryngoceles may contain air or fluid (mucus or salivary gland excretions) and may occasionally become infected. Laryngeal fissures and clefts are rare conditions, but 20% of posterior fissures or clefts are associated with tracheoesophageal fistulas.

(2) Dislocation of the cricothyroid or cricoarytenoid articulations may occur during a traumatic birth. The trauma may also produce unilateral or bilateral vocal cord paralysis because of damage to the recurrent laryngeal nerve. Unilateral paralysis is usually on the left and manifests as hoarseness and mild stridor. It may be positional. Trauma related to neonatal intubation may also cause webs or dislocation of the laryngeal cartilages.

(3) Both congenital and acquired hoarseness can accompany numerous neurologic disorders in the newborn and include myasthenia gravis, bulbar palsy, hydrocephalus, and subdural hematoma. Other causes of brainstem compression can be associated with hoarseness. Bilateral paralysis causes dyspnea and stridor rather than hoarseness and is more likely to be associated with neurologic syndromes (e.g., Dandy-Walker cysts, Arnold-Chiari malformations).

(4) In some rare conditions, laryngoscopic findings are poorly described.

(5) Congenital hypothyroidism is often not apparent until after the newborn period. Presenting signs include hoarseness, prolonged hyperbilirubinemia, constipation, hypotonia, and hypothermia.

(6) Hoarseness may accompany hypocalcemic tetany in newborn infants. These infants should be assessed for aortic arch and thymus abnormalities.

(7) Rarely, breast-fed infants of thiamine-deficient mothers may develop hoarseness and aphonia.

(8) In older infants and toddlers, croup (laryngotracheobronchitis) is the most common cause of transient hoarseness and stridor. In older children laryngitis due to viral upper respiratory infections is the most common cause of transient hoarseness. Sinus disease is another less common cause.

(9) Hoarseness commonly occurs as a result of overuse of the voice. Inquire about recent attendance at athletic events or rock concerts.

(10) Allergic angioneurotic edema of the larynx may occur acutely with hoarseness and respiratory distress. Urgent evaluation and treatment are indicated.

(11) Benign vocal cord nodules ("screamer's nodules") may also be a complication of vocal overuse. Further evaluation is indicated if rest does not result in resolution.

(12) Acquired vocal cord paralysis may occur as a result of polyneuropathy (Guillain-Barré syndrome), brainstem encephalitis, compression from a mass or tumor, or neck or thoracic surgery.

(13) Granulomatous lesions in the larynx due to syphilis, tuberculosis, and histoplasmosis may result in hoarseness. Immunologic disorders including HIV infection may predispose patients to fungal infections of the airways. Prolonged use of inhaled corticosteroids has been associated with Candida overgrowth. Diphtheria, rabies, and tetanus may cause vocal cord paralysis.

(14) Airway papillomatosis develops as a progressive hoarseness and cough over the first several months of life. The etiology is human papillomavirus (most commonly type eleven) transmitted at birth from the mother's genital tract. Cutaneous hemangiomas, especially of the head and neck, may be a marker for underlying airway hemangiomas that can occur as progressive hoarseness or stridor over the first few months of life. Lymphangiomas, rhabdomyosarcomas, and leukemic infiltrations are other etiologies.

(15) Connective tissue disorders including juvenile rheumatoid arthritis are rare causes of hoarseness in children. Metabolic disorders cause hoarseness because of the abnormal deposition of metabolites in the airways or vocal cords. Vincristine toxicity, laryngeal edema related to congestive heart failure, and dryness (sicca syndrome) due to ectodermal dysplasia, cystic fibrosis, and antihistamine therapy are other causes.

BIBLIOGRAPHY

Friedberg J: Hoarseness. In Bluestone CD, Stool SE, Kenna MA (eds): Pediatric Otolaryngology, 3rd ed, p 1253. Philadelphia, WB Saunders Company,1996.

Smith D: Hoarseness. In Schidlow D, Smith D (eds): A Practical Guide to Pediatric Respiratory Diseases, p 27. Philadelphia, Hanley & Belfus, Inc, 1994.

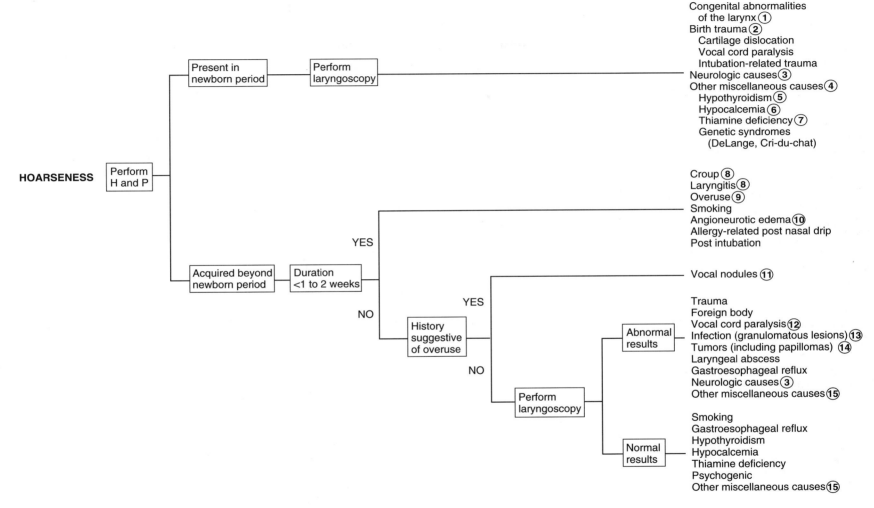

HOARSENESS

Perform H and P

Present in newborn period → Perform laryngoscopy →
Congenital abnormalities
of the larynx ①
Birth trauma ②
   Cartilage dislocation
   Vocal cord paralysis
   Intubation-related trauma
Neurologic causes ③
Other miscellaneous causes ④
   Hypothyroidism ⑤
   Hypocalcemia ⑥
   Thiamine deficiency ⑦
   Genetic syndromes
      (DeLange, Cri-du-chat)

Acquired beyond newborn period → **Duration <1 to 2 weeks**

YES →
Croup ⑧
Laryngitis ⑧
Overuse ⑨
Smoking
Angioneurotic edema ⑩
Allergy-related post nasal drip
Post intubation

NO → **History suggestive of overuse**

YES → Vocal nodules ⑪

NO → Perform laryngoscopy

Abnormal results →
Trauma
Foreign body
Vocal cord paralysis ⑫
Infection (granulomatous lesions) ⑬
Tumors (including papillomas) ⑭
Laryngeal abscess
Gastroesophageal reflux
Neurologic causes ③
Other miscellaneous causes ⑮

Normal results →
Smoking
Gastroesophageal reflux
Hypothyroidism
Hypocalcemia
Thiamine deficiency
Psychogenic
Other miscellaneous causes ⑮

Nelson chapters 388, 389
Practical Strategies chapter 10

Chapter 12 Stridor

Stridor is a predominantly inspiratory, coarse, crowing sound caused by obstruction in the upper airway.

① Inquire about risk factors for respiratory problems such as prematurity, intubation, chronic medical problems, and hospitalizations. The review of systems should include signs of infection, aggravating factors (such as position in infants), and any recent choking episodes. Signs of respiratory distress (e.g., nasal flaring, grunting, accessory muscle use, retractions) should be noted as well as chest wall asymmetry and chest excursion. More worrisome signs are cyanosis and altered mental status.

② X-rays may not be required in all cases of stridor. They will depend on the degree of respiratory distress and the specific clinical presentation. A child with a clinical picture consistent with croup who is stable and responding well to therapy may be managed without the need for a film. In contrast, a child with severe respiratory distress and a clinical picture suggesting epiglottitis (e.g., high fever, anxiety, drooling, cyanosis, tripod position) should be taken emergently to an operating room for intubation.

③ Croup (laryngotracheobronchitis) occurs most commonly in children under 2 years of age. It typically follows the onset of a cold by a few days and is characterized by a "barky" cough and inspiratory stridor. Low-grade fever is common. Occasional cases are complicated by severe upper airway obstruction and respiratory distress. In those cases bacterial tracheitis should be considered. Spasmodic croup refers to a clinically similar condition but without evidence of infection. Possible etiologies are allergic, psychologic, and viral, and gastroesophageal reflux. Croup is an unlikely etiology of stridor in children younger than 2 months of age.

④ Retropharyngeal abscesses usually occur as a complication of a bacterial pharyngitis. Patients become acutely ill with high fever, difficulty swallowing, hyperextension of the head, labored respiration, and drooling. Patients are usually less than 5 years of age.

⑤ Subglottic stenosis may be congenital or acquired. The latter may occur as a result of prolonged endotracheal intubation. Symptoms are exaggerated in an acute respiratory illness.

⑥ Diagnosis of foreign bodies can be difficult. Episodes of choking or gagging associated with the aspiration are often unobserved. Chest X-ray findings are frequently negative since many foreign bodies are not radiopaque. Associated chest X-ray findings are often subtle. Even fluoroscopy findings are negative in approximately 10% of patients. Computed tomography may be necessary for diagnosis. A history of recurrent or persistent pneumonia in a single lobe should arouse the clinician's suspicion for a retained foreign body.

⑦ Airway lesions (hemangioma, cyst) may cause airway obstruction due to rapid enlargement (hemorrhage, infection).

⑧ Laryngomalacia is a common cause of inspiratory stridor. It may appear at birth but most commonly appears at 2 to 4 weeks of age. Symptoms are characteristically worse when the infant is supine or agitated and typically resolve within the first year. Diagnosis is often clinical but may be confirmed by fluoroscopy or endoscopy. Laryngomalacia is often accompanied by tracheobronchomalacia that may cause cough and wheezing as well as stridor, which is more expiratory than inspiratory.

⑨ Hemangiomas may rarely occur in a subglottic location and are potentially life-threatening. They appear at several weeks to months of age as gradual enlargement causes progressive airway obstruction. Recurrent episodes of croup and concomitant cutaneous hemangiomas present in 50% of cases should prompt an evaluation for the condition.

⑩ Human papilloma viruses can cause recurrent respiratory tract papillomas. The larynx is the most common site for papillomas, although the entire respiratory tract may be affected. They can occur at any time from shortly after birth to several years of age as progressive hoarseness and dyspnea.

⑪ Vocal cord paralysis in the newborn is most commonly due to birth trauma secondary to recurrent laryngeal nerve trauma. Other causes include neurologic syndromes (e.g., Arnold-Chiari malformation) and neck or chest surgery.

BIBLIOGRAPHY

Pasterkamp H: The history and physical exam. In Chernick V, Boat TF (eds): Kendig's Disorders of the Respiratory Tract in Children, 6th ed, p 85. Philadelphia, WB Saunders Company, 1998.
Schidlow D, Smith D: Stridor and upper airway obstruction. In Schidlow D, Smith D (eds): A Practical Guide to Pediatric Respiratory Diseases, p 31. Philadelphia, Hanley & Belfus, Inc, 1994.

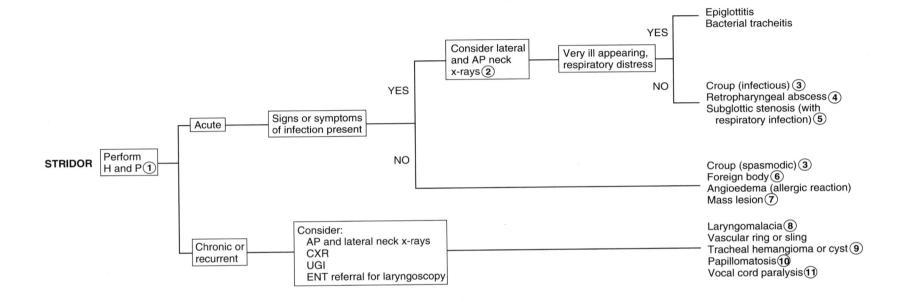

STRIDOR — Perform H and P ①

Acute → Signs or symptoms of infection present

YES → Consider lateral and AP neck x-rays ②

Very ill appearing, respiratory distress

YES → Epiglottitis
Bacterial tracheitis

NO → Croup (infectious) ③
Retropharyngeal abscess ④
Subglottic stenosis (with respiratory infection) ⑤

NO → Croup (spasmodic) ③
Foreign body ⑥
Angioedema (allergic reaction)
Mass lesion ⑦

Chronic or recurrent → Consider:
AP and lateral neck x-rays
CXR
UGI
ENT referral for laryngoscopy

→ Laryngomalacia ⑧
Vascular ring or sling
Tracheal hemangioma or cyst ⑨
Papillomatosis ⑩
Vocal cord paralysis ⑪

ENT= Otolaryngology

Nelson chapters 384, 386
Practical Strategies chapter 10

Chapter 13 **Wheezing**

Wheezing is a high-pitched musical sound caused by obstruction of the lower (intrathoracic) airways. The etiologies for wheezing are numerous. The clinical significance of the underlying problem can range from minimal to severe.

(1) Inquire about risk factors for respiratory problems such as prematurity, intubation, chronic medical problems, and hospitalizations. The review of systems should include signs and symptoms such as fever, weight loss, night sweats, and dysphagia. Inquire specifically about any recent choking episodes and about immunizations. Signs of respiratory distress (e.g., nasal flaring, grunting, accessory muscle use, retractions) should be noted as should chest wall asymmetry and chest excursion. More worrisome symptoms are cyanosis and altered mental status.

(2) In patients with an uncomplicated illness consistent with bronchiolitis, a chest X-ray is not indicated. One should be considered in other patients to rule out a treatable pneumonia.

(3) Bronchiolitis is a common lower respiratory tract infection in infants. Symptoms include profuse rhinorrhea, harsh cough, and tachypnea. Symptoms may progress to respiratory distress, especially in younger infants. Respiratory syncytial virus is the most common cause. Parainfluenza, influenza, and adenovirus can also cause bronchiolitis.

(4) *Mycoplasma* and *Chlamydia pneumoniae* are the exception to the "bacteria do not cause wheezing" generalization.

(5) Isolated episodes of wheezing or bronchospasm may occur with or without an associated respiratory illness. Allergic reactions and irritant inhalation can also be causes. A chest X-ray may be normal or show hyperinflation or atelectasis. A positive response to a trial of bronchodilator therapy confirms reversible airway obstruction. Until the wheezing manifests itself as a recurrent disorder of airway obstruction, the term asthma should not be used.

(6) Diagnosis of foreign bodies can be difficult. Episodes of choking or gagging associated with aspiration are often unobserved. Chest X-ray findings are frequently negative since many foreign bodies are not radiopaque. Associated chest X-ray findings are subtle. Even fluoroscopy findings are negative in approximately 10% of patients. Computed tomography may be necessary for diagnosis. A history of recurrent or persistent pneumonia in a single lobe should arouse the clinician's suspicion for a retained foreign body.

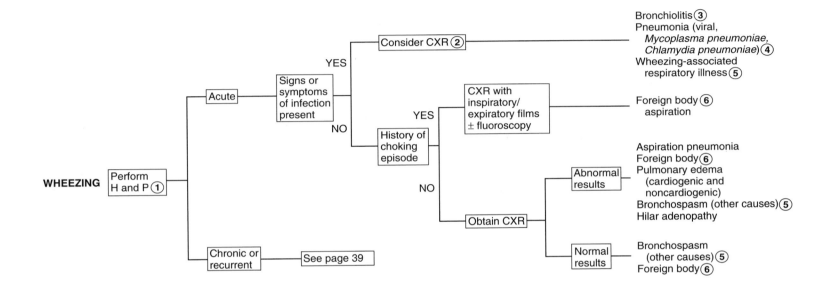

WHEEZING — Perform H and P ①

- **Acute**
  - **Signs or symptoms of infection present**
    - **YES** → Consider CXR ②
      - Bronchiolitis ③
      - Pneumonia (viral, *Mycoplasma pneumoniae*, *Chlamydia pneumoniae*) ④
      - Wheezing-associated respiratory illness ⑤
    - **NO** → **History of choking episode**
      - **YES** → CXR with inspiratory/expiratory films ± fluoroscopy
        - Foreign body ⑥ aspiration
      - **NO** → Obtain CXR
        - **Abnormal results**
          - Aspiration pneumonia
          - Foreign body ⑥
          - Pulmonary edema (cardiogenic and noncardiogenic)
          - Bronchospasm (other causes) ⑤
          - Hilar adenopathy
        - **Normal results**
          - Bronchospasm (other causes) ⑤
          - Foreign body ⑥
- **Chronic or recurrent**
  - See page 39

Nelson chapters 145, 384, 386, 415
Practical Strategies chapter 8

(7) Tracheobronchomalacia occurs with wheezing that is located more centrally then peripherally and is not responsive to bronchodilators. The lesion can be unilateral but is usually on the left. It can accompany laryngomalacia or occur as an isolated entity. (See Ch. 12.) Diagnosis is often clinically based, but it may be confirmed using endoscopy.

(8) Dyskinetic cilia syndrome is a rare cause of wheezing. Abnormal structure of the cilia leads to impaired clearance of endobronchial secretions resulting in chronic bronchitis. The clinical picture of recurrent wheezing, bronchitis, sinusitis, and otitis media is suspect for the disorder. It may also be present as a component of Kartagener syndrome (situs inversus totalis, chronic sinusitis, bronchiectasis, impaired sperm motility).

(9) Vocal cord dysfunction can mimic asthma by occurring with periodic wheezing and dyspnea that is unresponsive to inhaled bronchodilators. Even though the patients appear dyspneic, pulmonary gas exchange rate is normal. Pulmonary function tests during an episode demonstrate some degree of extrathoracic obstruction. Pulmonary function tests and supportive clinical history are adequate to make the diagnosis. Laryngoscopy (during an episode) may help to make the diagnosis in less clear cases. The disorder is most common in teenage girls, and underlying psychosocial stressors can often be identified.

(10) Several environmental contaminants including inorganic dusts (e.g., talcum, asbestos, silica), organic dusts, and chemical fumes can cause interstitial lung disease and wheezing. Inhalation of organic dusts can also cause hypersensitivity pneumonitis. This condition occurs as chronic or recurrent wheezing with characteristic chest X-ray and pulmonary function abnormalities.

(11) Gastroesophageal reflux (GER) can cause symptoms of wheezing from pulmonary aspiration or reflex bronchoconstriction occurring in response to esophageal acidification.

(12) Congenital malformations, including vascular anomalies, may appear with recurrent wheezing or stridor in young infants. Examples include tracheoesophageal fistulas, laryngeal or tracheal webs, stenoses, clefts, or atresias. Vascular anomalies include pulmonary slings and double aortic arches. Subtle characteristic chest X-ray findings may aid in diagnosis, but an esophagram, endoscopy, or bronchoscopy is often necessary.

BIBLIOGRAPHY

Kapoor S, Kurland G, Tunnessen W. Recurrent severe wheezing in a 17-year-old. Contemp Pediatr 17:27, 2000.

Pasterkamp H: The history and physical exam. In Chernick V, Boat TF (eds): Kendig's Disorders of the Respiratory Tract in Children, 6th ed, p 85. Philadelphia, WB Saunders Company, 1998.

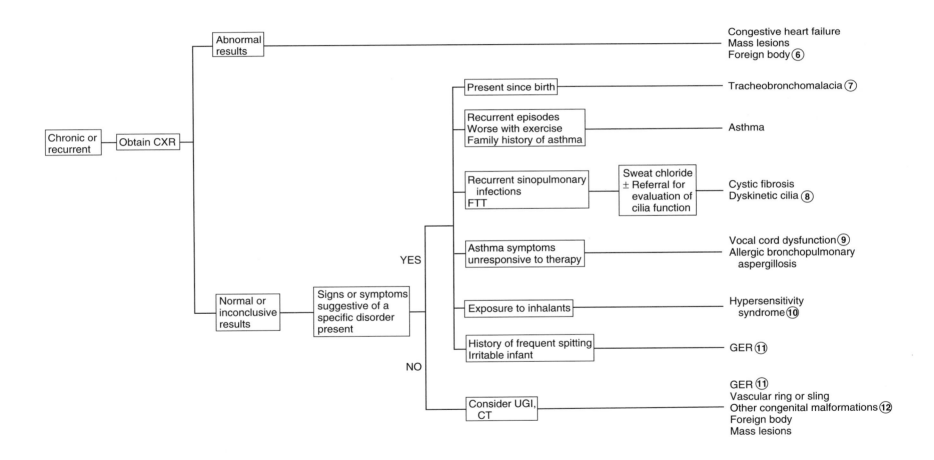

Chapter 14 *Cyanosis*

Cyanosis refers to a bluish discoloration of the skin or mucous membranes. Central cyanosis affects the skin, mucous membranes, lips, and conjunctiva. It occurs secondary to significant arterial oxygen desaturation. A minimum of 4 to 5 g/dl of desaturated hemoglobin must be present in order for cyanosis to be clinically evident. Cyanosis is due to pulmonary, cardiac, CNS (hypoventilation), neuromuscular (hypoventilation), or hematologic etiologies. Acrocyanosis is a benign bluish discoloration of the hands and feet that occurs due to peripheral vasoconstriction, usually in young infants. (The differential diagnosis of cyanosis in the neonate is not included in this algorithm.)

(1) Pertinent elements of the history of the cyanotic patient vary according to the age of the patient. For infants, the birth history and age of onset of cyanosis are important. For older children, a history of trauma, possible ingestion, or choking may be helpful. Physical signs suggestive of certain genetic syndromes may also be helpful in the evaluation of some infants. Older children should be assessed for signs of chronic or progressive illness, including growth parameters, clubbing, and stigmata of neuromuscular or hepatic disease. Obtaining an oxygen saturation value early in the assessment of a cyanotic patient is recommended. Arterial blood gases help to distinguish pulmonary from cardiac etiologies.

(2) Cyanotic congenital heart disease (CHD) is almost always diagnosed early in the newborn period. Some cardiac diseases, most commonly tetralogy of Fallot, can occur with cyanosis weeks to months after birth. If CHD is suspected, the hyperoxia test (i.e., obtaining an arterial blood gas value before and after the child breathes 100% FIO_2) can help distinguish respiratory causes of cyanosis from pulmonary causes. Clinical status and arterial PO_2 improve with respiratory disease. Minimal changes occur with cyanotic heart lesions. A pediatric cardiologist should be consulted whenever the diagnosis of CHD is suspected. An echocardiogram will quickly help to establish most diagnoses.

(3) Cyanosis commonly accompanies apnea in children of any age. Causes include infection (RSV, pertussis, sepsis, meningitis), seizures, gastroesophageal reflux, ALTE, and neuromuscular disorders causing hypoventilation. (See also Ch. 16.)

(4) Cyanotic breath-holding spells (cyanotic infant syncope) are common paroxysmal episodes characterized by sudden lack of inspiratory effort during crying. Cyanosis, opisthotonus, tonic posturing or clonic movements, and a brief loss of consciousness typically follow. The child is fully recovered within one minute. These spells typically occur between 6 months and 18 months, although they may be seen up to age 6 years. They are usually precipitated by an event that is frustrating, frightening, or painful to the child. No diagnostic evaluation is indicated.

(5) Cyanosis can occur with ingestion of agents that cause respiratory depression (e.g., narcotics and sedatives) or airway edema and obstruction (e.g., acid and alkali products).

(6) Methemoglobinemia may occur because of abnormal hemoglobin or deficiency of enzymes involved in the reduction of heme. Certain drugs or toxins (e.g., oxidizing agents in drugs or anesthesia, nitrates in well water) can also be responsible for the disorder, especially in young infants who have low levels of methemoglobin reductase activity and increased susceptibility to oxidation of hemoglobin F. Mild forms of congenital methemoglobinemia may appear later in infancy or childhood due to infections or exposure to precipitating agents. Obtain a methemoglobin level to confirm the diagnosis. Be aware that a blood gas test provides a calculated saturation value that may be misleading. A pulse oximetry provides an accurate value in the presence of methemoglobinemia. A low pulse oximetry saturation, dark brown arterial blood, and normal arterial PO_2 are highly suggestive.

BIBLIOGRAPHY

Dimaia AM, Singh J: The infant with cyanosis in the emergency room. Pediatr Clin North Am 39:987–1006, 1992.

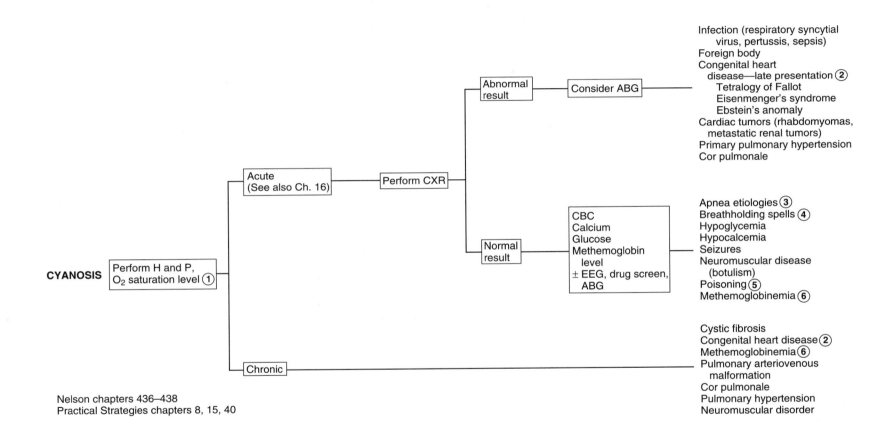

CYANOSIS — Perform H and P, O₂ saturation level ①

Acute (See also Ch. 16) → Perform CXR

Abnormal result → Consider ABG →
- Infection (respiratory syncytial virus, pertussis, sepsis)
- Foreign body
- Congenital heart disease—late presentation ②
  - Tetralogy of Fallot
  - Eisenmenger's syndrome
  - Ebstein's anomaly
- Cardiac tumors (rhabdomyomas, metastatic renal tumors)
- Primary pulmonary hypertension
- Cor pulmonale

Normal result →
- CBC
- Calcium
- Glucose
- Methemoglobin level
- ± EEG, drug screen, ABG

→
- Apnea etiologies ③
- Breathholding spells ④
- Hypoglycemia
- Hypocalcemia
- Seizures
- Neuromuscular disease (botulism)
- Poisoning ⑤
- Methemoglobinemia ⑥

Chronic →
- Cystic fibrosis
- Congenital heart disease ②
- Methemoglobinemia ⑥
- Pulmonary arteriovenous malformation
- Cor pulmonale
- Pulmonary hypertension
- Neuromuscular disorder

Nelson chapters 436–438
Practical Strategies chapters 8, 15, 40

Chapter 15 **Hemoptysis**

Hemoptysis, the expectoration of blood from the respiratory tract, is typically bright red, foamy, and mixed with sputum, and has an alkaline pH. It is associated with coughing and in some cases chest pain or sensation of gurgling or warmth. Hemoptysis must be distinguished from blood from the GI tract (hematemesis), which is often dark red or brown with an acidic pH. Hematemesis is also more likely to be associated with nausea or abdominal pain than with coughing. It must also be distinguished from blood that originates in one site but is expelled from another. For example, bleeding from epistaxis may result in blood that is swallowed and coughed out.

(1) The history should contain inquiries about associated respiratory symptoms, epistaxis, recent procedures (e.g., tonsillectomy, laryngoscopy), and the possibility of a bleeding disorder. Children with certain underlying conditions are predisposed to pulmonary hemorrhage that, in some cases, can be severe. Children with cystic fibrosis have the greatest risk of hemoptysis. Other at-risk disorders include cardiac disease, hemoglobinopathies, connective tissue disorders, coagulation abnormalities, and immunodeficiency states. A chest X-ray and specialty consultation should be urgently obtained when children with these conditions present with hemoptysis.

(2) Lung contusions may occur without evidence of external trauma. The chest X-ray may reveal a poorly defined density. Initial films, however, may appear normal.

(3) If the child has spit up a minimal amount of blood and if the clinical picture is consistent with a nonthreatening self-limiting upper respiratory illness, it may not be necessary to obtain a chest X-ray or perform any further evaluation. Severe coughing may cause a small amount of hemoptysis in even mild cases of viral respiratory infections (e.g., tracheobronchitis) because the mucosa is inflamed and friable.

(4) In approximately 20% of cases of hemoptysis no etiology will be found. These patients generally have a very good prognosis and minimal likelihood of recurrence.

(5) Infection is a common cause of hemoptysis. Children who have traveled internationally may be at risk for unusual parasitic infections. Uncomplicated pneumonias are unlikely to cause hemoptysis, but severe pneumonias, particularly in immunodeficient children, may result in hemoptysis due to erosion of bronchial wall vessels. Severe viral pneumonias (e.g., adenovirus, measles) and tuberculosis are other risk factors for hemoptysis.

(6) Bleeding from a foreign body may appear weeks to months after the aspiration. Often there is no recall of a choking episode. Organic foreign bodies are problematic because they cause an inflammatory reaction that can result in significant bleeding. They are radiolucent and typically yield only subtle X-ray findings, such as air trapping or atelectasis. In some cases, bronchoscopy may not be diagnostic if the object has worked its way into smaller airways. Diagnosis may be delayed until the infected area is removed surgically. Sharp foreign bodies may cause acute hemoptysis because of airway laceration.

(7) Cystic fibrosis is the most common chronic condition in children who experience hemoptysis. Bronchiectasis (i.e., dilation and weakening of the airway wall) occurs secondary to chronic inflammation and infection. Acute or chronic hemoptysis that is usually mild occurs due to leakage of these bronchial wall vessels. Anastomoses between pulmonary and bronchial arteries can occasionally result in significant bleeding. Coagulopathy due to vitamin K malabsorption may also be present.

(8) The most common vascular anomalies leading to hemoptysis are arteriovenous malformations. One half of children with pulmonary arteriovenous malformations have hereditary hemorrhagic telangiectasia (Osler-Weber-Rendu syndrome), an autosomal dominant condition. A history of recurrent epistaxis, positive family history, and development of mucocutaneous telangiectases at puberty support this diagnosis. Large fistulas may be seen on chest X-ray. Computed tomography, MRI, or fluoroscopy may be necessary to help to diagnose smaller lesions. Airway hemangiomas, unilateral pulmonary artery agenesis, and bronchial artery aneurysms are less common lesions.

(9) Pulmonary hemosiderosis is a rare condition that results from alveolar hemorrhage. Chest X-ray findings may or may not correlate with the severity of the disease. Four types of primary pulmonary hemosiderosis are recognized: idiopathic, hypersensitivity to cow's milk (Heiner syndrome), and association with myocarditis and with progressive glomerulonephritis (Goodpasture syndrome). Clinical manifestations of chronic lung disease develop over time and include cough, hemoptysis, dyspnea, wheezing, clubbing, and occasionally cyanosis. Iron deficiency anemia is also characteristic. Large numbers of hemosiderin-laden macrophages in gastric fluid, sputum, bronchial washings, or lung biopsy specimens are diagnostic indicators. Open lung biopsy may be necessary for the definitive diagnosis.

Hypersensitivity to cow's milk is suggested by high serum titers of precipitins to cow's milk proteins and symptomatic improvement on a milk-free diet. Goodpasture syndrome occurs mostly in young adult males and is characterized by immunoglobulin deposition on alveolar and glomerular basement membranes.

(10) Congenital or acquired heart lesions that cause chronically elevated pulmonary venous pressures result in hemoptysis due to dilation and angiomatoid changes of small pulmonary arteries. These changes occur slowly and appear with hemoptysis in adolescence or young adulthood.

(11) Rigid or flexible bronchoscopy may be indicated when bleeding is active to provide suction during the procedure. Bronchoscopy would also be the procedure of choice if aspiration of a

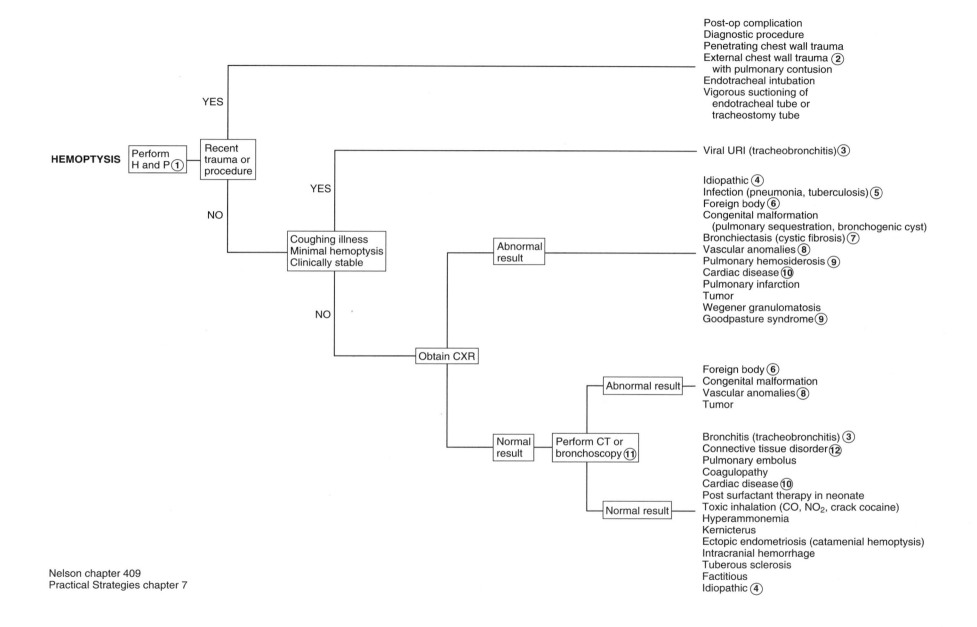

HEMOPTYSIS → Perform H and P ①

Recent trauma or procedure

YES →
Post-op complication
Diagnostic procedure
Penetrating chest wall trauma
External chest wall trauma ②
  with pulmonary contusion
Endotracheal intubation
Vigorous suctioning of
  endotracheal tube or
  tracheostomy tube

NO → Coughing illness / Minimal hemoptysis / Clinically stable

YES → Viral URI (tracheobronchitis) ③

NO → Obtain CXR

Abnormal result →
Idiopathic ④
Infection (pneumonia, tuberculosis) ⑤
Foreign body ⑥
Congenital malformation
  (pulmonary sequestration, bronchogenic cyst)
Bronchiectasis (cystic fibrosis) ⑦
Vascular anomalies ⑧
Pulmonary hemosiderosis ⑨
Cardiac disease ⑩
Pulmonary infarction
Tumor
Wegener granulomatosis
Goodpasture syndrome ⑨

Normal result → Perform CT or bronchoscopy ⑪

Abnormal result →
Foreign body ⑥
Congenital malformation
Vascular anomalies ⑧
Tumor

Normal result →
Bronchitis (tracheobronchitis) ③
Connective tissue disorder ⑫
Pulmonary embolus
Coagulopathy
Cardiac disease ⑩
Post surfactant therapy in neonate
Toxic inhalation (CO, NO_2, crack cocaine)
Hyperammonemia
Kernicterus
Ectopic endometriosis (catamenial hemoptysis)
Intracranial hemorrhage
Tuberous sclerosis
Factitious
Idiopathic ④

Nelson chapter 409
Practical Strategies chapter 7

foreign body is suspected because it provides the capability for extraction. Bronchoalveolar washings should be obtained if pulmonary hemosiderosis is a consideration. Chest CT with contrast or angiography is helpful in diagnosis of congenital or arteriovenous malformations.

 Hemoptysis can occur as a result of vasculitis associated with an immunologic or connective tissue disorder. Occasionally, this may be the first manifestation of a disorder, although other signs and symptoms (e.g., malaise, weight loss, unexplained fever) are often present.

BIBLIOGRAPHY

Boat TF: Pulmonary hemorrhage and hemoptysis. In Chernick V, Boat TF (eds): Kendig's Disorders of the Respiratory Tract in Children, 6th ed, p 623. Philadelphia, WB Saunders Company, 1998.

Panitch HB: Hemoptysis. In Schidlow D, Smith D (eds): A Practical Guide to Pediatric Respiratory Diseases, p 49. Philadelphia, Hanley & Belfus, Inc, 1994.

Sherman JM: When you see red. Contemp Pediatr 14:79, 1997.

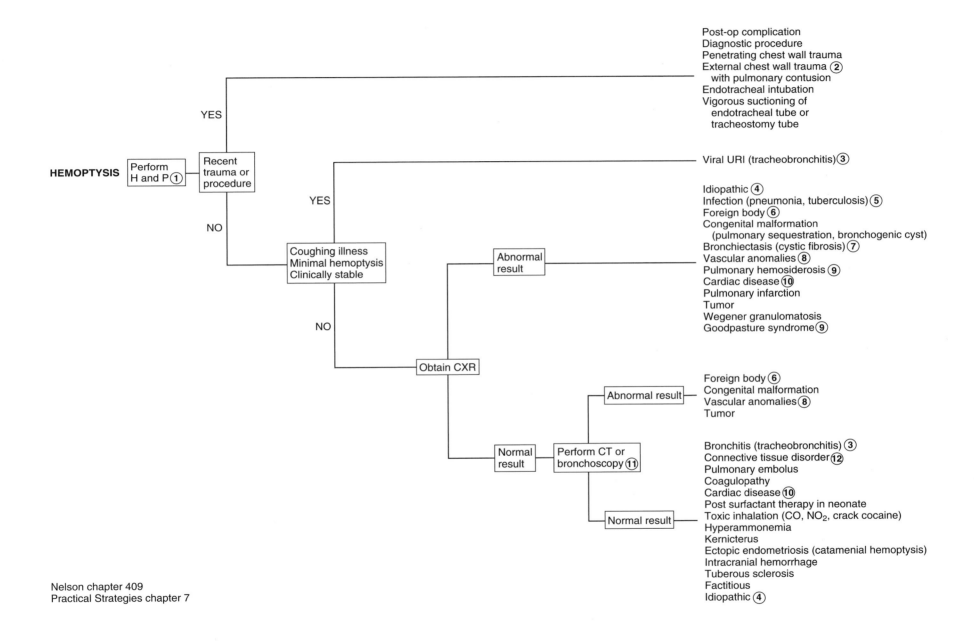

HEMOPTYSIS — Perform H and P ①

Recent trauma or procedure

YES →
Post-op complication
Diagnostic procedure
Penetrating chest wall trauma
External chest wall trauma ②
 with pulmonary contusion
Endotracheal intubation
Vigorous suctioning of
 endotracheal tube or
 tracheostomy tube

NO → Coughing illness / Minimal hemoptysis / Clinically stable

YES → Viral URI (tracheobronchitis) ③

Abnormal result →
Idiopathic ④
Infection (pneumonia, tuberculosis) ⑤
Foreign body ⑥
Congenital malformation
 (pulmonary sequestration, bronchogenic cyst)
Bronchiectasis (cystic fibrosis) ⑦
Vascular anomalies ⑧
Pulmonary hemosiderosis ⑨
Cardiac disease ⑩
Pulmonary infarction
Tumor
Wegener granulomatosis
Goodpasture syndrome ⑨

NO → Obtain CXR

Abnormal result →
Foreign body ⑥
Congenital malformation
Vascular anomalies ⑧
Tumor

Normal result → Perform CT or bronchoscopy ⑪

Abnormal result →
(see above)

Normal result →
Bronchitis (tracheobronchitis) ③
Connective tissue disorder ⑫
Pulmonary embolus
Coagulopathy
Cardiac disease ⑩
Post surfactant therapy in neonate
Toxic inhalation (CO, NO_2, crack cocaine)
Hyperammonemia
Kernicterus
Ectopic endometriosis (catamenial hemoptysis)
Intracranial hemorrhage
Tuberous sclerosis
Factitious
Idiopathic ④

Nelson chapter 409
Practical Strategies chapter 7

Chapter 16 Apnea

Apnea is the cessation of breathing for twenty seconds or for any period if accompanied by pallor, cyanosis, or bradycardia. Apnea may originate from a central or an obstructive cause or from a combination of both elements.

Apparent life-threatening event (ALTE) is a term used to describe any acute apneic event that is considered life-threatening. An ALTE includes some combination of apnea, bradycardia, cyanosis, and altered tone or consciousness. It may be caused by a number of etiologies.

When parents report that their child stopped breathing, benign conditions such as periodic breathing or breath-holding spells must be differentiated from true apnea. Periodic breathing is a nonpathologic breathing pattern of three or more respiratory pauses of three to five seconds separated by periods of respiration of less than twenty seconds. It is most common in premature infants but is also seen in full term infants until several months of age. Cyanotic breath-holding spells (cyanotic infant syncope) are characterized by a sudden lack of inspiratory effort during crying usually due to frustration or anger. Apnea, cyanosis, opisthotonus, tonic posturing or clonic movements, and brief loss of consciousness typically follow. In pallid breath-holding spells, pallor, tone loss, and occasionally a tonic seizure accompany the apneic event. Pallid spells are less common than cyanotic ones and are usually precipitated by a painful event. Breath-holding spells typically occur between ages 6 and 18 months, although they may be seen in children to age 6 years. Children recover quickly from these events, and no diagnostic evaluation is indicated.

The differential diagnosis of apnea in neonates is extensive and includes many conditions unique to the neonate. Neither neonatal apnea nor apnea of prematurity are discussed here.

(1) The history for an apneic event should include any associated illness, the relationship of the event to sleeping and eating, and the presence or absence of associated symptoms, such as cyanosis, bradycardia, altered level of consciousness, and posturing or abnormal tonic-clonic movements. Inquiries should be made about whether any intervention was needed and how quickly the child recovered from the event. For infants who were sleeping, inquire about position, bedding, and covering. The review of systems should include information about symptoms of airway obstruction, including chronic mouth breathing, noisy daytime respirations, snoring, and restlessness during sleep.

(2) Respiratory infections frequently associated with apnea include RSV (respiratory syncytial virus) bronchiolitis and pertusis. Both central and obstructive apnea can occur with RSV bronchiolitis. In RSV there may be minimal pulmonary findings. Localized upper airway infections (e.g., tonsillitis, peritonsillar or retropharyngeal abscesses, croup, epiglottitis) can result in obstructive apnea.

(3) Urine toxicology screens are simple to perform, and in 10% to 15% of cases reveal a drug contributing to the episode. Barbiturates, salicylates, ipecac, boric acid, and cocaine are examples. Carbon monoxide poisoning can also be an etiology.

(4) Obstructive sleep apnea is a sleep-related airway obstruction. The diagnosis can be made based on certain anatomic abnormalities; however, the physical examination is often normal, and symptoms of airway obstruction are not always present. Children are less likely to experience frequent awakenings and daytime hypersomnolence than adults with obstructive sleep apnea. They are also less likely to be obese. They are more likely to exhibit poor growth or failure to thrive. Parents typically describe their children's cycle of loud snoring followed by a pause, then a snorting with some level of arousal, and resumption of the snoring. If the diagnosis is not obvious, polysomnography in a sleep laboratory with experience with children is necessary for diagnosis.

(5) Nasal obstruction may occur due to polyps, choanal stenosis, or severe allergies.

(6) Laryngeal and subglottic abnormalities detected by upper airway evaluation include cysts, webs, hemangiomas, laryngomalacia, and vocal cord paralysis. Airway hemangiomas are often associated with hemangiomas on the face, neck, or upper trunk.

(7) Children with neurologic problems (e.g., birth asphyxia, Chiari malformation, neuromuscular disease) often experience pharyngeal hypotonia, which contributes to airway obstruction.

(8) Gastroesophageal reflux (GER) can be the cause of apnea both with and without an association with feeding and spitting. An upper gastrointestinal series (UGI) is not a sensitive test for GER. In the child with clinical reflux, the UGI is done primarily to rule out causes of outlet obstruction. In the case in which the reflux is not clinically apparent, further evaluation may be deferred if the UGI reveals severe reflux. A pH probe performed as part of polysomnography (i.e., an overnight study assessing multiple cardiorespiratory parameters) is a more sensitive diagnostic test for GER, plus it can distinguish between obstructive and nonobstructive apnea.

(9) Electroencephalograms are performed most commonly at this point in the evaluation of a child with apnea, but the diagnostic yield is very low. The diagnosis of a seizure is more likely in children who are experiencing recurrent apneic episodes or having associated abnormal movements.

Rarely, certain metabolic disorders occur with apnea, but clinical stigmata, such as recurrent emesis, lethargy, hepatomegaly, and developmental delays or regression, are usually apparent. A serum ammonia is considered an adequate screen for metabolic disorders. More extensive evaluation may be necessary in infants with a family history of metabolic disorders or unexplained infant deaths and with frequent severe apneic events or apneic events after 7 months of age.

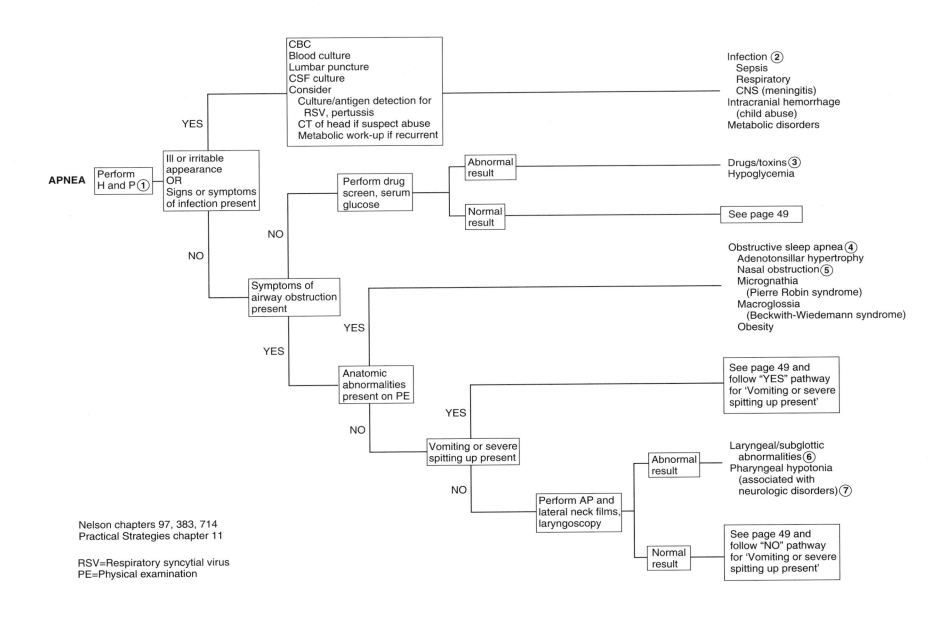

APNEA → Perform H and P ①

Ill or irritable appearance OR Signs or symptoms of infection present

YES →
CBC
Blood culture
Lumbar puncture
CSF culture
Consider
    Culture/antigen detection for
      RSV, pertussis
    CT of head if suspect abuse
    Metabolic work-up if recurrent

→ Infection ②
  Sepsis
  Respiratory
  CNS (meningitis)
Intracranial hemorrhage
  (child abuse)
Metabolic disorders

NO → Perform drug screen, serum glucose

Abnormal result → Drugs/toxins ③
Hypoglycemia

Normal result → See page 49

NO → Symptoms of airway obstruction present

YES → Obstructive sleep apnea ④
  Adenotonsillar hypertrophy
  Nasal obstruction ⑤
  Micrognathia
    (Pierre Robin syndrome)
  Macroglossia
    (Beckwith-Wiedeman syndrome)
  Obesity

NO → Anatomic abnormalities present on PE

YES → See page 49 and follow "YES" pathway for 'Vomiting or severe spitting up present'

NO → Vomiting or severe spitting up present

NO → Perform AP and lateral neck films, laryngoscopy

Abnormal result → Laryngeal/subglottic abnormalities ⑥
Pharyngeal hypotonia (associated with neurologic disorders) ⑦

Normal result → See page 49 and follow "NO" pathway for 'Vomiting or severe spitting up present'

Nelson chapters 97, 383, 714
Practical Strategies chapter 11

RSV=Respiratory syncytial virus
PE=Physical examination

Apnea *(continued)*

If a child who experiences apnea also presents with evidence of cranial nerve dysfunction (stridor, hoarseness, weak cry) or weakness or hyperreflexia, neuroimaging should be performed to rule out a Chiari II malformation. Progressive hydrocephalus and myelomeningocele are usually evident in children with this disorder.

(10) Apnea of infancy is an idiopathic sleep-dependent episode accompanied by bradycardia, cyanosis, and hypotonia. Although it is the major subcategory of ALTEs, it remains a diagnosis of exclusion.

(11) Central hypoventilation syndrome (CHS) is a rare but serious disorder of decreased central respiratory drive. It may occur with apnea at birth, although milder cases may not occur until later, with the development of cor pulmonale or acute respiratory infection. A sleep laboratory evaluation that documents central apnea or hypoventilation and an abnormal response to hypercarbia are necessary to make the diagnosis.

BIBLIOGRAPHY

Arens R, Gozai D, Williams JC, et al: Recurrent apparent life-threatening events during infancy. J Pediatr 123:415, 1993.

Keens TG: Apnea spells, sudden death and the role of the apnea monitor. Pediatr Clin North Am 40:897–911, 1993.

Varlotta L, Allen J: Apnea. In Schidlow D, Smith D (eds): A Practical Guide to Pediatric Respiratory Diseases, p 149. Philadelphia, Hanley & Belfus, Inc, 1994.

APNEA (continued)

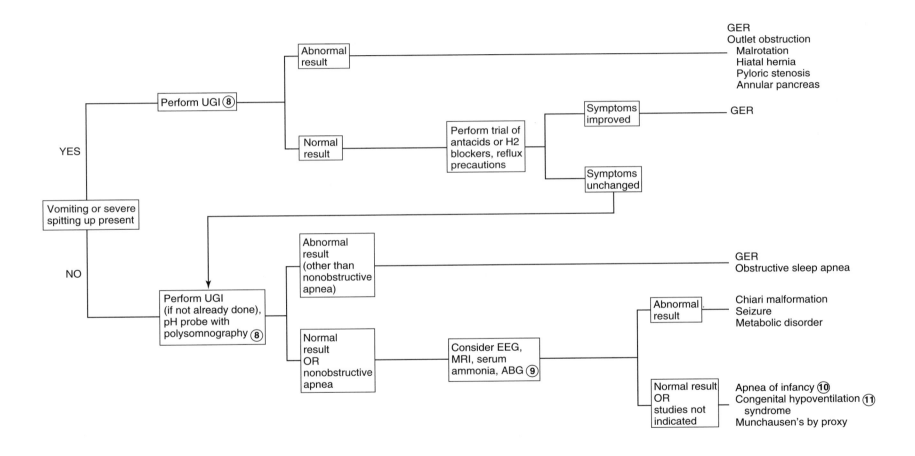

CARDIOLOGY

Chapter 17 Chest Pain

Chest pain is common in children and adolescents. Despite the degree of concern that it generates, the symptom is rarely associated with a serious illness. Between 20% and 45% of pediatric cases of chest pain are labeled idiopathic. Cardiac etiologies of pediatric chest pain are less than 5% of all identifiable etiologies.

(1) A properly done history and physical are often the only tools required in the evaluation of chest pain. Screening tests are not considered helpful unless specifically indicated.

A medical history of asthma, sickle cell disease, or recent coughing illness may be helpful. Long-standing diabetes mellitus and chronic anemias are risk factors for ischemic chest pain. Inquire about a history of Kawasaki disease, including the possibility of an undiagnosed case. The review of systems should include inquiries about associated acute and chronic symptoms and any precipitating factors. Associated syncope is very worrisome and mandates an urgent cardiac evaluation. Identify medications (e.g., cisapride, antihistamine, erythromycin) and investigate the possibility of substance abuse, including that of cocaine. Evaluation of psychosocial factors in the child's life is very important. Ask about school attendance and performance, relationships with friends and family, and any current stresses or conflicts.

The family history should include references to hypercholesterolemia, Marfan syndrome, and cardiomyopathy. A family history of recurrent syncope or unexplained sudden death may suggest hypertrophic obstructive cardiomyopathy or long Q-T syndrome. Heart disease in an adult may provoke anxiety-related chest pain in a younger person (i.e., they may worry that they too have a problem).

(2) Costochondritis is pain of the costal cartilages and a common cause of chest pain. More rare is Tietze syndrome that includes visible swelling at the costochondral junction in addition to the pain and tenderness associated with costochondritis.

(3) Musculoskeletal chest wall pain is characterized by areas of localized tenderness involving the ribs, costochondral junctions, costal cartilages, intercostal muscles, sternum, clavicles, or spine. Exertion is the likely cause if the patient recently began a new activity or sport. Intense or persistent coughing may produce this type of pain. The carrying of heavy books is another frequent cause. Overuse due to excessive or repetitive truncal or upper extremity action can also be responsible.

(4) Early puberty may cause chest pain related to breast nodule development in males and females. Other breast disorders including infections, cystic disorders, pregnancy, and menstrual swelling may cause chest pain in females.

(5) Sharp pain in the intercostal muscles is frequently due to infection with Coxsackie virus or other enteroviruses. This pain (pleurodynia) is sudden in onset, paroxysmal, and accompanied by fever and other systemic signs. Sometimes the illness occurs in a biphasic pattern.

(6) Pain related to shingles (herpes zoster) may precede the appearance of the rash.

(7) Chest pain is frequently attributed to psychogenic causes. An exclusively psychologic basis is rare. More commonly, a patient has a physiologic type of pain (usually benign, like chest wall pain) that is exacerbated by psychologic issues. Anxiety and panic disorders manifest with a variety of symptoms including chest pain and hyperventilation that are usually related temporally to a stressful event. Do not use psychogenic chest pain as a diagnosis of exclusion. Criteria that support the diagnosis must be identified.

(8) Hyperventilation typically occurs with over-breathing, dyspnea, and anxiety, and sometimes with palpitations, chest pain, paresthesias, lightheadedness, and confusion. Anxiety or underlying psychiatric problems are frequently revealed. No additional work-up is required when the history is consistent with hyperventilation.

(9) Precordial catch syndrome or Texidor twinge is a benign condition characterized by brief paroxysms (30 seconds to 3 minutes) of sharp pains in the left parasternal region near the cardiac apex. It is more likely to occur if a patient's posture is slouched or bent over, and it is likely to correct with improved posture.

(10) Chest pain from esophageal motility disorders is usually substernal but may radiate to the infrascapular area and neck. It is nonexertional but may be associated with bending forward. Achalasia occurs with the classic triad of dysphagia, nocturnal regurgitation, and chest pain. It may be difficult to diagnose because of an insidious onset.

(11) Mitral valve prolapse (MVP) is not more common in children with chest pain than in the general pediatric population. Most children with MVP do not complain of chest pain.

(12) Referral to a cardiologist is generally considered a more cost-effective alternative than obtaining an echocardiogram without consultation.

(13) Hypertrophic obstructive cardiomyopathy is an autosomal dominant condition, although 40% of cases will not be associated with evidence of genetic transmission. The cardiac examination typically reveals a left ventricular lift and an ejection murmur that is heard best over the left sternal border and apex and is exaggerated with a Valsalva maneuver.

(14) Infections are rare but serious causes of chest pain in children. Pericarditis is more symptomatic than myocarditis. The latter may occur with a more subtle but progressive illness, including fever, chest pain, vomiting, and shortness of breath. Electrocardiograms are abnormal in each of these conditions, and chest X-rays show cardiomegaly.

(15) Asthma, cystic fibrosis, and Marfan syndrome are risk factors for pneumothorax.

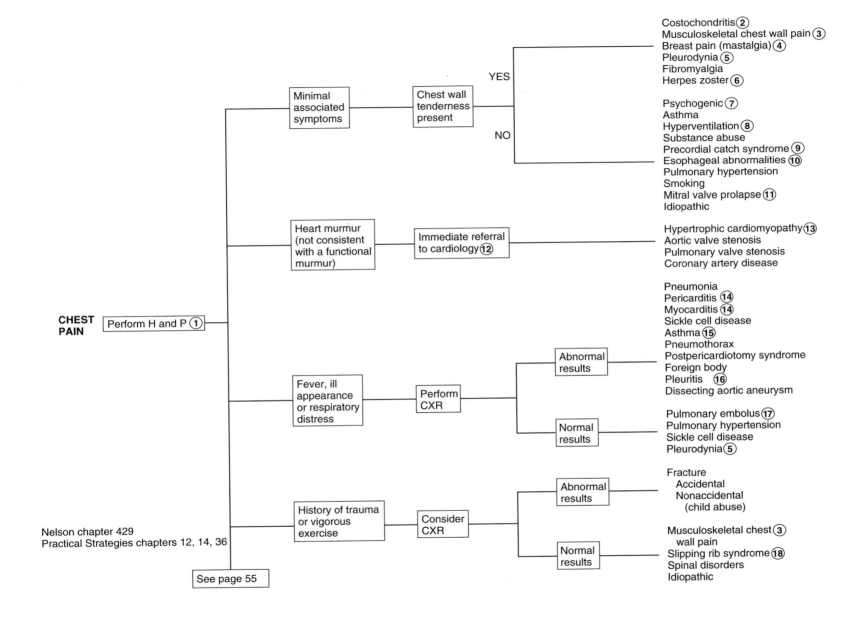

CHEST
PAIN — Perform H and P ①

Minimal associated symptoms → **Chest wall tenderness present**

YES →
Costochondritis ②
Musculoskeletal chest wall pain ③
Breast pain (mastalgia) ④
Pleurodynia ⑤
Fibromyalgia
Herpes zoster ⑥

NO →
Psychogenic ⑦
Asthma
Hyperventilation ⑧
Substance abuse
Precordial catch syndrome ⑨
Esophageal abnormalities ⑩
Pulmonary hypertension
Smoking
Mitral valve prolapse ⑪
Idiopathic

Heart murmur (not consistent with a functional murmur) → **Immediate referral to cardiology ⑫**
Hypertrophic cardiomyopathy ⑬
Aortic valve stenosis
Pulmonary valve stenosis
Coronary artery disease

Fever, ill appearance or respiratory distress → **Perform CXR**

Abnormal results →
Pneumonia
Pericarditis ⑭
Myocarditis ⑭
Sickle cell disease
Asthma ⑮
Pneumothorax
Postpericardiotomy syndrome
Foreign body
Pleuritis ⑯
Dissecting aortic aneurysm

Normal results →
Pulmonary embolus ⑰
Pulmonary hypertension
Sickle cell disease
Pleurodynia ⑤

History of trauma or vigorous exercise → **Consider CXR**

Abnormal results →
Fracture
  Accidental
  Nonaccidental
    (child abuse)

Normal results →
Musculoskeletal chest ③
  wall pain
Slipping rib syndrome ⑱
Spinal disorders
Idiopathic

Nelson chapter 429
Practical Strategies chapters 12, 14, 36

See page 55

Healthy children may also experience pneumothorax. Cocaine use is a risk factor.

(16) Movement and deep breathing often aggravate the pain associated with pleuritis or pleural effusions. Bacterial pneumonias are the most common cause of pleuritis in children.

(17) Risk factors for venous thrombosis (e.g., oral contraceptives; recent abortion or surgery; immobilization; genetic, hypercoagulable states) should raise suspicion for pulmonary emboli. Associated symptoms include dyspnea, cough, hypoxia, and occasionally hemoptysis. If emboli are suspected, a ventilation perfusion scan or spiral CT should be performed.

(18) Slipping rib syndrome is characterized by pain and a slipping sensation sometimes with a popping or clicking sound at the lower costal margin. Trauma to the eighth, ninth, or most commonly tenth rib causes a sprainlike injury which increases the mobility of the rib. The pain may be elicited by hooking the fingers under the anterior costal margins and pulling the ribs forward.

(19) If syncope has accompanied the palpitations, a more urgent evaluation is indicated. (See also Ch. 19.)

(20) Exercise testing is recommended when symptoms are primarily associated with exercise. The patient's EKG is monitored during incremental increases in exercise in an attempt to uncover an arrhythmia.

(21) Holter monitoring or transtelephonic event recording are options for further evaluation of presumed arrhythmias. When the EKG is normal and the episodes are believed to be secondary to premature beats or bradycardia, additional work-up is optional or determined by the severity of the symptoms or complaint. Although not painful per se, the sensation of premature beats or bradycardia may be described as chest pain or discomfort by some patients.

CHEST PAIN (continued)

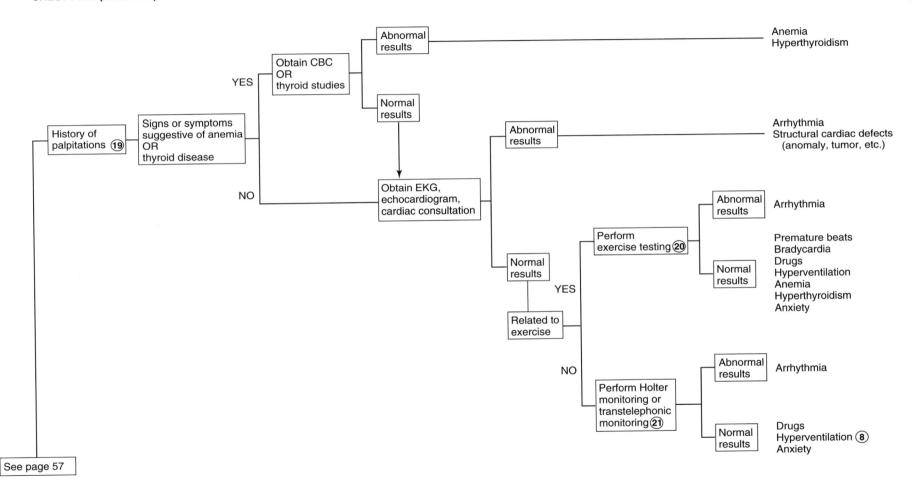

Chest Pain *(continued)*

(22) Ischemic or anginal type chest pain typically increases gradually during exercise or other stress, lasts 1 to 5 minutes, and is relieved by rest. The pain is described as having a tight or squeezing quality and a retrosternal location, although it may be diffuse or epigastric and radiate to the neck, jaw, arms, or interscapular region. In addition to syncope, diaphoresis, tachycardia, tachypnea, and hypotension may occur.

(23) Coronary artery anomalies are rare but can be associated with severe ischemia. The physical examination may be normal or may reveal a soft murmur or gallop rhythm suggesting myocardial dysfunction. Angiography may be necessary to make the diagnosis.

(24) Reflux esophagitis in older children and adolescents is classically typified by substernal pain, increased pain after meals or when recumbent, and relief with antacids.

(25) Peptic ulcer disease is more likely to occur with a chronic intermittent history of dull or aching pain and often includes nighttime complaints. The pain may be relieved by food or antacids.

BIBLIOGRAPHY

Kocis KC: Chest pain in pediatrics. Pediatr Clin North Am. 46:189–203, 1999.

Pasterkamp H: The history and physical exam. In Chernick V, Boat TF (eds): Kendig's Disorders of the Respiratory Tract in Children, 6th ed, p 85. Philadelphia, WB Saunders Company, 1998.

Selbst S: Consultation with the specialist: Chest pain in children. Pediatr Rev 18:169, 1997.

Selbst S: Evaluation of chest pain in children. Pediatr Rev 8:56, 1986.

CHEST PAIN (continued)

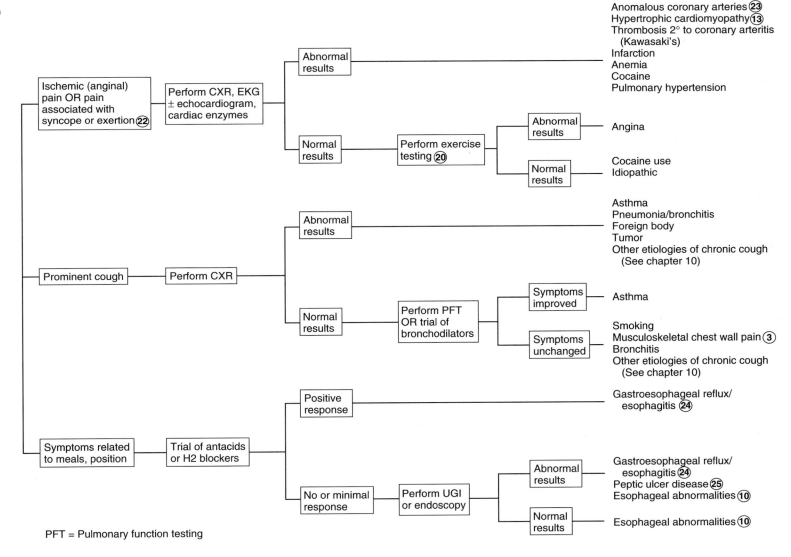

PFT = Pulmonary function testing

Chapter 18 Syncope

Syncope is the temporary loss of consciousness and tone that occurs as a result of inadequate cerebral perfusion. It is a common complaint in older children and adolescents but is unusual in younger children less than 6 years of age. Syncope is usually benign but must be carefully addressed since it may occasionally herald a life-threatening condition. When recurrent, it can generate a significant amount of stress for a patient and family.

Presyncope is the sense that one is about to pass out but without a loss of consciousness. Presyncope should be approached in the same diagnostic manner as syncope.

1 When obtaining a history of the event, witnesses can be especially helpful. Inquire about events and position prior to the episode, duration of loss of consciousness, associated symptoms, and time since the last meal. Syncope associated with exertion or exercise is ominous because it may indicate a serious cardiac etiology. A thorough evaluation is always indicated.

A family history of sudden death, sudden infant death syndrome (SIDS), congenital heart disease, arrhythmias, deafness, seizures, and metabolic disorders may be helpful in the diagnosis. A history of fainting is often common in cases of benign (vasovagal) syncope.

The social history should investigate the possibility of ingestion or illicit drug use. Inquire about medications and potential ingestion, including medications of other family members that might be accessible. Medications that can cause syncope through a mechanism of decreased venous tone include nitroglycerin, ganglionic blocker, and guanethidine.

The physical examination findings are usually normal in children who experience syncope.

2 All children with syncope need an electrocardiogram (EKG). Printed automated measurements should not be relied on. Careful interval measurements should be done manually. Abnormal PR, QRS, and QT/QTc intervals suggest an underlying conduction or electrolyte abnormality. The EKG also indicates chamber enlargement or hypertrophy. Testing of glucose and electrolytes is usually not helpful, especially in children who present for evaluation hours to days after the episode.

3 Depending on the symptomatology, further evaluation may include a Holter monitor (24-hour ambulatory EKG), an echocardiogram, or an exercise stress test. Cardiac catheterization and electrophysiologic studies with invasive monitoring may be necessary in some severe cases.

4 Supraventricular tachycardia (SVT), ventricular tachycardia, and heart block are the most common arrhythmias causing syncope. Heart block can be congenital, postsurgical, acquired (Lyme disease), or medication related.

5 Wolff-Parkinson-White (WPW) syndrome and long QT syndrome are primary conduction abnormalities that should be diagnosed using the EKG. Wolff-Parkinson-White is characterized by an accessory conduction pathway that results in SVT. Atrial flutter may also occur. Patients with long QT syndrome are at risk for lethal ventricular arrhythmias. The heterozygous form of congenital long QT (Romano-Ward) syndrome is most common and milder than the homozygous form (Jervell and Lange-Nielsen). The latter is also associated with congenital deafness. Acquired long QT syndrome can occur secondary to myocarditis, mitral valve prolapse, electrolyte abnormalities, and medications.

6 Idiopathic hypertrophic subaortic stenosis (IHSS) is a rare but serious cause of syncope. The obstruction causes an outflow tract murmur. An immediate evaluation is indicated whenever a murmur is present in a patient with syncope. A positive family history should always prompt an evaluation because the inheritance risk is high.

7 Worrisome elements of the history include syncope that either occurs in a recumbent position or is associated with exercise, chest pain, or palpitations. (See also Ch. 19.) A history of heart disease (operated or unoperated) or a family history of unexplained death, hypertrophic cardiomyopathy (IHSS), or long QT syndrome is worrisome. Patients with abnormal cardiac examination findings should be referred for an urgent cardiac evaluation.

8 Seizures are the most likely neurologic cause of syncope in children; however, overall neurologic causes are rare in children and adolescents. A few tonic-clonic contractions are normal in cases of vasovagal syncope. They should not be considered true seizure activity. To distinguish a seizure from a syncopal event, consider that a postictal phase, a rigid rather than limp posture, and incontinence are more suggestive of a seizure. Patients with seizures do not experience presyncopal symptoms, and they are usually unconscious after the episode for a longer period. Loss of consciousness with syncope is usually less than one minute. Seizures should also be suspected when the loss of consciousness occurs in the supine position.

9 Hysterical syncope is a diagnosis of exclusion. It is most common in adolescents. Hemodynamic changes, sweating, pallor, and subsequent psychologic distress regarding the episode are absent.

10 Vasovagal or neurocardiogenic or vasodepressor syncope is the most common type of syncope in normal children and adolescents. Vasovagal syncope is preceded by a prodrome of warning signs (e.g., dizziness, lightheadedness, pallor, nausea, diaphoresis, hyperventilation). Children usually can recognize these presyncopal signs at least after the first episode, prompting them to recline or sit with their heads between their knees to prevent the episode. Factors that may predispose children to syncope include a warm environmental temperature, a confined or crowded space, and anxiety or sudden surprise. Fright, blood drawing or the sight of blood, and prolonged and motionless standing are

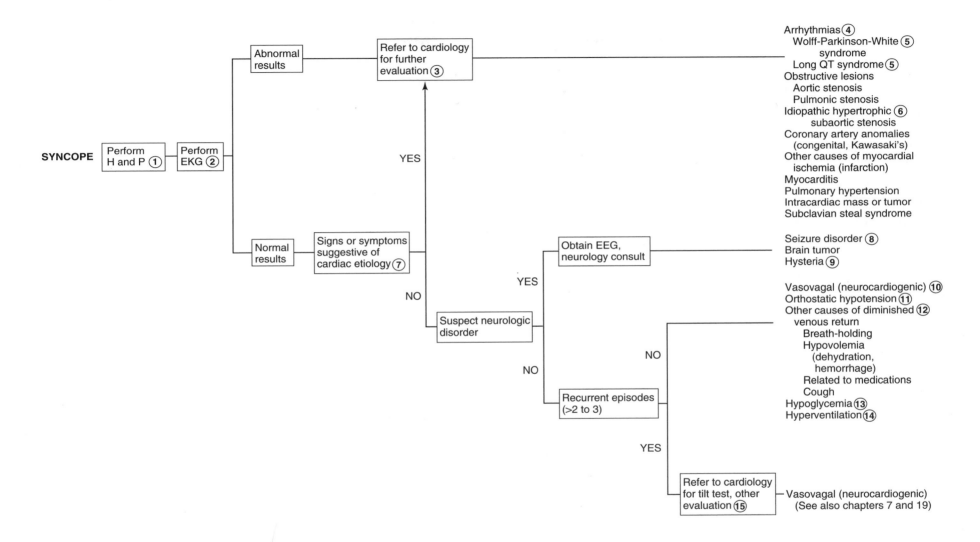

SYNCOPE — Perform H and P ①　Perform EKG ②

- Abnormal results → Refer to cardiology for further evaluation ③ →
  - Arrhythmias ④
    - Wolff-Parkinson-White ⑤ syndrome
    - Long QT syndrome ⑤
  - Obstructive lesions
    - Aortic stenosis
    - Pulmonic stenosis
  - Idiopathic hypertrophic ⑥ subaortic stenosis
  - Coronary artery anomalies (congenital, Kawasaki's)
  - Other causes of myocardial ischemia (infarction)
  - Myocarditis
  - Pulmonary hypertension
  - Intracardiac mass or tumor
  - Subclavian steal syndrome

- Normal results → Signs or symptoms suggestive of cardiac etiology ⑦
  - YES → Refer to cardiology for further evaluation ③
  - NO → Suspect neurologic disorder
    - YES → Obtain EEG, neurology consult →
      - Seizure disorder ⑧
      - Brain tumor
      - Hysteria ⑨
    - NO → Recurrent episodes (>2 to 3)
      - NO →
        - Vasovagal (neurocardiogenic) ⑩
        - Orthostatic hypotension ⑪
        - Other causes of diminished ⑫ venous return
          - Breath-holding
          - Hypovolemia (dehydration, hemorrhage)
          - Related to medications
          - Cough
        - Hypoglycemia ⑬
        - Hyperventilation ⑭
      - YES → Refer to cardiology for tilt test, other evaluation ⑮ — Vasovagal (neurocardiogenic) (See also chapters 7 and 19)

Nelson chapter 603
Practical Strategies chapter 43

Syncope (continued)

contributory. The absence of a prodromal or pre-syncopal sensation is not consistent with a vasovagal etiology.

(11) Syncope due to orthostatic hypotension has no prodromal symptoms. Patients may report feeling lightheaded prior to fainting, but no autonomic symptoms (e.g., pallor, diaphoresis) occur. Prolonged bed rest, prolonged standing, intravascular depletion (e.g., bleeding, dehydration), and certain drugs are precipitants. Blood pressure should be measured supine and after standing for 5 to 10 minutes.

(12) Breath-holding spells are the most common mechanism of syncope in children younger than 6 years of age. Children who are startled or upset hold their breath in expiration, collapse, and become cyanotic for a brief period. Cough syncope occasionally occurs in children with asthma during prolonged paroxysms. Increased intrathoracic pressure is responsible for the diminished venous return in both cases.

Medications that increase the risk of decreased venous return and syncope include diuretics, antihypertensive drugs, and phenothiazines.

(13) Hunger, weakness, sweating, agitation, and confusion may accompany hypoglycemia. Supine position does not provide relief.

(14) A history of preceding psychologic distress, sensations of shortness of breath, chest pain, visual changes, and numbness and tingling of the extremities may be reported in children with syncope due to hyperventilation. The patient may be able to reproduce the episode when requested to hyperventilate.

(15) A tilt table evaluation may aid in the diagnosis of vasovagal syncope and in the selection of therapy.

BIBLIOGRAPHY

Lewis DA, Chala A: Syncope in the pediatric patient: The cardiologist's perspective. Pediatr Clin North Am 46:205–219, 1999.
Park MK: Pediatric Cardiology for Practitioners. St. Louis: Mosby, 1996.

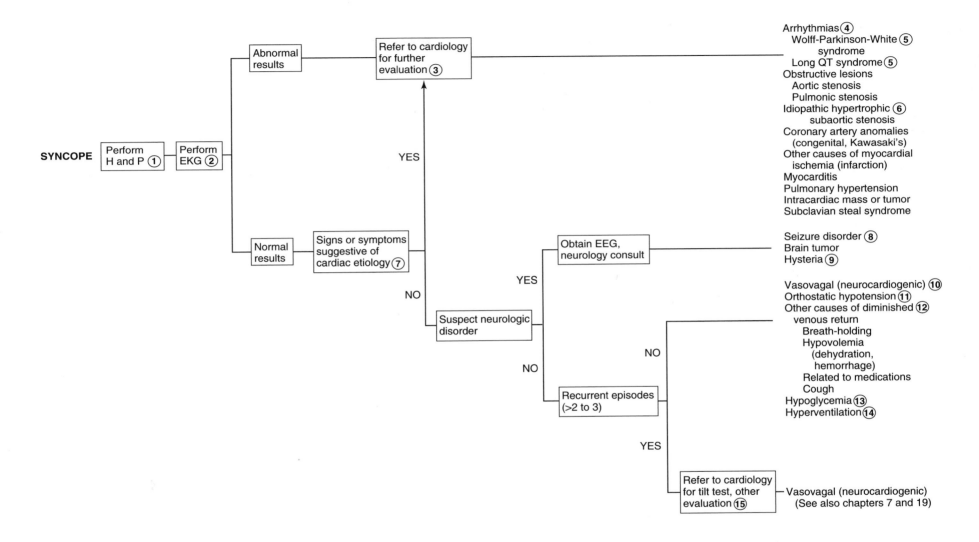

SYNCOPE → Perform H and P ① → Perform EKG ②

Abnormal results → Refer to cardiology for further evaluation ③ →

Arrhythmias ④
  Wolff-Parkinson-White ⑤
    syndrome
  Long QT syndrome ⑤
Obstructive lesions
  Aortic stenosis
  Pulmonic stenosis
Idiopathic hypertrophic ⑥
  subaortic stenosis
Coronary artery anomalies
  (congenital, Kawasaki's)
Other causes of myocardial
  ischemia (infarction)
Myocarditis
Pulmonary hypertension
Intracardiac mass or tumor
Subclavian steal syndrome

Normal results → Signs or symptoms suggestive of cardiac etiology ⑦

YES → Refer to cardiology for further evaluation ③

NO → Suspect neurologic disorder

YES → Obtain EEG, neurology consult →
Seizure disorder ⑧
Brain tumor
Hysteria ⑨

NO → Recurrent episodes (>2 to 3)

NO →
Vasovagal (neurocardiogenic) ⑩
Orthostatic hypotension ⑪
Other causes of diminished ⑫
  venous return
    Breath-holding
    Hypovolemia
      (dehydration,
      hemorrhage)
    Related to medications
    Cough
Hypoglycemia ⑬
Hyperventilation ⑭

YES → Refer to cardiology for tilt test, other evaluation ⑮ → Vasovagal (neurocardiogenic) (See also chapters 7 and 19)

Nelson chapter 603
Practical Strategies chapter 43

Palpitations are the sensations of the heart's actions. They may be described as rapid or slow, skipping or stopping, and regular or irregular. Some asymptomatic rhythm abnormalities are detected during routine physical examination. Most cases are not due to serious cardiac etiologies. The goal of the evaluation is to identify the small proportion of patients who are at risk for serious cardiac disease.

(1) An accurate description of the sensation may aid in the diagnosis. Racing, heart stopping, or skipping beats are common descriptors. Inquire about the duration of symptoms, whether the onset and termination of symptoms are subtle or abrupt, and the factors associated with onset (e.g., exercise) or termination (e.g., Valsalva). Instruct the parents on how to take the child's pulse during future episodes.

A medical history of structural cardiac abnormalities increases the risk of arrhythmias. Certain medications can be responsible for arrhythmias. Symptoms suggestive of endocrine disorders may also indicate etiologies. A social history should investigate stress levels, caffeine intake, and tobacco use.

Familial disorders that may be a cause of palpitations include Wolff-Parkinson-White syndrome, prolonged QT syndrome (deafness is associated with one of the inherited syndromes), and Kearns-Sayre syndrome (retinal degeneration, ophthalmoplegia, muscle weakness).

(2) The most ominous signs suggestive of a serious cardiac etiology associated with an arrhythmia are syncope or near syncope. Other worrisome history components include severe chest pain, family history of prolonged QT syndrome, unexplained sudden death, or aborted sudden death. If the history reveals any of these risk factors, an urgent cardiac evaluation is recommended.

(3) A resting electrocardiogram (EKG) may reveal an arrhythmia that is likely responsible for the palpitations. It may reveal a condition that could be associated with an arrhythmia. In the latter case, cardiology consultation for an echocardiogram and possibly further investigation is indicated. T-wave changes may indicate a myocardial disorder. Dilated or hypertrophic cardiomyopathy may be suggested by ventricular hypertrophy on the EKG. Wolff-Parkinson-White syndrome with its characteristic delta wave may be associated with an Ebstein anomaly.

(4) Sinus arrhythmia is a normal variation of the heart rate with a slowing during expiration and acceleration during inspiration. It is normal in children of all ages.

(5) Sinus tachycardia should be distinguished from supraventricular tachycardia (SVT). Both are narrow complex tachycardias. Sinus tachycardia is characterized by a normal P-wave axis, a gradual onset and termination, and a rate less than 250 beats per minute (bpm). Sinus tachycardia demonstrates some variability in the rate. Fever, pain, anemia, and dehydration are common causes of sinus tachycardia.

(6) SVTs are characterized by an abrupt onset and cessation and tend to occur when the patient is at rest. They demonstrate a narrow QRS complex, an abnormal P-wave axis, and an unvarying rate that usually exceeds 180 bpm. It may be as high as 300 bpm. Congenital heart disease and use of over-the-counter decongestants are common causes of SVTs.

(7) Premature ventricular complexes (PVCs) may be unifocal in origin with identical contours or multifocal with varying contours. PVCs usually are followed by a compensatory pause preceding the next beat. They are often asymptomatic, although patients may describe a skipped beat or a sensation of the heart turning over. Anxiety, fever, and certain drugs, especially stimulants may increase the occurrence of PVCs.

PVCs are usually a benign entity. Worrisome exceptions include two or more PVCs in a row, multifocal origin, increased frequency with exercise, occurrence following a recently converted ventricular tachycardia, repeated occurrence on the early part of the T wave of the preceding beat (i.e., the "R on T" phenomenon), underlying heart disease, and unusual awareness or anxiety regarding the beats.

(8) A junctional (escape or ectopic) beat from the atrioventricular node may occur when the sinus rate is slow enough in sinus arrhythmia. Escape beats or extrasystoles can occur because of discharge of an ectopic focus anywhere in the atrial, junctional, or ventricular tissue. They are usually insignificant unless associated with an underlying cardiac condition (e.g., inflammation, ischemia) or drug toxicity, especially digitalis.

(9) Complete heart block may be congenital or acquired. Congenital block is usually associated with congenital heart disease or maternal connective tissue disorders, in particular systemic lupus erythematosus. Acquired block may occur following surgery and with other conditions, such as Lyme disease and Kearns-Sayre syndrome. Complete dissociation between atrial and ventricular rhythms occurs.

(10) In neonates, sinus bradycardia may be associated with some type of fetal or neonatal stress (e.g., hypoxia, apnea of prematurity). In older children and adolescents it may be associated with an athletic cardiac condition or increased vagal tone. Increased intracranial pressure, abdominal distension, anorexia nervosa, and certain drugs and toxins (e.g., digoxin, propranolol, organophosphates) are also causes.

(11) In atrial flutter, an atrial rate of 250 to 400 bpm causes a regular or regularly irregular tachycardia. It usually occurs in children with congenital heart disease but may occur in neonates with normal hearts. The EKG shows characteristic rapid and regular, atrial saw-toothed flutter waves.

(12) In atrial fibrillation, chaotic atrial excitation at a rapid rate (300 to 500 bpm) produces an irregular ventricular rhythm. It usually occurs in

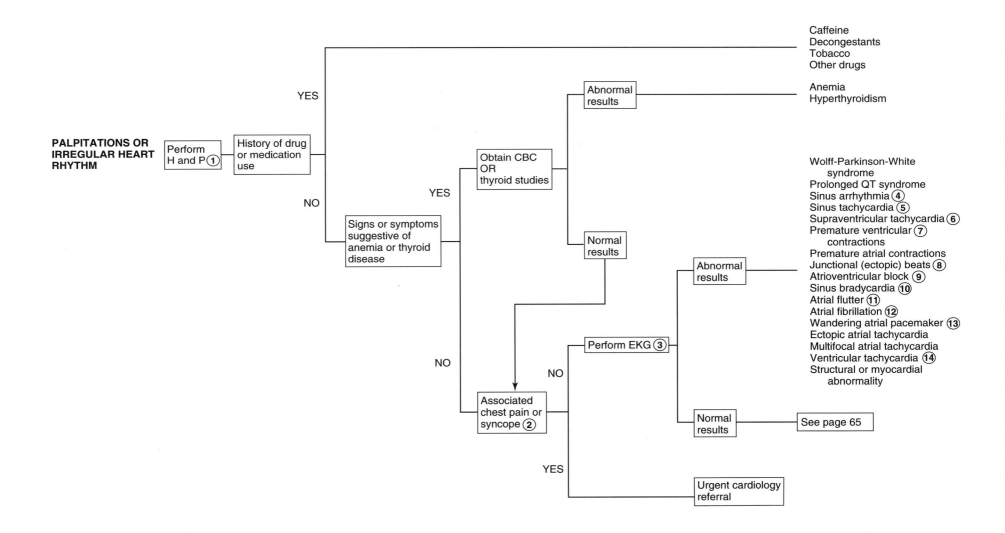

PALPITATIONS OR IRREGULAR HEART RHYTHM

Perform H and P ①

History of drug or medication use

YES → Caffeine
Decongestants
Tobacco
Other drugs

NO → Signs or symptoms suggestive of anemia or thyroid disease

YES → Obtain CBC OR thyroid studies

Abnormal results → Anemia
Hyperthyroidism

Normal results

NO → Associated chest pain or syncope ②

NO → Perform EKG ③

Abnormal results →
Wolff-Parkinson-White syndrome
Prolonged QT syndrome
Sinus arrhythmia ④
Sinus tachycardia ⑤
Supraventricular tachycardia ⑥
Premature ventricular ⑦ contractions
Premature atrial contractions
Junctional (ectopic) beats ⑧
Atrioventricular block ⑨
Sinus bradycardia ⑩
Atrial flutter ⑪
Atrial fibrillation ⑫
Wandering atrial pacemaker ⑬
Ectopic atrial tachycardia
Multifocal atrial tachycardia
Ventricular tachycardia ⑭
Structural or myocardial abnormality

Normal results → See page 65

YES → Urgent cardiology referral

Nelson chapter 442
Practical Strategies chapter 12

the presence of cardiac abnormalities. Otherwise healthy children experiencing atrial fibrillation should be evaluated for thyrotoxicosis, pulmonary emboli, and pericarditis.

(13) Variability in the shape of the P-waves indicates a wandering atrial pacemaker. This shift of the pacemaker from the sinus node to another area of the atrium is usually a normal variant in childhood. It can also be seen in central nervous system disorders.

(14) Ventricular (i.e., wide QRS complex) tachycardia necessitates prompt treatment. It needs to be distinguished from supraventricular tachycardia with aberrant or rapid conduction over an accessory pathway.

(15) Holter monitoring is a 24-hour rhythm recording recommended to attempt to capture an abnormal rhythm when the patient experiences frequent symptoms. If events are more intermittent, an incident or event recorder is recommended. Some models require patients to connect to an interfacing device when their symptoms start. Others are worn continuously, and recording starts when the patient touches a button.

(16) Drugs that may be responsible for palpitations include tobacco, caffeine, tricyclic antidepressants, decongestants, digitalis, albuterol, and aminophylline. Cocaine, amphetamines, carbon monoxide, atropine, terbutaline, and amyl nitrite are also causes. Proarrhythmia agents that have been associated with a prolonged QT interval, resulting in ventricular tachycardia, include erythromycin, terfenadine, astemizole, quinidine, amiodarone, flecainide, and encainide.

BIBLIOGRAPHY

Case LC: Diagnosis and treatment of pediatric arrhythmias. Pediatr Clin North Am 46:347–354, 1999.

PALPITATIONS (continued)

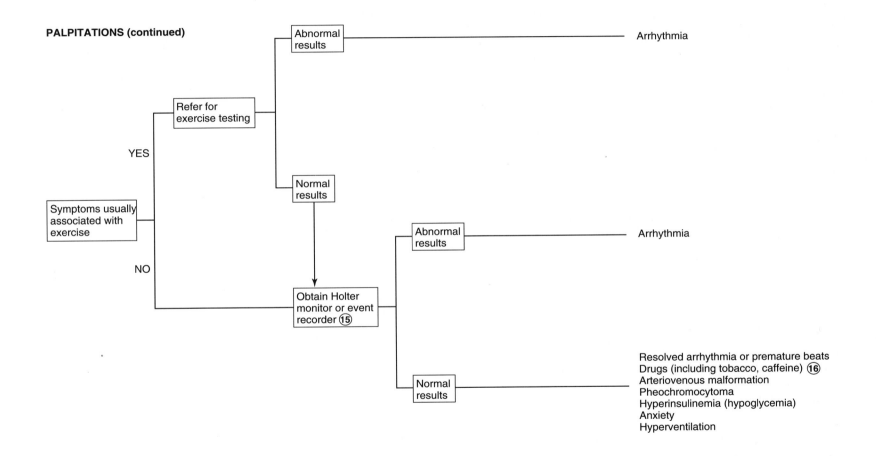

Chapter 20 Heart Murmurs

Most normal children (50% to 90%) have an audible heart murmur at some point prior to school age. The challenge to the practitioner is to ascertain which of these murmurs warrants additional evaluation. The clinical diagnosis of a normal or innocent murmur should be made only in the presence of a normal history and physical examination, with characteristics consistent with a normal murmur. Despite the increased availability of echocardiography, the history and physical examination remain the accepted means of diagnosing normal murmurs. When the diagnosis of a murmur is unclear, it is generally more cost-effective to refer to a pediatric cardiologist than to order an echocardiogram.

① A maternal history of gestational diabetes, infection, or drug use may be risk factors for congenital heart disease.

The feeding history in young infants can reveal signs or symptoms suggestive of congestive heart failure. Inquire about the quantity and quality of feeds. Limited intake, prolonged feeding times, and tachypnea associated with the feeds are worrisome. Ask about the development of cyanosis with feeding. In older children, exercise or exertion can be assessed by inquiring about level of activity, tolerance to extended playtimes, and walking or climbing stairs. Inquiring how well older children keep up with their peers or siblings regarding exercise tolerance is also helpful.

A history of fevers, lethargy, and recent dental work suggests possible endocarditis. A history of chronic mouth breathing, snoring, or obstructive sleep apnea may suggest pulmonary hypertension.

A family history of sudden death, rheumatic fever, sudden infant death syndrome, and structural cardiac defects in a first-degree relative may be significant. A family history of hypertrophic cardiomyopathy is sufficient to mandate an echocardiogram because of the autosomal dominant pattern of inheritance.

When assessing the child with a murmur, pressures in both arms and a leg should be obtained. Lower extremity blood pressure is usually 10 mm Hg higher than upper extremity pressure. Diminished femoral pulses or a delay between the brachial and femoral pulses suggests coarctation of the aorta. The simple presence of a femoral pulse does not rule out coarctation. In infants and children, liver size is assessed as an indicator of systemic congestion. Splenomegaly occurs in endocarditis but is usually not seen with congestive heart failure.

② Systemic disorders that can cause a systolic outflow murmur include anemia, hyperthyroidism, and arteriovenous malformations (AVM). In addition to thyromegaly, tachycardia, a hyperdynamic precordium, slightly bounding pulses, and mild hypertension suggest hyperthyroidism. An AVM can cause similar findings. Localized continuous bruits over the head, neck, or liver suggest the diagnosis. Pulmonary AVMs are generally not associated with bruits or murmurs. Anemia is suggested by pallor, tachycardia, and exercise intolerance or weakness.

③ Other elements of the history that may be suggestive of a pathologic murmur include feeding difficulties, diaphoresis with feeds, failure to thrive, and impaired growth. A family history of idiopathic hypertrophic subaortic stenosis (IHSS) and sudden death in an adolescent are suggestive. On physical examination, abnormal rhythm, suprasternal thrill, prominent apical thrust, and digital clubbing are also worrisome, as are wide or bounding pulses and absent or weak femoral pulses. Signs of systemic disease should prompt consideration of acquired conditions, such as rheumatic heart disease and endocarditis.

④ When the diagnosis of a murmur is unclear, referral to a pediatric cardiologist is recommended. Obtaining an EKG, a chest X-ray, or an echocardiogram is less cost-effective than a referral.

⑤ Ventricular septal defects (VSDs) are the most common congenital heart lesions. Symptoms depend on the size of the defect and pulmonary vascular resistance. Most VSDs are small and asymptomatic and close spontaneously in the first year of life. The murmur is classically described as a loud harsh or blowing systolic murmur at the left sternal border, often obscuring the first heart sound. Small defects may have soft murmurs that become softer over time as the lesion closes. In large defects, the left-to-right shunting increases over the first few weeks of life as pulmonary vascular resistance falls. Clinical symptoms of congestive heart failure develop gradually over this period. Referral for definitive diagnosis is recommended.

⑥ Atrial septal defects (ASD) are usually asymptomatic in infants and tend to be detected on routine physical examinations in the toddler or preschooler. They are characterized by a hyperdynamic right ventricular impulse, a characteristic fixed and widely split second heart sound, and a pulmonary flow murmur. A mid-diastolic rumble may be present if the defect is large. Early detection of an ASD may be masked by a peripheral pulmonic stenosis (PPS) murmur (see 20). When ASD is suspected, a cardiology evaluation is warranted to identify the type of defect and the need for repair and counseling.

⑦ Coarctation of the aorta may be diagnosed in infancy with congestive heart failure and lower extremity hypoperfusion. Children not diagnosed in infancy may remain asymptomatic, even with severe coarctation. The classic physical findings are delayed or diminished arterial pulses in the lower extremities compared with the upper extremities. Blood pressures in the upper extremities are higher than in the lower extremities in coarctation. It may even be difficult to obtain the blood pressure in the lower extremities. A short systolic murmur at the third or fourth left intercostal spaces may be detected with transmission to the left infrascapular area. A systolic ejection click or suprasternal thrill is consistent with a bicuspid aortic valve that occurs in 40% to 50% of patients with coarctation of the aorta.

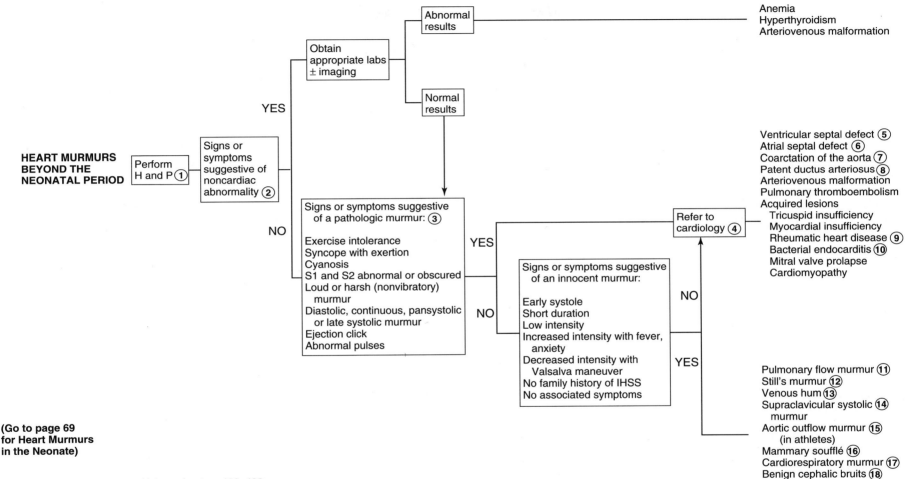

HEART MURMURS BEYOND THE NEONATAL PERIOD

Perform H and P ①

Signs or symptoms suggestive of noncardiac abnormality ②

YES → Obtain appropriate labs ± imaging

Abnormal results → Anemia
Hyperthyroidism
Arteriovenous malformation

Normal results

NO

Signs or symptoms suggestive of a pathologic murmur: ③

Exercise intolerance
Syncope with exertion
Cyanosis
S1 and S2 abnormal or obscured
Loud or harsh (nonvibratory) murmur
Diastolic, continuous, pansystolic or late systolic murmur
Ejection click
Abnormal pulses

YES →

Signs or symptoms suggestive of an innocent murmur:

Early systole
Short duration
Low intensity
Increased intensity with fever, anxiety
Decreased intensity with Valsalva maneuver
No family history of IHSS
No associated symptoms

NO

NO → Refer to cardiology ④

Ventricular septal defect ⑤
Atrial septal defect ⑥
Coarctation of the aorta ⑦
Patent ductus arteriosus ⑧
Arteriovenous malformation
Pulmonary thromboembolism
Acquired lesions
  Tricuspid insufficiency
  Myocardial insufficiency
  Rheumatic heart disease ⑨
  Bacterial endocarditis ⑩
  Mitral valve prolapse
  Cardiomyopathy

YES →

Pulmonary flow murmur ⑪
Still's murmur ⑫
Venous hum ⑬
Supraclavicular systolic ⑭ murmur
Aortic outflow murmur ⑮ (in athletes)
Mammary soufflé ⑯
Cardiorespiratory murmur ⑰
Benign cephalic bruits ⑱

(Go to page 69 for Heart Murmurs in the Neonate)

Nelson chapters 429, 433
Practical Strategies chapter 16
IHSS = idiopathic hypertrophic subaortic stenosis

8 A small patent ductus arteriosus (PDA) in infants may be asymptomatic. Large ones tend to be symptomatic, causing congestive heart failure and failure to thrive. The lesion is one of the cardiac anomalies frequently associated with prenatal maternal rubella infection. Classic findings of large PDA shunts are a wide peripheral pulse pressure, a prominent apical impulse, a systolic thrill, and a continuous harsh machinery-like murmur at the left upper sternal border. Referral to cardiology is indicated for definitive diagnosis and treatment.

9 Rheumatic fever is an immunologically mediated inflammatory disorder following infection with group A streptococcus. The modified Jones criteria are used for diagnosis. Pancarditis, most commonly appearing as valvulitis, is common. The patient presents with murmurs of aortic or mitral regurgitation. A history of fevers in the presence of a new or changing heart murmur should raise the suspicion for rheumatic fever and for endocarditis.

10 Infective endocarditis is most common in children with congenital heart disease or rheumatic heart disease but can occur in children with normal hearts. Cases occur acutely or insidiously, with intermittent fevers and vague symptoms of fatigue, myalgias, joint pain, and headache. New or changing murmurs, splenomegaly, and petechiae are common. Echocardiography is helpful in identifying vegetations, although results may be normal early in the disease. Blood cultures are necessary to identify the pathogen. Three to five cultures from separate sites are recommended. Laboratories should be notified when endocarditis is suspected so that enriched media and prolonged incubation times are used.

11 The normal turbulence of ejection into the pulmonic root frequently generates an audible murmur of no hemodynamic significance. These murmurs are usually grade 1 to 3, short systolic murmurs heard best over the left upper sternal border. They may or may not transmit to the neck and apex. Clicks and thrills associated with pulmonary valve stenosis are absent. The murmur can be accentuated by full exhalation and the supine position, and diminished by the upright posture and holding the breath. It can occur in any age group but is most likely in older children and adolescents. The main differential is an ASD.

12 The Still murmur is a common normal murmur heard in children. It is typically heard in the preschool period. The murmur is usually a grade 1 to 3 short systolic murmur heard best at the left sternal border. It has a characteristic vibratory or musical quality compared with a vibrating tuning fork or twanging cello string. Rarely, it can be surprisingly loud and ominous-sounding with transmission throughout the precordium. It is usually loudest when the patient is supine and tends to diminish with an upright or a sitting position. This murmur is also exacerbated by fever, anxiety, excitement, or exercise.

13 Venous hums are another common, normal murmur of childhood. These are medium frequency continuous murmurs usually best heard at the right upper sternal border, although they may be heard on the left and radiate to the neck. The murmur typically is heard when the patient is sitting up, and it diminishes significantly or disappears when the patient turns the head far to the left (or right if the murmur is left-sided) and when supine. They are thought to be caused by the turbulence created as the internal jugular and subclavian veins enter the superior vena cava. The main differential diagnoses are PDA and arteriovenous malformation.

14 A supraclavicular or brachiocephalic systolic murmur is a short systolic murmur heard best above the clavicles with minimal radiation to the neck. It is distinguished from aortic or pulmonary valve stenosis when it disappears as the patient raises the head and throws back the shoulders, and by the absence of an associated click and significant radiation to the neck.

15 Adolescents who are very athletic may demonstrate a systolic murmur over the aortic outflow tract (right upper sternal border) due to a slower heart rate and increased stroke volume. A loud S3 and occasional S4 can also occur because of the increased filling phase. The most serious murmurs to rule out diagnostically in this clinical setting are aortic stenosis and IHSS. The absence of a positive family history, rapid cardiac upstroke, and diminished intensity of the murmur with a Valsalva maneuver support an innocent murmur. In IHSS, a Valsalva maneuver increases the intensity of the murmur because decreased cardiac filling worsens the left ventricular outflow tract obstruction. Referral is recommended when the diagnosis is not clear.

16 The mammary soufflé murmur is usually heard in young women who are pregnant or lactating due to increased blood flow in the developing breast tissue. It can occasionally be heard in adolescents. The murmur is systolic, starting distinctly after S1 but may extend into diastole. It is high-pitched and heard best on the anterior chest wall over the breast. This murmur characteristically varies significantly from day to day.

17 The cardiorespiratory murmur is a rare, innocent, late systolic murmur occasionally heard in older children. It is heard at the apex only during inspiration.

18 Benign cephalic bruits are common in children. These bruits are low intensity, bilateral, and continuous or systolic, and do not require additional evaluation in the absence of other worrisome symptoms.

19 Congenital heart disease usually appears in the first few days or weeks of life, depending on the lesion. The development of a significant murmur in the neonatal period accompanied by cyanosis or congestive heart failure, or both, warrants an urgent evaluation. Congestive heart failure may manifest as poor feeding, disinterest in feeding, excessive fatigue, diaphoresis, and tachyphea or dyspnea. Cyanosis only occurs in one third of infants with serious congenital heart disease. In cyanotic heart defects, a sudden deterioration in the first few days of life occurs coincident with the closing of the ductus. (See also Ch. 14.) Many syndromes (e.g., Down, Turner, Williams) have characteristic cardiac anomalies.

(20) Despite the concern they generate, murmurs in the newborn are often normal. The most common newborn murmur is PPS. It is an ejection murmur caused by flow through the sharp angulation of branches off the main pulmonary artery. The murmur is heard best at the left and right upper sternal borders with good transmission to each axilla and the back. The murmur generally disappears in the first few months of life. Persistence beyond 12 months is abnormal and should be evaluated by a cardiologist. The occurrence and duration of the murmur is greater in premature infants.

(21) In addition to PPS murmurs, pulmonary flow murmurs can occur in neonates. These innocent murmurs are grade 2 or less, systolic ejection murmurs with a left sternal border location and normal heart sounds.

Allen HD, Golinko RJ: Heart murmurs in children: When is a work-up needed? Contemp Pediatr 11:29, 1994.
Feit LR: The heart of the matter: Evaluating murmurs in children. Contemp Pediatr 14:97, 1997.
Park MK: Pediatric Cardiology for Practitioners. St. Louis: Mosby, 1996.
Pelech AN: Evaluation of the pediatric patient with a cardiac murmur. Pediatr Clin North Am 46:167–188, 1999.
Rosenthal A: How to distinguish between innocent and pathologic murmurs in children. Pediatr Clin North Am 31:1229–1240, 1984.

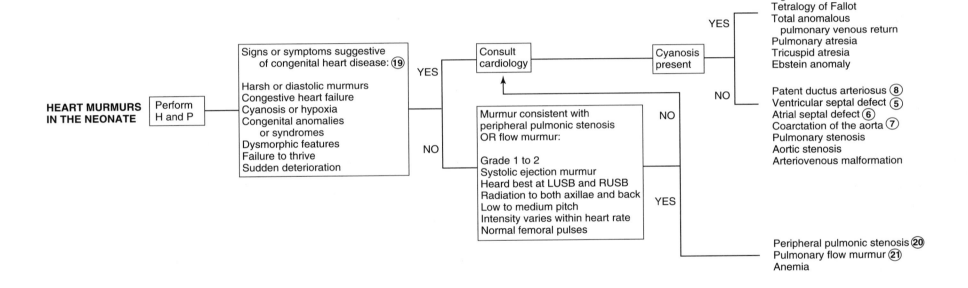

RUSB = Right upper sternal border
LUSB = Left upper sternal border

Nelson chapters 429, 433
Practical Strategies chapter 16

GASTROINTESTINAL SYSTEM

Abdominal pain is a symptom of multiple disorders; this chapter includes disorders in which it is a predominant symptom. In children younger than 2 years of age, an organic cause of recurrent pain is more likely than a nonorganic cause.

1 A history of the nature and progression of abdominal pain is very helpful in arriving at a diagnosis but often difficult to obtain, especially in young children. Young patients may assume a protective posture and protect themselves from movement or cough, which may exacerbate the pain. The history should include a thorough review of symptoms, including a complete medication and diet history.

A thorough unhurried physical examination is essential in the evaluation of the child with abdominal pain. Inspection may reveal pallor, distention, jaundice, or pain with movement. A pelvic examination should be done in any sexually active female (and may be helpful regardless of the patient's sexual history). A rectal examination should be performed unless the diagnosis is obvious.

Certain underlying medical conditions predispose a child to problems that may present primarily as abdominal pain. A child with sickle cell anemia is at risk for vasoocclusive crises, splenic sequestration, and cholelithiasis. Bacterial peritonitis should be carefully considered with nephrotic syndrome or cirrhosis. Children with previous surgeries may have strictures or adhesions that may cause obstructive symptoms.

2 The first challenge to the practitioner is to identify those cases that may be surgical or life threatening. Certain historical and physical criteria suggest an acute or surgical problem and mandate immediate surgical consultation. Worrisome signs and symptoms include sudden, excruciating pain; point or diffuse severe tenderness on examination; bilious vomiting; involuntary guarding; a rigid voluntary wall; and rebound tenderness. After ruling out potential emergencies, the chronicity and location of the complaint should be considered to narrow the diagnosis.

3 Ultrasound is a useful diagnostic aid for suspected disorders related to the gallbladder, pancreas, and urinary tract and for any abdominal mass. It provides a good assessment of the female reproductive organs and can also be used to visualize the appendix.

4 Acute pancreatitis presents as an intense, steady epigastric and periumbilical pain that may radiate to the back or scapula. Bilious vomiting and fever may occur. Affected children look ill and often assume a knee-to-chest posture while sitting or lying on their side. The etiology may include trauma (including abuse), infection, congenital anomalies, medications, or systemic disorders (cystic fibrosis, diabetes mellitus, hemoglobinopathies); children dependent on total parenteral nutrition are also at risk due to gallstones. Diagnosis may be confirmed by an elevated amylase or lipase level; amylase may be normal initially (in 10% to 15%); it normalizes sooner than lipase. Ultrasound and CT are helpful imaging studies for confirming the diagnosis and in follow-up.

5 Cholelithiasis is characterized by episodic severe right upper quadrant pain that may radiate to the angle of the scapula or back. Risk factors include total parenteral nutrition, hemolytic disease, and cholestatic liver disease. Patients appear agitated and uncomfortable and may exhibit pallor, jaundice, tachycardia, nausea, weakness, and diaphoresis. On examination the tenderness is localized deep in the right upper quadrant. If superficial tenderness is present, an accompanying cholecystitis is suggested. Laboratory findings include elevated direct bilirubin and serum alkaline phosphatase levels. Ultrasound is the preferred diagnostic imaging study.

6 Lower lobe pneumonia may present as abdominal pain and occasional vomiting. Cough may or may not be significant. In these cases the abdominal examination is nonspecific but the lung examination should suggest the diagnosis.

7 Always consider obtaining a pregnancy test in an adolescent female with lower or diffuse abdominal pain.

8 X-ray studies are of limited usefulness in the routine evaluation of abdominal pain. Kidney-ureter-bladder views (upright and lateral) are most likely to be helpful when suspected diagnoses include intestinal obstruction, renal or biliary tract calculi, calcified fecaliths, or intestinal perforation (e.g., pneumoperitoneum, free air). Ileus (i.e., diminished peristalsis in the absence of obstruction) occurs with infection, abdominal surgery, and metabolic abnormalities; it is demonstrated as multiple air-fluid levels on plain films. Plain films may also reveal large amounts of stool in the colon (this is often an incidental finding and should not always be presumed to be the cause of the pain).

9 Appendicitis is a difficult diagnosis. It often presents as a nonspecific intermittent periumbilical pain. Nausea, anorexia, low-grade fever, and vomiting may occur. Diarrhea (small volume) and urinary frequency or dysuria may also occur. The pain gradually intensifies and shifts to the right lower quadrant (McBurney point) usually within several hours of the onset (but may take up to 3 days). Be aware that an atypical location of the appendix may cause pain in sites other than the right lower quadrant. The occurrence of emesis before pain makes the diagnosis of appendicitis unlikely. The total white blood cell count may be normal or elevated; a left shift is supportive of the diagnosis. Urinalysis may be normal or reveal some red and white blood cells. Ultrasound or CT may aid in the diagnosis, although in many cases observation and serial examinations will be the most useful diagnostic entities.

10 Mesenteric adenitis mimics appendicitis. Inflamed abdominal lymph nodes occur as a result of viral (adenovirus, measles) or bacterial (*Yersinia*) infections; diagnosis may be aided by accompanying upper respiratory symptoms, conjunctivitis, or pharyngitis. Ultrasound or CT may make the diagnosis.

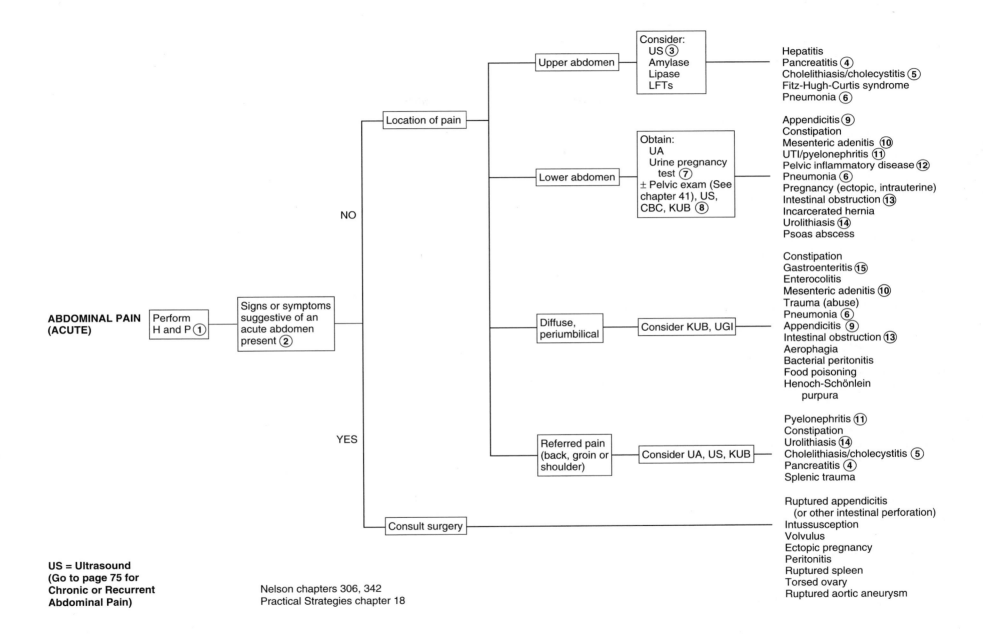

ABDOMINAL PAIN (ACUTE)

Perform H and P ①

Signs or symptoms suggestive of an acute abdomen present ②

NO

Location of pain

Upper abdomen

Consider:
US ③
Amylase
Lipase
LFTs

Hepatitis
Pancreatitis ④
Cholelithiasis/cholecystitis ⑤
Fitz-Hugh-Curtis syndrome
Pneumonia ⑥

Lower abdomen

Obtain:
UA
Urine pregnancy test ⑦
± Pelvic exam (See chapter 41), US, CBC, KUB ⑧

Appendicitis ⑨
Constipation
Mesenteric adenitis ⑩
UTI/pyelonephritis ⑪
Pelvic inflammatory disease ⑫
Pneumonia ⑥
Pregnancy (ectopic, intrauterine)
Intestinal obstruction ⑬
Incarcerated hernia
Urolithiasis ⑭
Psoas abscess

Diffuse, periumbilical

Consider KUB, UGI

Constipation
Gastroenteritis ⑮
Enterocolitis
Mesenteric adenitis ⑩
Trauma (abuse)
Pneumonia ⑥
Appendicitis ⑨
Intestinal obstruction ⑬
Aerophagia
Bacterial peritonitis
Food poisoning
Henoch-Schönlein
     purpura

YES

Referred pain (back, groin or shoulder)

Consider UA, US, KUB

Pyelonephritis ⑪
Constipation
Urolithiasis ⑭
Cholelithiasis/cholecystitis ⑤
Pancreatitis ④
Splenic trauma

Consult surgery

Ruptured appendicitis
   (or other intestinal perforation)
Intussusception
Volvulus
Ectopic pregnancy
Peritonitis
Ruptured spleen
Torsed ovary
Ruptured aortic aneurysm

US = Ultrasound
(Go to page 75 for Chronic or Recurrent Abdominal Pain)

Nelson chapters 306, 342
Practical Strategies chapter 18

Abdominal Pain (continued)

(11) Acute unilateral back or flank pain, fever, dysuria, pyuria, and urinary frequency suggest pyelonephritis. An ultrasound obtained acutely may suggest pyelonephritis or identify obstructions or abscesses. A dimercaptosuccinic acid (DMSA) scan is a more sensitive test for pyelonephritis. CT is also helpful, but the urinalysis and urine culture are the most important first tests.

(12) The minimal diagnostic criteria for pelvic inflammatory disease include lower abdominal pain, adnexal tenderness, and cervical motion tenderness. Additional diagnostic criteria include fever (>38.3°C [101F°]), abnormal cervical or vaginal discharge, elevated C-reactive protein or erythrocyte sedimentation rate, and positive cervical cultures for *Neisseria gonorrhoeae* or *Chlamydia trachomatis*. The role of ultrasound is not so much for definitive diagnosis but rather to identify tuboovarian abscesses, a common complication of pelvic inflammatory disease.

(13) In intestinal obstruction, vomiting is usually a predominant symptom. Pain is a later finding and is crampy or colicky, and rushes of high-pitched "tinkling" bowel sounds may be noted. Plain x-ray films (kidney-ureter-bladder view) may reveal air-fluid levels or distended bowel loops above the obstruction; free air indicates an intestinal perforation. Contrast medium studies may aid in definitive diagnosis if malrotation or volvulus, distal small bowel obstruction, or intussusception is suspected.

(14) Urolithiasis (i.e., kidney stones) presents as hematuria and acute colicky abdominal, flank, or back pain. The pain may radiate to the upper leg and groin. Ultrasound and helical CT will detect both radiopaque and radiolucent stones.

(15) When acute gastroenteritis is suggested based on a clinical presentation of vomiting and diarrhea preceding the complaint of diffuse abdominal pain and in the absence of any signs or symptoms of an acute abdomen, no additional workup is indicated. Parents should be counseled about worrisome signs and symptoms and supportive measures.

(16) Chronic or recurrent abdominal pain is defined by recurrent or persistent bouts of pain that occur over a minimum of 3 months and may or may not interfere with daily activities. Chronic pain may be organic, nonorganic, or psychogenic.

(17) Practitioners should have a low threshold for obtaining an abdominal film because constipation is the most common cause of chronic and recurrent abdominal pain in children.

(18) Elements of the history and physical examination that suggest an organic cause of abdominal pain include fever, weight loss or growth deceleration, joint symptoms, emesis, especially if blood or bile-stained, abnormal findings on physical examination (e.g., abdominal mass, perianal disease), and blood in the stool or other abnormal results of laboratory studies. An organic cause should be considered for pain or diarrhea that awakens a child from sleep, pain that is well localized away from the umbilicus, and pain that is referred to the back, flank, or shoulders.

(19) Inflammatory bowel disease is an important diagnosis to exclude when faced with the child with chronic abdominal pain. A thorough evaluation, including history, physical examination, and screening laboratory studies will often suggest the disorder. Additional signs and symptoms that suggest inflammatory bowel disease are anorexia, growth failure, perianal disease, hematochezia, and diarrhea. The pain and diarrhea may awaken the child at night. Supportive laboratory results include anemia, increased ESR or CRP, thrombocytosis, hypoalbuminemia, and heme-positive stools. Contrast medium studies (upper GI series with small bowel follow-through) and endoscopy will aid in making a definitive diagnosis.

(20) Gastroesophageal reflux esophagitis presents as substernal pain, increased pain after meals or when recumbent, and relief from pain with use of antacids.

(21) Peptic ulcer disease includes gastric and duodenal ulcers, gastritis, and duodenitis. Unlike the classic adult presentation of epigastric pain, exacerbation with meals, and early morning occurrence, in children the pain is more diffuse (epigastric or periumbilical) and unrelated to meals or time of day. If it is suggested, then improvement with a trial of therapy is often diagnostic. If symptoms do not respond to treatment, a search for *Helicobacter pylori* with a urea breath test or serum antibodies or endoscopy may be indicated. An upper GI series is not reliable to diagnose peptic ulcer disease in children.

(22) Nonulcer dyspepsia is characterized by epigastric pain accompanied by early satiety, bloating, belching, and nausea or occasionally vomiting. Diagnosis is based on the presence of these symptoms of peptic ulcer disease in the presence of normal findings on upper endoscopy.

(23) Chronic pancreatitis is a rare cause of recurrent abdominal pain in children. Children experience intermittent epigastric abdominal pain, often with associated nausea and vomiting; symptoms are frequently precipitated by a large meal or stress. Serum lipase and amylase levels are not as likely to be elevated as with acute cases. Ultrasound and CT may aid in diagnosis; X-ray studies may reveal calcifications consistent with chronic pancreatitis.

(24) Irritable bowel syndrome is characterized by a variable defecation pattern at least 25% of the time and three or more of the following: (1) altered stool consistency or frequency, (2) abdominal distention or bloating, (3) straining or urgency, and (4) passage of mucus. The disorder is recognized in middle school and high school students. Either diarrhea or constipation may predominate in the disorder; the abdominal pain is usually relieved by defecation.

(25) Lactose malabsorption causes symptoms of abdominal pain and cramping, bloating, diar-

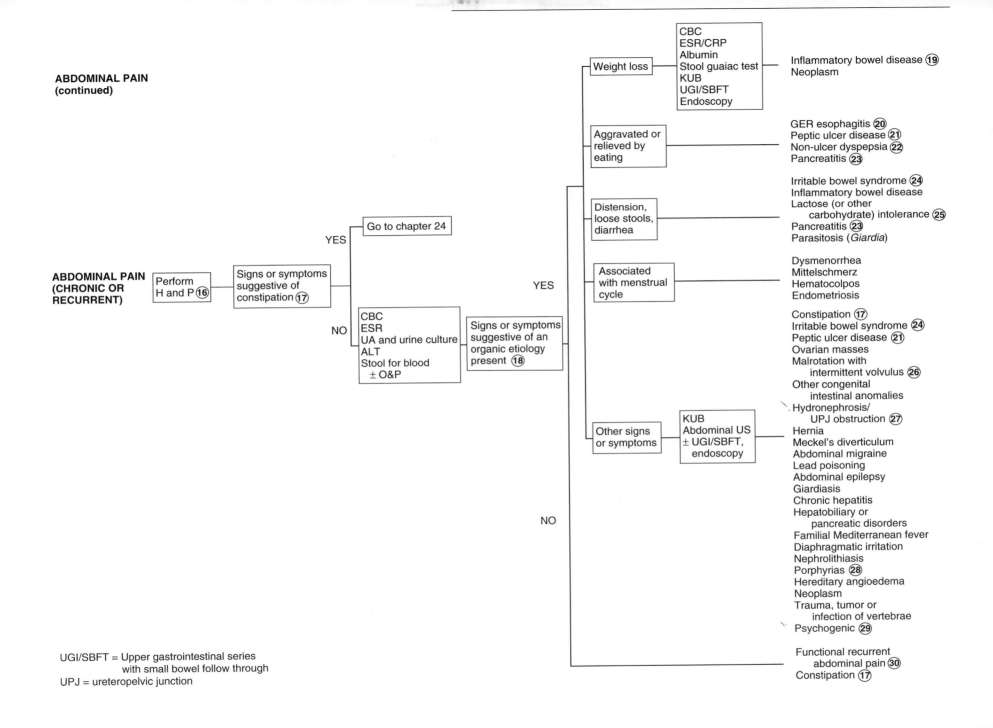

ABDOMINAL PAIN
(continued)

**ABDOMINAL PAIN
(CHRONIC OR
RECURRENT)**

Perform H and P ⑯

Signs or symptoms suggestive of constipation ⑰

YES — Go to chapter 24

NO

CBC
ESR
UA and urine culture
ALT
Stool for blood
± O&P

Signs or symptoms suggestive of an organic etiology present ⑱

YES

Weight loss —
CBC
ESR/CRP
Albumin
Stool guaiac test
KUB
UGI/SBFT
Endoscopy
— Inflammatory bowel disease ⑲
Neoplasm

Aggravated or relieved by eating —
GER esophagitis ⑳
Peptic ulcer disease ㉑
Non-ulcer dyspepsia ㉒
Pancreatitis ㉓

Distension, loose stools, diarrhea —
Irritable bowel syndrome ㉔
Inflammatory bowel disease
Lactose (or other carbohydrate) intolerance ㉕
Pancreatitis ㉓
Parasitosis (*Giardia*)

Associated with menstrual cycle —
Dysmenorrhea
Mittelschmerz
Hematocolpos
Endometriosis

Other signs or symptoms —
KUB
Abdominal US
± UGI/SBFT, endoscopy
—
Constipation ⑰
Irritable bowel syndrome ㉔
Peptic ulcer disease ㉑
Ovarian masses
Malrotation with intermittent volvulus ㉖
Other congenital intestinal anomalies
Hydronephrosis/ UPJ obstruction ㉗
Hernia
Meckel's diverticulum
Abdominal migraine
Lead poisoning
Abdominal epilepsy
Giardiasis
Chronic hepatitis
Hepatobiliary or pancreatic disorders
Familial Mediterranean fever
Diaphragmatic irritation
Nephrolithiasis
Porphyrias ㉘
Hereditary angioedema
Neoplasm
Trauma, tumor or infection of vertebrae
Psychogenic ㉙

NO

Functional recurrent abdominal pain ㉚
Constipation ⑰

UGI/SBFT = Upper gastrointestinal series with small bowel follow through
UPJ = ureteropelvic junction

rhea, and excess flatulence. In primary (genetic) cases, symptoms may not develop until 3 to 5 years of age when lactase levels begin to decline. Breath hydrogen testing after an oral lactose load will make the diagnosis, although resolution of symptoms after dietary restriction of lactose is strongly suggestive. Malabsorption of fructose and sorbitol may also cause symptoms of GI distress; a history of high fruit juice ingestion suggests the former, and frequent use of "sugar-free" products (sorbitol-containing) should raise suspicion of the latter.

(26) An upper GI series with small bowel follow-through is required to diagnosis most cases of malrotation.

(27) Ureteropelvic junction obstruction is an uncommon disorder, often presenting as abdominal pain in children and adolescents. Diagnosis in infants is often assisted by the presence of an abdominal mass or occurrence of a urinary tract infection. In older children, the physical examination and urinalysis may be normal or may reveal a unilateral abdominal mass or hematuria. The chief complaint in over 70% of children older than 6 years old with ureteropelvic junction obstruction is abdominal pain that is frequently referred to the groin or flank. In older children the disorder most commonly occurs in males and is on the left side. Symptoms tend to predominate during periods of fluid loading and diuresis. Ultrasound is recommended if obstruction is suspected.

(28) Acute intermittent porphyria is the most common of the porphyrias. It generally presents as abdominal pain; peripheral neuropathies are also common. In severe cases the urine may turn a port wine color. The diagnosis is made by demonstrating decreased porphobilinogen deaminase in erythrocytes and increased urinary levels of aminolevulinic acid and porphobilinogen.

(29) Psychogenic pain is not the same as functional pain; it is believed to be perceived pain or imaginary pain occurring in the absence of physical stimuli.

(30) Nonorganic chronic abdominal pain or "functional recurrent abdominal pain" is the most common diagnosis after organic causes have been ruled out. It describes a pain that does not have a clear structural or biochemical basis but is recognized as genuine pain. Characteristics include onset at age older than 5 years, intermittent or episodic nature, periumbilical location, and a lack of association with activity, meals, and bowel pattern. The physical examination is always normal (although patients may appear tired or pale during episodes), and results of laboratory studies are normal. The entity remains a common yet poorly explained affliction of childhood.

BIBLIOGRAPHY

Wyllie R, Mahajan LA: Chronic abdominal pain of childhood and adolescence. In Wyllie R, Hyams J (eds): Pediatric Gastrointestinal Disease: Pathophysiology, Diagnosis, Management, 2nd ed, p 3. Philadelphia: WB Saunders Company, 1999.

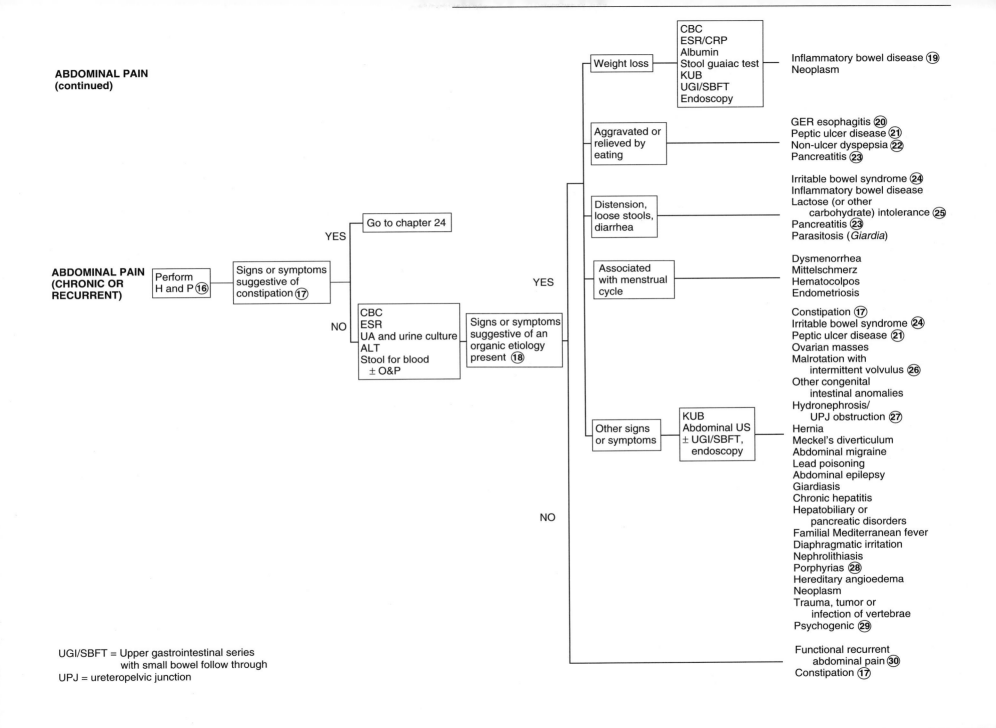

ABDOMINAL PAIN
(continued)

ABDOMINAL PAIN
(CHRONIC OR
RECURRENT)

Perform H and P ⑯

Signs or symptoms suggestive of constipation ⑰

YES — Go to chapter 24

NO

CBC
ESR
UA and urine culture
ALT
Stool for blood
± O&P

Signs or symptoms suggestive of an organic etiology present ⑱

YES

NO

Weight loss

CBC
ESR/CRP
Albumin
Stool guaiac test
KUB
UGI/SBFT
Endoscopy

Inflammatory bowel disease ⑲
Neoplasm

Aggravated or relieved by eating

GER esophagitis ⑳
Peptic ulcer disease ㉑
Non-ulcer dyspepsia ㉒
Pancreatitis ㉓

Distension, loose stools, diarrhea

Irritable bowel syndrome ㉔
Inflammatory bowel disease
Lactose (or other carbohydrate) intolerance ㉕
Pancreatitis ㉓
Parasitosis (Giardia)

Associated with menstrual cycle

Dysmenorrhea
Mittelschmerz
Hematocolpos
Endometriosis

Other signs or symptoms

KUB
Abdominal US
± UGI/SBFT, endoscopy

Constipation ⑰
Irritable bowel syndrome ㉔
Peptic ulcer disease ㉑
Ovarian masses
Malrotation with intermittent volvulus ㉖
Other congenital intestinal anomalies
Hydronephrosis/ UPJ obstruction ㉗
Hernia
Meckel's diverticulum
Abdominal migraine
Lead poisoning
Abdominal epilepsy
Giardiasis
Chronic hepatitis
Hepatobiliary or pancreatic disorders
Familial Mediterranean fever
Diaphragmatic irritation
Nephrolithiasis
Porphyrias ㉘
Hereditary angioedema
Neoplasm
Trauma, tumor or infection of vertebrae
Psychogenic ㉙

Functional recurrent abdominal pain ㉚
Constipation ⑰

UGI/SBFT = Upper gastrointestinal series with small bowel follow through
UPJ = ureteropelvic junction

True vomiting is a forceful ejection of stomach or esophageal contents from the mouth. Regurgitation is an effortless or near-effortless ejection.

(1) Vomiting should be approached by first identifying the pattern. The review of systems should include other abdominal, respiratory, and neurologic complaints. Inquire about diet and medication use. In cases of chronic recurrent vomiting, the frequency averages about two episodes per week and abdominal pain and diarrhea are frequently associated; children are generally not acutely ill and vomit with a low intensity. In cyclic recurrent vomiting, episodes are infrequent but are characterized by acute severity and illness and forceful vomiting occurring at a high frequency (i.e., more than four times per hour). Autonomic signs and symptoms such as pallor, lethargy, nausea, and abdominal pain are frequent. Initially, chronic and cyclic vomiting appear as acute problems until the pattern becomes evident.

(2) When acute vomiting occurs in the context of an acute abdomen, immediate surgical consultation should be obtained. Signs and symptoms of an acute abdomen include sudden severe pain, bilious vomiting, point or diffuse tenderness on examination, diarrhea with abdominal distention, absent bowel sounds, involuntary guarding, rebound tenderness, a rigid abdomen, and pain with movement or cough.

(3) Volvulus, the twisting of bowel on the mesentery, generally occurs in the context of congenital intestinal malrotation. Many cases of malrotation present as volvulus (e.g., bilious vomiting, severe clinical toxicity) in the newborn period. Other cases present many years later as intermittent vomiting.

(4) Obstruction can occur at any level of the GI tract and can appear as a surgical emergency or a chronic complaint of abdominal pain or vomiting. Congenital lesions (esophageal stenosis, volvulus, duodenal webs, annular pancreas) usually occur acutely in the newborn period but may occur later if the obstruction is partial. Many disorders (e.g., inflammatory bowel disease, mucosal disease, postoperative adhesions) may result in acquired obstructive lesions. Plain abdominal X-rays are recommended initially. Ultrasound, CT, or fluoroscopy may provide a more definitive diagnosis but may not be necessary or recommended if a need for surgery has already been established.

(5) Superior mesenteric artery syndrome describes a condition of transient duodenal obstruction due to a trapping or compression in the duodenum by the superior mesenteric artery anteriorly and the aorta posteriorly. Clinically, bilious vomiting and epigastric pain occur and are relieved by a prone or knee-chest position. The condition is most commonly seen in cases of recent weight loss, lordosis, prolonged bed rest, or body casting.

(6) Abdominal trauma occasionally results in an obstructive duodenal hematoma. Child abuse and seat belt injuries are recognized causes.

(7) Signs or symptoms suggestive of increased intracranial pressure include early morning occurrence, progressive headaches, absence of nausea, abnormal funduscopic examination, or a bulging fontanel in infants.

(8) In a child with acute-onset, large-volume emesis, fever, and/or diarrhea—a picture consistent with acute gastroenteritis—additional workup may not be necessary. With rotavirus in particular, vomiting often precedes diarrhea by 1 to 2 days. In other cases of acute severe vomiting, laboratory tests and a urinalysis may aid in the assessment of dehydration and possible diagnosis. Further studies should be ordered based on suspected diagnoses.

(9) Pyloric stenosis presents as nonbilious vomiting in the first few weeks of life and progresses in frequency and intensity. Clinical characteristics include projectile vomiting, later onset of "coffee ground" emesis (hematemesis), and poor weight gain. Patients are often dehydrated, with a metabolic alkalosis and hypochloremia by the time they present. Diagnosis is by physical examination and by ultrasound or an upper GI study that shows the "string sign" of contrast medium through the narrowed pylorus.

(10) Sinusitis may cause an acute, chronic, or cyclic pattern of vomiting. Associated nausea, congestion, postnasal drip, and early morning occurrence often preceded by coughing suggest the diagnosis. Diagnosis is made by sinus films or CT and confirmed by improvement with antibiotics.

(11) Mental status changes and abnormal respirations may indicate ingestion of a toxic drug or poison.

(12) Ureteropelvic junction obstruction results in hydronephrosis during fluid loading and diuresis. Congenital cases appear as an abdominal mass or urinary tract infection. Older children tend to present with intermittent abdominal or flank pain and often with vomiting. The physical examination and urinalysis may be normal or may reveal a unilateral abdominal mass or hematuria. A history of spontaneous resolution after several hours due to relief of the renal pelvic distention as dehydration develops is suggestive. Ultrasound during an acute episode or after furosemide or an intravenous pyelogram should help provide the diagnosis.

(13) Most inborn errors of metabolism appear early in the newborn period with vomiting and failure to thrive. Some disorders, especially partial errors or disorders of fatty acid metabolism, occur as chronic or cyclic vomiting at later ages after the addition of certain foods to the diet or in the context of acute stresses or illnesses. These children may experience acute intermittent episodes of vomiting accompanied by acidosis, mental deterioration, and coma. There may be a family history of the disorder or of unexplained mental retardation, failure to thrive, or neonatal deaths.

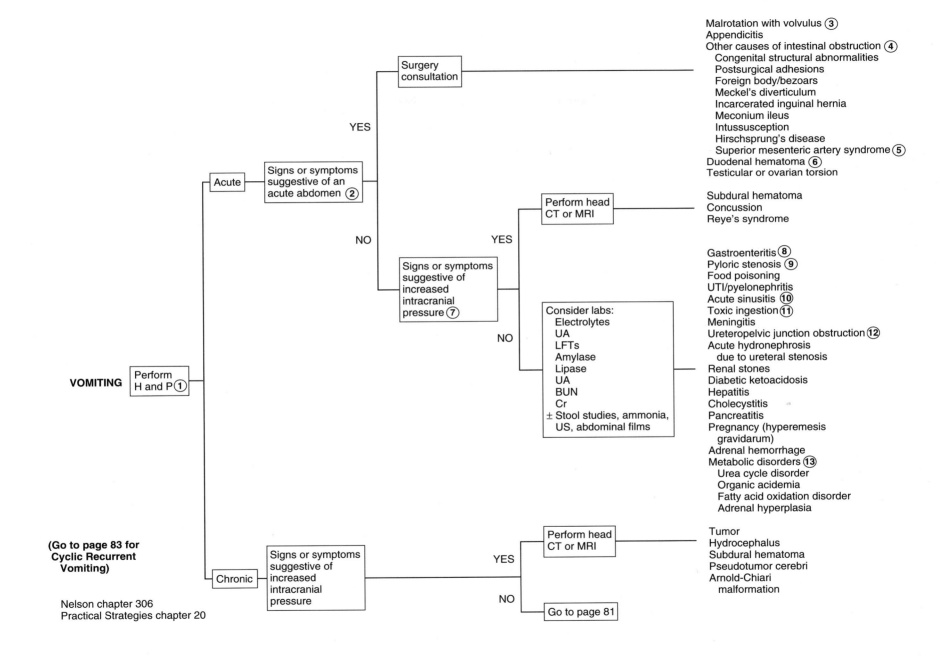

VOMITING — Perform H and P ①

Acute

Signs or symptoms suggestive of an acute abdomen ②

YES — Surgery consultation

Malrotation with volvulus ③
Appendicitis
Other causes of intestinal obstruction ④
   Congenital structural abnormalities
   Postsurgical adhesions
   Foreign body/bezoars
   Meckel's diverticulum
   Incarcerated inguinal hernia
   Meconium ileus
   Intussusception
   Hirschsprung's disease
   Superior mesenteric artery syndrome ⑤
Duodenal hematoma ⑥
Testicular or ovarian torsion

NO

Signs or symptoms suggestive of increased intracranial pressure ⑦

YES — Perform head CT or MRI

Subdural hematoma
Concussion
Reye's syndrome

NO — Consider labs:
   Electrolytes
   UA
   LFTs
   Amylase
   Lipase
   UA
   BUN
   Cr
   ± Stool studies, ammonia, US, abdominal films

Gastroenteritis ⑧
Pyloric stenosis ⑨
Food poisoning
UTI/pyelonephritis
Acute sinusitis ⑩
Toxic ingestion ⑪
Meningitis
Ureteropelvic junction obstruction ⑫
Acute hydronephrosis
   due to ureteral stenosis
Renal stones
Diabetic ketoacidosis
Hepatitis
Cholecystitis
Pancreatitis
Pregnancy (hyperemesis gravidarum)
Adrenal hemorrhage
Metabolic disorders ⑬
   Urea cycle disorder
   Organic acidemia
   Fatty acid oxidation disorder
   Adrenal hyperplasia

Chronic

Signs or symptoms suggestive of increased intracranial pressure

YES — Perform head CT or MRI

Tumor
Hydrocephalus
Subdural hematoma
Pseudotumor cerebri
Arnold-Chiari malformation

NO — Go to page 81

(Go to page 83 for Cyclic Recurrent Vomiting)

Nelson chapter 306
Practical Strategies chapter 20

Consider a metabolic workup whenever neurologic symptoms (e.g., altered mental status, hypotonia, seizures, unexplained mental retardation), hepatosplenomegaly, or unusual odors (e.g., from breath, urine, ear wax) are present. For a metabolic workup, blood and urine should be obtained during episodes of suggestive symptoms. Blood tests should include a CBC, electrolytes, pH, glucose, ammonia, lactate, carnitine, and serum amino acids. Urine should be analyzed for ketones, reducing substances, organic acids, amino acids, and carnitine.

(14) The presentation of peptic ulcer disease (gastritis, duodenitis, and gastric and duodenal ulcers) may be classic, including epigastric pain, nocturnal awakening, evidence of GI bleeding, relief or exacerbation with meals, or nonspecific, especially in young children. A history of peptic ulcer disease or similar symptoms in family members should prompt a urea breath test to look for *Helicobacter pylori. H. pylori* antibodies can be tested for but are less useful than the urea breath test for diagnosis. Endoscopy should be considered if symptoms are atypical or there is no response to therapy.

(15) In infants, gastroesophageal reflux appears as a near effortless regurgitation. Infants may be irritable and demonstrate poor weight gain, apnea, or Sandifer syndrome (arching). Older children may complain of effortless vomiting, substernal pain, dysphagia, exacerbation with certain foods, and relief with liquid antacids. When clinical suspicion is present without life-threatening symptoms (i.e., apnea), a trial of an H_2-blocker or proton pump inhibitor may be diagnostic. The occurrence of apnea often prompts additional study.

(16) Vomiting may be a sign of food allergy or intolerance, most commonly due to cow's milk or soy protein. It may also occur as a sign of a specific disorder (hereditary fructose intolerance, celiac disease) that becomes evident after the introduction of certain foods.

(17) Gastric stasis and paralytic ileus may be postsurgical, owing to a neuropathy or drugs, electrolyte disturbances, endocrinopathies, or injuries. Pseudoobstruction is a rare chronic disorder of intermittent episodes of ileus. Causes are primarily neuropathic or myopathic. There is often a family history. Manometry and biopsy may be necessary for definitive diagnosis.

(18) Psychogenic vomiting should only be diagnosed after organic causes have been ruled out. Diagnostic advances (e.g., endoscopy with biopsy, motility studies) are responsible for a declining number of diagnoses of psychogenic causes. Patients are often anxious, affected by familial conflict, and not bothered by the vomiting.

(19) Nausea, dizziness, vertigo, and nystagmus characterize vestibular disorders, including motion sickness.

CHRONIC VOMITING (continued)

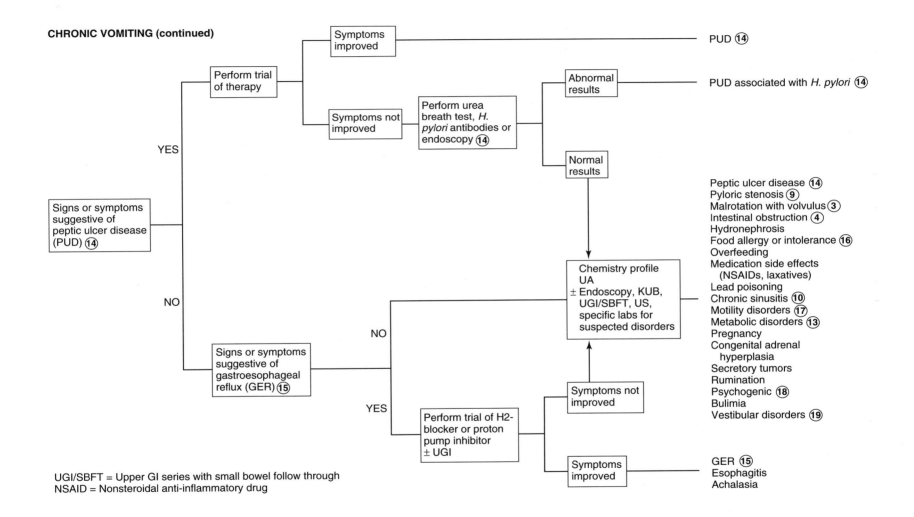

UGI/SBFT = Upper GI series with small bowel follow through
NSAID = Nonsteroidal anti-inflammatory drug

20 Other characteristics of abdominal migraine include recurrent stereotypical episodes of midline abdominal pain lasting more than 6 hours, associated pallor, lethargy, anorexia, nausea, and normal laboratory values, as well as radiographic and endoscopic studies. The typical migraine symptoms of headache and photophobia only occur in 30% to 40% of children with the abdominal symptoms. The vomiting pattern is replaced by the more typical headaches as the child gets older.

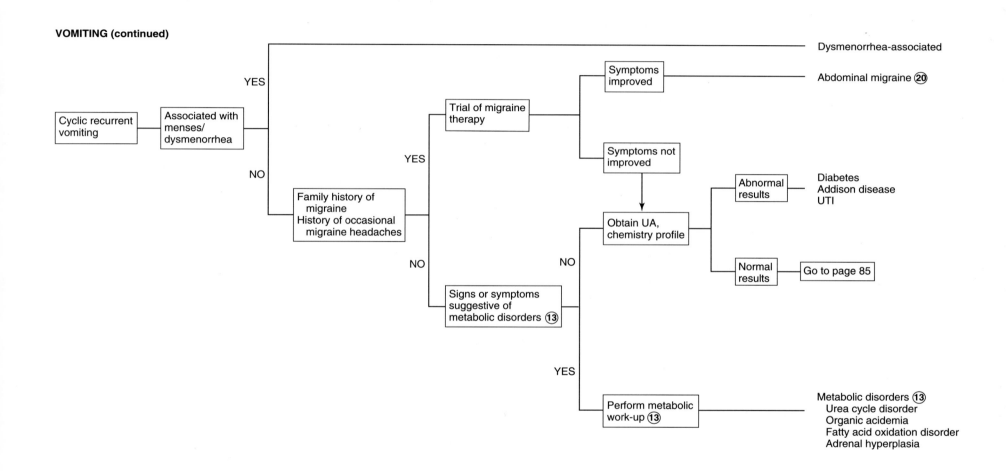

21 Cyclic vomiting syndrome is characterized by recurrent stereotypical episodes of prolonged vomiting accompanied by pallor, lethargy, anorexia, nausea, retching, and abdominal pain. These children present with a recurrent history of these episodes with normal health in between. A family history of migraine may be absent, and results of laboratory, radiographic, and endoscopic studies are normal. An overlap between the cyclic vomiting syndrome and abdominal migraine may complicate the diagnosis; some believe cyclic vomiting syndrome and abdominal migraine are the same entity.

BIBLIOGRAPHY

Burton BK: Inborn errors of metabolism in infancy: A guide to diagnosis. Pediatrics 102:69, 1998.

Li BUK, Sferra TJ: Vomiting. In Wyllie R, Hyams J (eds): Pediatric Gastrointestinal Disease: Pathophysiology, Diagnosis, Management, 2nd ed, p 14. Philadelphia: WB Saunders Company, 1999.

**CYCLIC RECURRENT
VOMITING (continued)**

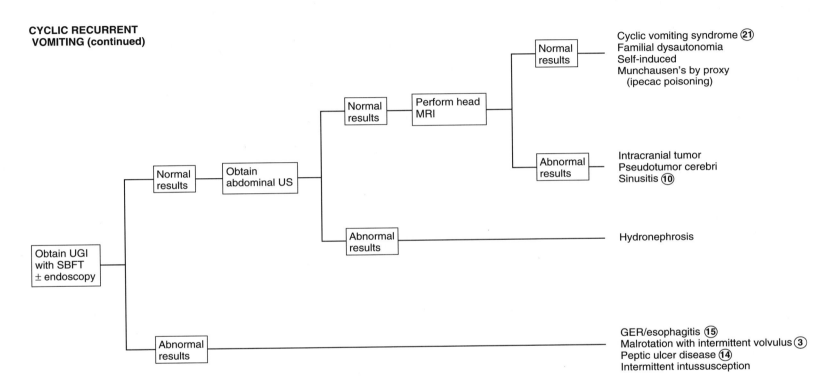

UGI/SBFT = Upper GI series with small bowel follow through
NSAID = Nonsteroidal anti-inflammatory drug

Chapter 23 **Diarrhea**

Diarrhea is defined as stools of increased frequency, fluidity, and volume. Diarrhea lasting longer than 2 to 3 weeks may be considered chronic.

(1) The history should include associated symptoms as well as the child's growth pattern. Hematuria and abnormal renal function suggest an enterohemorrhagic strain of *Escherichia coli;* an associated *severe dermatitis* (perioral, acral, perineal) should suggest acrodermatitis enteropathica. The social history should inquire about recent travel, exposure to unsanitary conditions, daycare attendance, risk factors for HIV, and sick contacts.

A diet history that includes seafood, unwashed vegetables, unpasteurized milk, contaminated water, or uncooked meats may suggest a foodborne or waterborne agent in acute cases of diarrhea. In chronic cases, assessing type and quantity of oral intake, especially fluid selection, is helpful because certain selections may exacerbate diarrhea symptoms by an osmotic load. Inquire whether the onset of symptoms coincided with a change in diet (e.g., discontinuation of breast milk or formula, addition of jar foods or cereals, addition of sugar-free or other sorbitol containing compounds).

(2) Sudden vomiting and explosive diarrhea within several hours of ingestion of a contaminated food suggests food poisoning from preformed toxins produced by *Staphylococcus aureus* or *Bacillus cereus.* Causes of foodborne illness include not only certain bacteria and viruses but also heavy metals, fish or shellfish poisoning, and mushrooms. Paresthesias, paralysis, or mental status changes are associated with some of these causes.

(3) High fevers and seizures have been associated with *Shigella. E. coli* 0157:H7 (an enterohemorrhagic strain) causes a hemorrhagic colitis that is followed by hemolytic-uremic syndrome in approximately 10% of cases. In hemolytic-uremic syndrome, watery diarrhea precedes the grossly bloody stools; abdominal cramping with minimal or absent fevers is characteristic. Undercooked beef is the most commonly identified source of outbreaks. Specific testing must be requested when the 0157:H7 strain is suspected. *Yersinia* and *Campylobacter* may be associated with a prolonged course of diarrhea.

(4) Infection with *Clostridium difficile* should be considered whenever diarrhea develops within several weeks of antibiotic treatment. It may manifest as mild or severe illness with or without grossly bloody diarrhea, abdominal pain, fever, or systemic toxicity. Definitive diagnosis is by culture or detection of the *C. difficile* toxin in the stool.

(5) Rotavirus is primarily a wintertime virus that affects infants and small children most often. Vomiting and diarrhea occur abruptly after a 2- to 3-day incubation period; the vomiting generally lasts 1 to 2 days, and loose watery stools last from 2 to 8 days. Fever commonly occurs; gross or occult blood is uncommon.

(6) Giardiasis (from infection with *Giardia lamblia*) often results from contaminated food or water, but person-to-person spread is common, especially in daycare centers and other crowded institutions. It should be considered as an etiology in acute cases of diarrhea, although it is most frequently considered a pathogen in chronic diarrhea (i.e., watery, without blood or mucus) with associated weight loss and abdominal pain. Symptoms may also be intermittent and may even include constipation. Diagnosis may be difficult. Sensitivity of stool examination for ova and parasites increases with a greater number of samples. Examination of a single specimen is approximately 70% sensitive. Antigen tests are more sensitive but will not aid in identifying other protozoans. Small intestinal biopsy or aspiration of duodenal or jejunal contents for examination are other more sensitive means of diagnosis.

Cryptosporidium may cause an acute diarrheal illness, including large watery stools, flatulence, malaise, and abdominal pain, lasting 3 to 30 days in a normal host. It causes a severe, chronic diarrheal illness in immunocompromised patients. It is associated with contact with farm animals or contaminated water but is also spread through person-to-person contact. The organism may be identified in the stool, although intestinal biopsy may be required.

(7) Parenteral diarrhea refers to diarrhea accompanying an infection outside the GI tract. Diarrhea is frequently associated with upper respiratory infections, otitis media, and urinary tract infections. The mechanism is not clear.

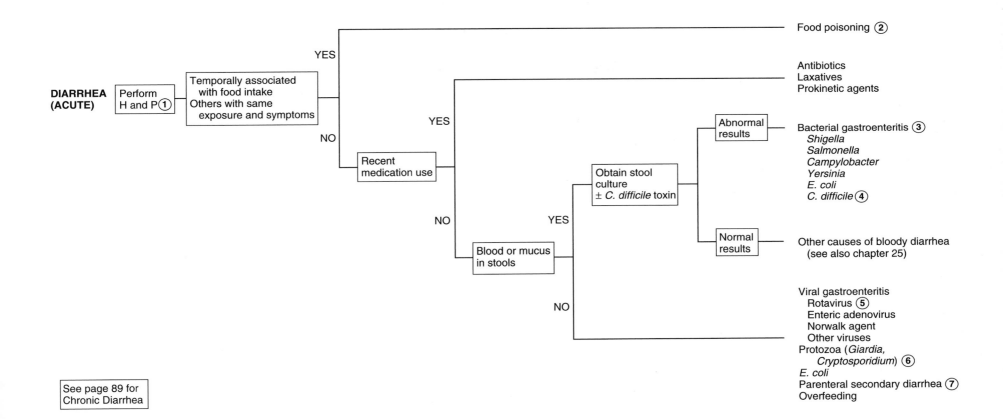

DIARRHEA (ACUTE)

Perform H and P ①

Temporally associated with food intake
Others with same exposure and symptoms

YES → Food poisoning ②

NO → Recent medication use

YES → Antibiotics / Laxatives / Prokinetic agents

NO → Blood or mucus in stools

YES → Obtain stool culture ± *C. difficile* toxin

Abnormal results → Bacterial gastroenteritis ③
Shigella
Salmonella
Campylobacter
Yersinia
E. coli
C. difficile ④

Normal results → Other causes of bloody diarrhea (see also chapter 25)

NO → Viral gastroenteritis
Rotavirus ⑤
Enteric adenovirus
Norwalk agent
Other viruses
Protozoa (*Giardia, Cryptosporidium*) ⑥
E. coli
Parenteral secondary diarrhea ⑦
Overfeeding

See page 89 for Chronic Diarrhea

Nelson chapters 176, 306
Practical Strategies chapter 19

(8) Formula protein (cow's milk and/or soy) allergy or intolerance may manifest as an enterocolitis with bloody diarrhea in the first few months of life. Clinical improvement with a trial of a casein or whey hydrolysate formula or elimination of cow's milk from a breast-feeding mother's diet may be therapeutic and eliminate the need for any further evaluation. After 6 months of age the same etiology may present as a protein-losing enteropathy with diarrhea, occult blood loss, and hypoproteinemia.

(9) Commercial reagents (Clinitest) are available to test for reducing substances; pH testing with Nitrazine paper should be performed on a fresh stool specimen. Positive reducing substances or a pH less than 5.5 suggests carbohydrate malabsorption. Be aware of two caveats: (1) the test for reducing substances is only reliable when the child is being fed adequate amounts of carbohydrates, and (2) sucrose is not a reducing sugar and must be digested or split by bacteria to produce a positive test. Adding hydrochloric acid before the analysis should have the same result.

(10) Postinfectious enteritis after acute enteritis is a common cause of prolonged diarrhea. Low-grade mucosal injury is responsible for the malabsorption. In young infants, a secondary lactase deficiency is considered a contributing factor; in older infants and children a hypocaloric, high-carbohydrate diet is often responsible for the persistent malabsorption.

(11) Approximately 10% of children with Hirschsprung disease develop enterocolitis. Historical "red flags" include a history of delayed passage of meconium, preceding constipation, Down syndrome, and a positive family history. Absent stool on rectal examination and immediate passage of stool after the rectal examination are suggestive. A rectal suction biopsy demonstrating absent ganglion cells is necessary for diagnosis.

(12) In chronic diarrhea a finding of leukocytes or occult blood is more suggestive of inflammatory bowel disease than bacterial infection. A Sudan stain for fat will confirm steatorrhea but does not specify whether the abnormality is of bowel, pancreatic, or biliary origin. Many causes of chronic diarrhea demonstrate an acidic pH or positive reducing substances consistent with some element of carbohydrate malabsorption.

(13) Cystic fibrosis is characterized by frequent large, foul-smelling fatty stools not classic loose, watery diarrheal stools. When accompanied by a history of recurrent respiratory infections and failure to thrive, a sweat chloride test should be done. Infants younger than 6 months tend to present with failure to thrive; diarrhea (steatorrhea) is more common in older infants and toddlers.

(14) Chronic neutropenia, pancreatic insufficiency, and short stature characterize Shwachman-Diamond syndrome.

(15) Congenital chloride-losing diarrhea is a rare congenital disorder diagnosed by abnormally high levels of stool chloride.

(16) If Munchausen by proxy or laxative abuse is suspected, determine the osmotic gap of a fresh stool specimen:

$$\text{Osmotic gap} = \text{stool osmolality}$$
$$- 2[\text{stool sodium} + \text{stool potassium}]$$

An osmotic gap greater than 50 mOsm/kg in the absence of reducing substances suggesting malabsorption of carbohydrate should raise suspicion for laxative abuse.

(17) When the cause of diarrhea and weight loss is not evident after a preliminary evaluation, consultation with a gastroenterologist should be obtained for further evaluation of less common causes (e.g., anatomic defects, congenital malabsorption defects, other enteropathies). Consider a urinary tract infection in chronic cases of diarrhea even though it is often difficult to distinguish it as a cause versus a consequence of diarrhea. Specialty consultation should be considered in any case of prolonged diarrhea, even in the absence of weight loss.

DIARRHEA (continued)

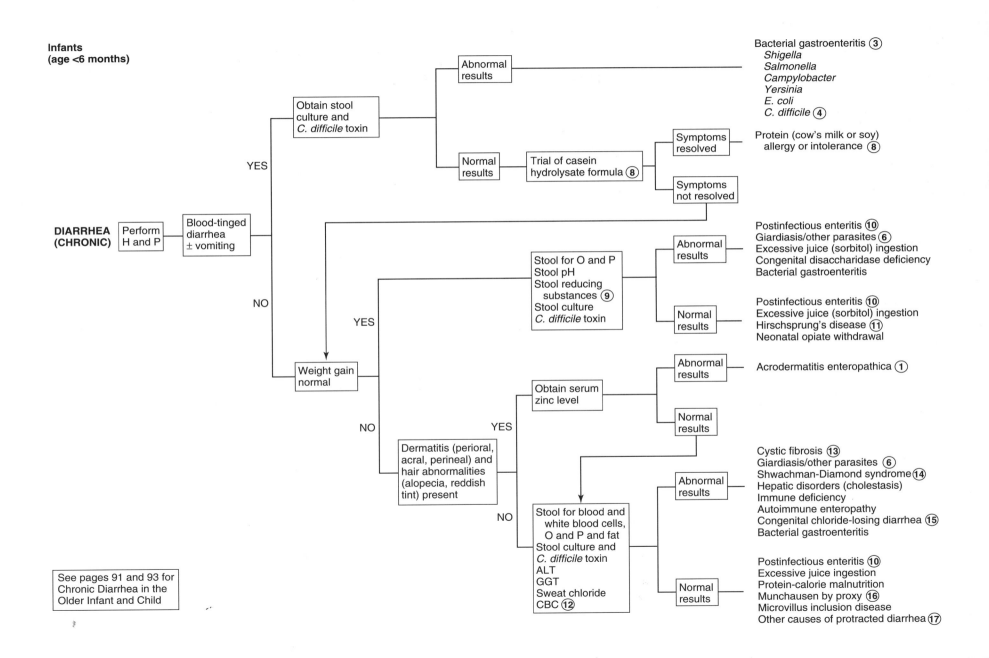

Infants (age <6 months)

DIARRHEA (CHRONIC) → Perform H and P → Blood-tinged diarrhea ± vomiting

YES → Obtain stool culture and *C. difficile* toxin

- Abnormal results → Bacterial gastroenteritis ③
  - *Shigella*
  - *Salmonella*
  - *Campylobacter*
  - *Yersinia*
  - *E. coli*
  - *C. difficile* ④

- Normal results → Trial of casein hydrolysate formula ⑧
  - Symptoms resolved → Protein (cow's milk or soy) allergy or intolerance ⑧
  - Symptoms not resolved →

NO → Weight gain normal

YES → Stool for O and P / Stool pH / Stool reducing substances ⑨ / Stool culture / *C. difficile* toxin
- Abnormal results → Postinfectious enteritis ⑩ / Giardiasis/other parasites ⑥ / Excessive juice (sorbitol) ingestion / Congenital disaccharidase deficiency / Bacterial gastroenteritis
- Normal results → Postinfectious enteritis ⑩ / Excessive juice (sorbitol) ingestion / Hirschsprung's disease ⑪ / Neonatal opiate withdrawal

NO → Dermatitis (perioral, acral, perineal) and hair abnormalities (alopecia, reddish tint) present

YES → Obtain serum zinc level
- Abnormal results → Acrodermatitis enteropathica ①
- Normal results →

NO → Stool for blood and white blood cells, O and P and fat / Stool culture and *C. difficile* toxin / ALT / GGT / Sweat chloride / CBC ⑫
- Abnormal results → Cystic fibrosis ⑬ / Giardiasis/other parasites ⑥ / Shwachman-Diamond syndrome ⑭ / Hepatic disorders (cholestasis) / Immune deficiency / Autoimmune enteropathy / Congenital chloride-losing diarrhea ⑮ / Bacterial gastroenteritis
- Normal results → Postinfectious enteritis ⑩ / Excessive juice ingestion / Protein-calorie malnutrition / Munchausen by proxy ⑯ / Microvillus inclusion disease / Other causes of protracted diarrhea ⑰

See pages 91 and 93 for Chronic Diarrhea in the Older Infant and Child

18 Immune-mediated damage of the small intestine in response to gluten occurs in celiac disease (gluten-sensitive enteropathy). Symptoms of malabsorption and failure to thrive develop between 6 months and 3 years; symptom onset follows the addition of cereal grains (e.g., wheat, oat, barley, rye) to the diet. Diarrhea is often a late manifestation of the disorder, which may also include failure to thrive, anorexia, digital clubbing, anemia, abdominal distention, apathy, frequent fatty stools, and symptoms suggestive of specific nutrient deficiencies. Antibody screens for anti-gliadin IgA and IgG antibodies, anti-reticular, and anti-endomysium are sensitive screening tests. Biopsy is considered necessary for definitive diagnosis.

19 Inflammatory bowel disease (Crohn, ulcerative colitis) is very important in the differential diagnosis of chronic diarrhea in the school-aged child. Although rare, inflammatory bowel disease may present in younger children. Ulcerative colitis is more common than Crohn disease in the toddler age group. Weight loss and growth retardation are the cardinal symptoms. Gastrointestinal manifestations include diarrhea, abdominal pain, bloody stools, perianal disease, and malabsorption. Multiple extraintestinal manifestations (fever, oral ulcers, uveitis, rash, arthralgias) may also occur. Laboratory evaluation usually reveals anemia, an elevated sedimentation rate, leukocytosis, and some degree of hypoalbuminemia, thrombocytosis, and elevated acute phase-reactive proteins depending on the severity of the disease. Radiologic studies (barium enema, upper gastrointestinal series) aid in determining the extent of the disease. Colonoscopy and biopsy are necessary for definitive diagnosis.

20 Chronic nonspecific diarrhea or "toddler's diarrhea" is a frustrating but benign disorder most often affecting normally nourished children between 1 and 5 years of age. Children have up to 6 to 10 loose, watery, foul-smelling stools per day, often with food particles present. The pattern and consistency of the stools may vary considerably from day to day. In some cases they may be well formed in the morning and become looser throughout the day. In others the diarrhea may alternate with periods of constipation. Normal growth and an absence of stool passage at night suggest the diagnosis; stool examination is negative for blood, mucus, and excessive fat.

Previously, most of these cases were probably due to excessive fruit juice intake. As the role of fruit juices has been increasingly recognized, the disorder is diagnosed less frequently today.

Older infant/toddler

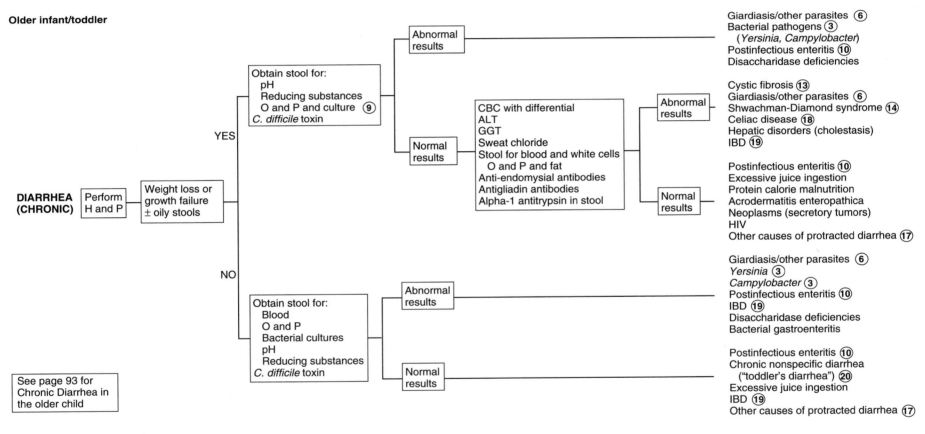

DIARRHEA (CHRONIC)

Perform H and P

Weight loss or growth failure ± oily stools

YES

Obtain stool for:
pH
Reducing substances
O and P and culture (9)
C. difficile toxin

Abnormal results

Giardiasis/other parasites (6)
Bacterial pathogens (3)
   (*Yersinia, Campylobacter*)
Postinfectious enteritis (10)
Disaccharidase deficiencies

Normal results

CBC with differential
ALT
GGT
Sweat chloride
Stool for blood and white cells
   O and P and fat
Anti-endomysial antibodies
Antigliadin antibodies
Alpha-1 antitrypsin in stool

Abnormal results

Cystic fibrosis (13)
Giardiasis/other parasites (6)
Shwachman-Diamond syndrome (14)
Celiac disease (18)
Hepatic disorders (cholestasis)
IBD (19)

Normal results

Postinfectious enteritis (10)
Excessive juice ingestion
Protein calorie malnutrition
Acrodermatitis enteropathica
Neoplasms (secretory tumors)
HIV
Other causes of protracted diarrhea (17)

NO

Obtain stool for:
Blood
O and P
Bacterial cultures
pH
Reducing substances
C. difficile toxin

Abnormal results

Giardiasis/other parasites (6)
Yersinia (3)
Campylobacter (3)
Postinfectious enteritis (10)
IBD (19)
Disaccharidase deficiencies
Bacterial gastroenteritis

Normal results

Postinfectious enteritis (10)
Chronic nonspecific diarrhea
   ("toddler's diarrhea") (20)
Excessive juice ingestion
IBD (19)
Other causes of protracted diarrhea (17)

See page 93 for
Chronic Diarrhea in
the older child

IBD = Inflammatory bowel disease

Diarrhea (continued)

(21) Lactase levels gradually decrease between 3 and 5 years of age in children with primary or genetic, late-onset lactase deficiency. Subtle increases in malabsorptive symptoms (flatulence, abdominal pain, loose stools) occur after milk ingestion. Breath hydrogen testing after an oral lactose load may make the diagnosis, although resolution of symptoms after dietary restriction of lactose is strongly suggestive. Postinfectious secondary lactase deficiency can occur in older children but is not as common or as severe as in younger children.

(22) Irritable bowel syndrome is a functional GI disorder that is being increasingly recognized in older children and adolescents. Patients report a variable pattern of diarrhea and constipation plus abdominal pain, bloating, urgency, a sense of incomplete stool evacuation, or passage of mucus.

(23) Soiling associated with chronic constipation (i.e., encopresis) may be described as diarrhea by parents. The history and rectal examination usually make a rapid diagnosis.

BIBLIOGRAPHY

Branski D, Lerner A, Lebenthal E: Chronic diarrhea and malabsorption. Pediatr Clin North Am 43:307–331, 1996.

Vanderhoof JA: Diarrhea. In Wyllie R, Hyams J (eds): Pediatric Gastrointestinal Disease: Pathophysiology, Diagnosis, Management, 2nd ed, p 32. Philadelphia: WB Saunders Company, 1999.

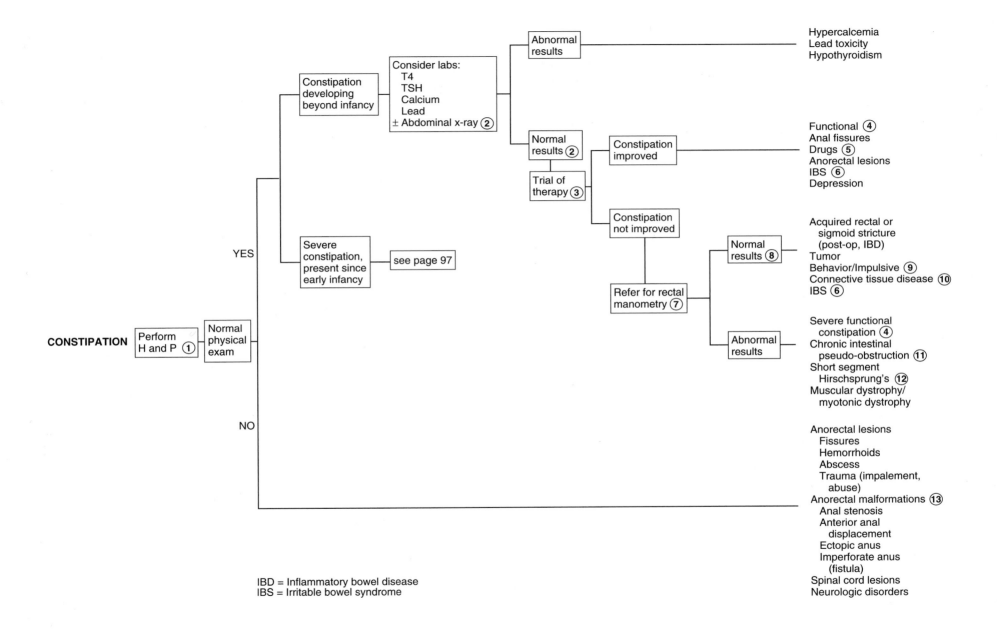

CONSTIPATION

Perform H and P ①

Normal physical exam

YES

Constipation developing beyond infancy

Consider labs:
T4
TSH
Calcium
Lead
± Abdominal x-ray ②

Abnormal results

Hypercalcemia
Lead toxicity
Hypothyroidism

Normal results ②

Trial of therapy ③

Constipation improved

Functional ④
Anal fissures
Drugs ⑤
Anorectal lesions
IBS ⑥
Depression

Constipation not improved

Refer for rectal manometry ⑦

Normal results ⑧

Acquired rectal or
   sigmoid stricture
   (post-op, IBD)
Tumor
Behavior/Impulsive ⑨
Connective tissue disease ⑩
IBS ⑥

Abnormal results

Severe functional
   constipation ④
Chronic intestinal
   pseudo-obstruction ⑪
Short segment
   Hirschsprung's ⑫
Muscular dystrophy/
   myotonic dystrophy

Severe constipation, present since early infancy

see page 97

NO

Anorectal lesions
   Fissures
   Hemorrhoids
   Abscess
   Trauma (impalement,
      abuse)
Anorectal malformations ⑬
   Anal stenosis
   Anterior anal
      displacement
   Ectopic anus
   Imperforate anus
      (fistula)
Spinal cord lesions
Neurologic disorders

IBD = Inflammatory bowel disease
IBS = Irritable bowel syndrome

Constipation (continued)

layed passage of meconium in 40% of affected infants, followed by lower intestinal obstruction in young infants. Milder presentations include severe constipation since birth, narrow-caliber stools, abdominal distention, and failure to thrive. Fecal soiling is almost unheard of in Hirschsprung cases. Patients with short segment disease may not present until older childhood, adolescence, or even adulthood.

A rectal mucosal suction biopsy revealing an absence of ganglion cells is necessary for diagnosis of Hirschsprung disease.

(13) Simple anterior displacement of the anus may contribute to constipation because of the anterior angle of the canal that stool must be expelled through, although this concept is not universally accepted. An anteriorly located anus must be distinguished from an ectopic anus in which the anal canal and internal anal sphincter are displaced anteriorly. The external anal sphincter remains in its normal posterior position. An ectopic anus should be suspected if an anal wink can be elicited posterior to the opening of the anal canal.

(14) Children with neurologic impairment of any cause (e.g., cerebral palsy, polyneuritis, spina bifida, muscular dystrophy) are at risk for constipation from poor intestinal motility, inadequate dietary fiber, and impaired sensation.

(15) In very young infants, an unprepared barium enema may be the preferred initial study in the evaluation of severe constipation. The test will identify Hirschsprung disease as well as congenital anomalies. If not done diagnostically, the barium enema should be performed after manometry or biopsy to assist in surgical planning.

(16) Meconium ileus (i.e., small bowel obstruction) appears in the newborn period in approximately 10% of infants with cystic fibrosis. In contrast to the meconium ileus, meconium plug syndrome is an obstruction of the colon with inspissated plugs. The condition may occur in the infant of a diabetic mother, and in cystic fibrosis, rectal aganglionosis, maternal drug abuse, and after maternal magnesium sulfate therapy for pre-eclampsia. A Gastrografin enema is usually diagnostic and therapeutic. Many cases are benign, but a sweat chloride test is recommended.

BIBLIOGRAPHY

Abi-Hanna A, Lake AM: Constipation and encopresis in childhood. Pediatr Rev 19:23, 1998.

Baker SS, Liptak GS, Colleti RB, et al: Constipation in infants and children: Evaluation and treatment. (A medical position statement for Pediatric Gastroenterology and Nutrition.) J Pediatr Gastroenterol 29:612, 1999.

Loening-Baucke V: Encopresis and soiling. Pediatr Clin North Am 43:279, 1996.

Steffen R, Loening-Baucke V: Constipation and encopresis. In Wyllie R, Hyams J (eds): Pediatric Gastrointestinal Disease: Pathophysiology, Diagnosis, Management, 2nd ed, p 43. Philadelphia: WB Saunders Company, 1999.

**CONSTIPATION
(continued)**

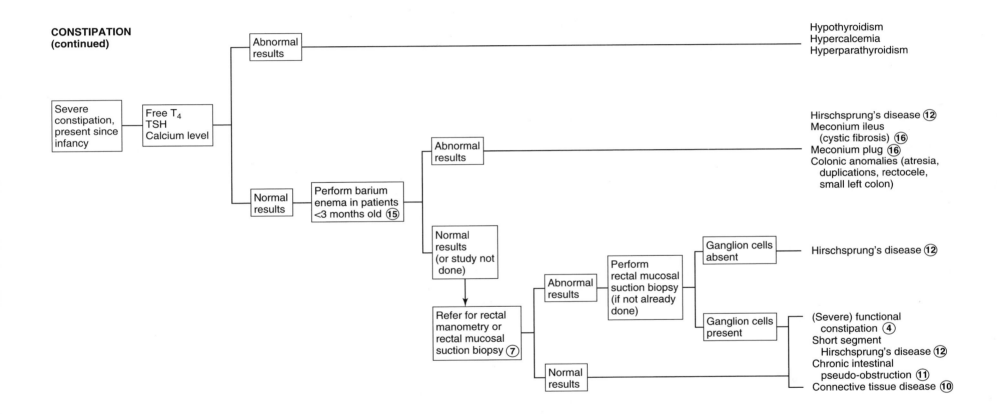

Severe constipation, present since infancy

Free T$_4$
TSH
Calcium level

Abnormal results → Hypothyroidism
Hypercalcemia
Hyperparathyroidism

Normal results → Perform barium enema in patients <3 months old ⑮

Abnormal results → Hirschsprung's disease ⑫
Meconium ileus (cystic fibrosis) ⑯
Meconium plug ⑯
Colonic anomalies (atresia, duplications, rectocele, small left colon)

Normal results (or study not done) → Refer for rectal manometry or rectal mucosal suction biopsy ⑦

Abnormal results → Perform rectal mucosal suction biopsy (if not already done)

Ganglion cells absent → Hirschsprung's disease ⑫

Ganglion cells present → (Severe) functional constipation ④
Short segment Hirschsprung's disease ⑫
Chronic intestinal pseudo-obstruction ⑪
Connective tissue disease ⑩

Normal results → (Severe) functional constipation ④
Short segment Hirschsprung's disease ⑫
Chronic intestinal pseudo-obstruction ⑪
Connective tissue disease ⑩

Hematemesis (i.e., vomiting of bright red blood or "coffee grounds") is generally associated with an upper GI hemorrhage proximal to the ligament of Treitz. Hematochezia (rectal passage of bright red or maroon-colored blood mixed in with the stool) is usually associated with lower GI or colonic bleeding, although brisk upper GI hemorrhages may also present in this way. Melena (i.e., dark, tarry-appearing stool) represents bleeding from any site above the ileocecal valve. Occult blood may originate from upper or lower GI sources. Blood originating in the rectum generally maintains a bright red color.

(1) The history should include any previous GI problems (e.g., jaundice, liver disease, ulcers, gastroesophageal reflux, other GI hemorrhages), blood transfusions, coagulopathies, and iron deficiency. A neonatal history of total parenteral nutrition, omphalitis, or umbilical vein catheterization is a risk factor for portal vein thrombosis. For infants, inquire about maternal idiopathic thrombocytopenic purpura and maternal use of nonsteroidal antiinflammatory drugs (NSAIDs). Aspirin, NSAIDs, and probably corticosteroids may play a contributing role in the development of gastritis.

A family history may be helpful in cases of suspected peptic ulcer disease, inflammatory bowel disease, liver disease, Meckel diverticulum, polyps, or milk allergy. Inquire about a family history of coagulopathies and Hirschsprung disease. A history of nosebleeds raises the possibility of swallowed blood presenting as hematemesis. Hemoptysis may need to be ruled out in cases in which severe coughing is present. Ask about ingestion of undercooked meat, recent medications, and the possibility of other ingestions (e.g., toxins, foreign bodies). Kool-Aid, gelatin, food coloring, antibiotics, bismuth, beets, licorice, cranberries, spinach, and blueberries can all mimic GI bleeding. Large iron ingestions can cause hematemesis due to mucosal injury. Therapeutic doses of iron will cause black stools, but they will remain guaiac negative.

(2) Confirming the presence of blood is important to avoid an unnecessary evaluation. A stool guaiac test must be part of the initial evaluation. False-positive test results can occur in young women around the time of their menses and after recent ingestion of rare red meat or fresh peroxidase-containing foodstuffs, such as broccoli, radishes, cauliflower, cantaloupe, or turnips. False-negative test results can occur in inappropriately collected stool samples (obtained from the toilet bowl), after ingestion of large doses of vitamin C, or in the presence of delayed transit time or bacterial overgrowth in the intestinal tract. Munchausen by proxy should be considered if a history of significant bleeding is not supported by any documentation of actual blood loss. Fecal leukocytes are consistent with an invasive infectious organism or an inflammatory condition.

GI bleeding warrants a CBC, differential, and reticulocyte count. If bleeding is significant or the history is suggestive of a bleeding disorder, obtain a PT, PTT, and bleeding time. Liver function tests, electrolytes, creatinine, and BUN may identify hepatic, renal, and metabolic problems. Hypoalbuminemia is consistent with long-standing liver dysfunction with portal hypertension, inflammatory bowel disease, or protein-losing enteropathies. In cases in which there was a limited amount of bleeding and a clinical picture consistent with a benign, self-limited condition (swallowed blood, a Mallory-Weiss tear), laboratory tests may not be indicated.

(3) Upper endoscopy is successful in identifying upper GI bleeding sites in 80% to 90% of cases. Radiographic contrast studies are less sensitive but may be used if endoscopy is not available. They are contraindicated in cases of active bleeding. Small bowel follow-through examinations offer the advantage of evaluation from the ligament of Treitz to the ileocecal valve and may be helpful in identifying atretic lesions, strictures, and rotation abnormalities.

(4) Bleeding scans can help locate bleeding sites not accessible with endoscopy. Angiography is most useful when bleeding is moderately brisk, but it is of limited value for lower GI hemorrhages.

(5) Peptic ulcer disease includes gastric and duodenal ulcers, gastritis, and duodenitis. Gastritis and peptic ulcers are common causes of upper GI bleeding in sick or stressed neonates or infants; they are more likely to present acutely as perforation or hemorrhage in this young age group than in older children. Less severe cases may present as irritability, vomiting, and regurgitation. Ulcers in older children and adolescents are more likely to appear in a history of long-standing intermittent abdominal pain. Frequent NSAID use is a risk factor in adolescents. Epigastric pain, especially if nocturnal or relieved with meals, is suggestive of peptic ulcer disease, although for children this "classic" constellation of symptoms is less reliable than for adults.

(6) Esophagitis as a complication of gastroesophageal reflux is a common cause of GI bleeding in infants. Gastroesophageal reflux may be present even in the absence of regurgitation.

(7) Mallory-Weiss tears are common. Forceful recurrent vomiting causes a tear in the distal esophageal mucosa that results in a limited amount of bright red hematemesis. In light of a stable clinical picture consistent with a self-limited vomiting illness and no evidence of obstruction, a diagnostic workup is not indicated.

(8) Varices are commonly due to portal vein hypertension secondary to intrinsic liver disease. Portal vein thrombosis is the next most likely etiology. Thrombus formation can occur as the result of sepsis, pancreatitis, omphalitis, or umbilical vein catheterization. A series of tortuous collateral veins develop to bypass the obstructing thrombus and may appear years later as bleeding esophageal varices. Ultrasound or endoscopy may be used to assess for varices when the patient is not actively bleeding.

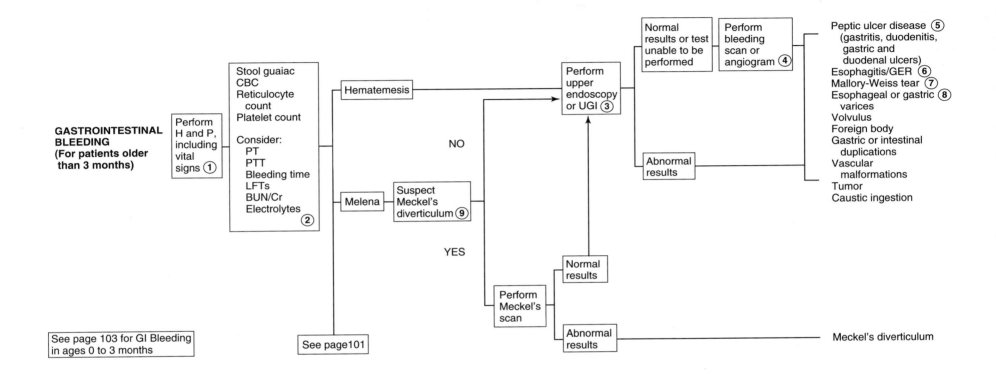

GASTROINTESTINAL BLEEDING
(For patients older than 3 months)

Perform H and P, including vital signs ①

Stool guaiac
CBC
Reticulocyte count
Platelet count

Consider:
  PT
  PTT
  Bleeding time
  LFTs
  BUN/Cr
  Electrolytes ②

Hematemesis

Melena

Suspect Meckel's diverticulum ⑨

NO

YES

See page 103 for GI Bleeding in ages 0 to 3 months

See page101

Perform Meckel's scan

Normal results

Abnormal results

Perform upper endoscopy or UGI ③

Normal results or test unable to be performed

Abnormal results

Perform bleeding scan or angiogram ④

Peptic ulcer disease ⑤
  (gastritis, duodenitis, gastric and duodenal ulcers)
Esophagitis/GER ⑥
Mallory-Weiss tear ⑦
Esophageal or gastric ⑧
  varices
Volvulus
Foreign body
Gastric or intestinal duplications
Vascular malformations
Tumor
Caustic ingestion

Meckel's diverticulum

Nelson chapters 306, 336
Strategies chapters 20, 21, 51

(9) Approximately two thirds of Meckel's diverticula occur as a painless but significant lower GI hemorrhage before 2 years of age. The bleeding occurs due to ulceration from gastric mucosa contained in the diverticulum.

(10) Intussusception is the "telescoping" of one segment of the intestine into a distal segment. It can occur between 3 months and 6 years of age, but most cases occur before age 36 months. Severe episodes of abdominal pain due to obstruction or ischemia and crying occur, accompanied initially by periods of normal behavior between paroxysms. Progression to vomiting (sometimes bilious or bloody), lethargy, and shock may occur. "Currant jelly" stools are observed in approximately 60% of cases.

The barium enema, the traditional diagnostic and therapeutic modality, has been replaced in many centers by ultrasound for diagnosis and fluoroscopy-guided reduction with hydrostatic or pneumatic pressure ("air enema"). Any method of reduction should always be performed with surgical back-up. Nonsurgical reduction should not be attempted if there is any evidence of shock or intestinal perforation (e.g., peritonitis).

(11) Barium enemas with air contrast can reveal mucosal abnormalities but overall are not very specific. Colonoscopy is more likely to yield a definitive cause for bloody stools and allows biopsy samples and cultures to be taken. Some practitioners use flexible sigmoidoscopy as a first study, even though the extent of the examination is limited. Barium enema may be indicated if an endoscopic examination was incomplete or a stricture or lesion limited the insertion of the scope.

(12) Fissures are a common cause of bright red streaks coating the stool. They can occur even in the absence of constipation. If the perianal region is erythematous, obtain a culture for group A *Streptococcus* to rule out a perianal cellulitis, which can predispose patients to fissures and bleeding. Hemorrhoids involving veins above the anorectal line may not be visible on examination.

(13) Familial adenomatous polyposis and Gardner syndrome are chronic polyposis syndromes that carry a risk of malignant transformation later in life. Peutz-Jeghers syndrome is characterized by diffuse intestinal hamartomas and hyperpigmented macules of the oral mucosa.

(14) Bloody diarrhea is a common manifestation of bacterial pathogens *(Yersinia, Salmonella, Shigella, Campylobacter)* and parasites (ameba). Colitis accompanied by anemia, thrombocytopenia, or renal insufficiency (consistent with hemolytic-uremic syndrome) should prompt a specific investigation for *Escherichia coli* serotype 0157:H7. Recent antibiotic use should raise suspicions for *Clostridium difficile*. Occult blood may occur with acute diarrhea due to any cause as a result of minor anal or perineal irritation.

(15) Milk protein allergy or milk intolerance typically presents as a history of bloody mucous stools and increasing stool frequency. Some infants will also have vomiting. The diagnosis may be delayed in breast-fed infants until the time they ingest formula. The family history is often positive. Some infants fed soy-based formula can develop an identical clinical picture. Breast-fed infants can develop allergic symptoms from cow's milk ingested by the mother.

(16) Most causes of upper and lower GI bleeding can manifest as occult bleeding. Careful history-taking may narrow the differential diagnosis and guide the appropriate workup. Current consensus is that significant blood loss due to whole cow's milk ingestion does not occur in the absence of colitis.

**GI BLEEDING
OLDER THAN 3 MONTHS
(continued)**

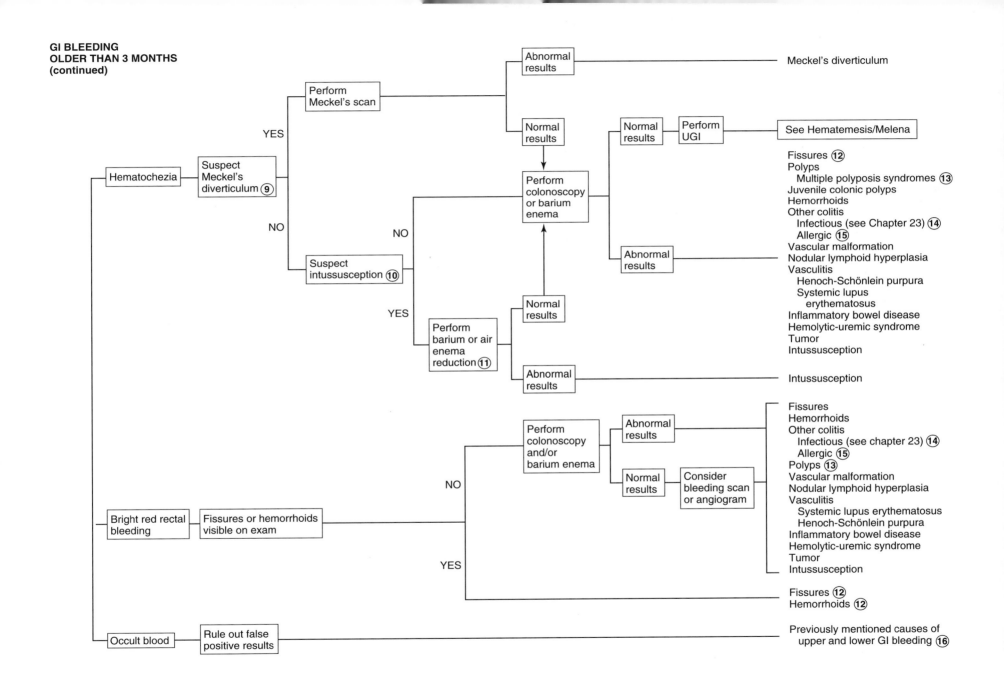

17 Although neonates are susceptible to most of the same problems as older age groups, some conditions tend to present almost exclusively in the neonatal period. Necrotizing enterocolitis should always be considered in the presence of prematurity. Hirschsprung disease typically occurs as an obstruction, but it may appear as an entero-colitis with bleeding. An unsuspected coagulopathy is more likely to occur in the newborn period than at older ages. Be aware of increased risk in breast-fed infants, especially those who did not receive vitamin K at birth.

18 A history of maternal mastitis or chapped, cracked nipples is suggestive of swallowed maternal blood. Definitive diagnosis can be made by an Apt-Downey test. The test is performed by diluting a sample of the grossly bloody (red) emesis with enough water to create a pink supernatant.

One part 0.25% N (1%) sodium hydroxide should then be added to 5 parts of the supernatant. If maternal hemoglobin is present, a yellow-brown color change will occur within a few minutes. If fetal hemoglobin is present, no color change occurs.

19 Pyloric stenosis presents classically between 3 and 6 weeks of age as nonbilious vomiting that rapidly progresses to frequent projectile vomiting often complicated by dehydration, weight loss, and metabolic alkalosis. The emesis may develop a "coffee-ground" appearance and may test positive for blood. Ultrasound is the preferred diagnostic test.

20 In infants with a clinical presentation for milk allergy or intolerance, a trial of a casein or whey hydrolysate formula or elimination of cow's milk from a breast-feeding mother's diet may be therapeutic and eliminate the need for any further evaluation.

21 Infectious colitis is a rare cause of bleeding in neonates. Be aware of positive tests for *C. difficile* toxin; *C. difficile* may not be a pathogen in the newborn.

BIBLIOGRAPHY

Heitlinger LA, McClung HJ: Gastrointestinal hemorrhage. In Wyllie R, Hyams J (eds): Pediatric Gastrointestinal Disease: Pathophysiology, Diagnosis, Management, 2nd ed, p 64. Philadelphia: WB Saunders Company, 1999.

Mezoff AG, Preud'Homme DL: How serious is that GI bleed? Contemp Pediatr 11:60, 1994.

Stanley P: The child with life-threatening gastrointestinal hemorrhage. In Von Waldenburg Hilton S, Edwards D: Practical Pediatric Radiology, p.287. Philadelphia, WB Saunders Company, 1994.

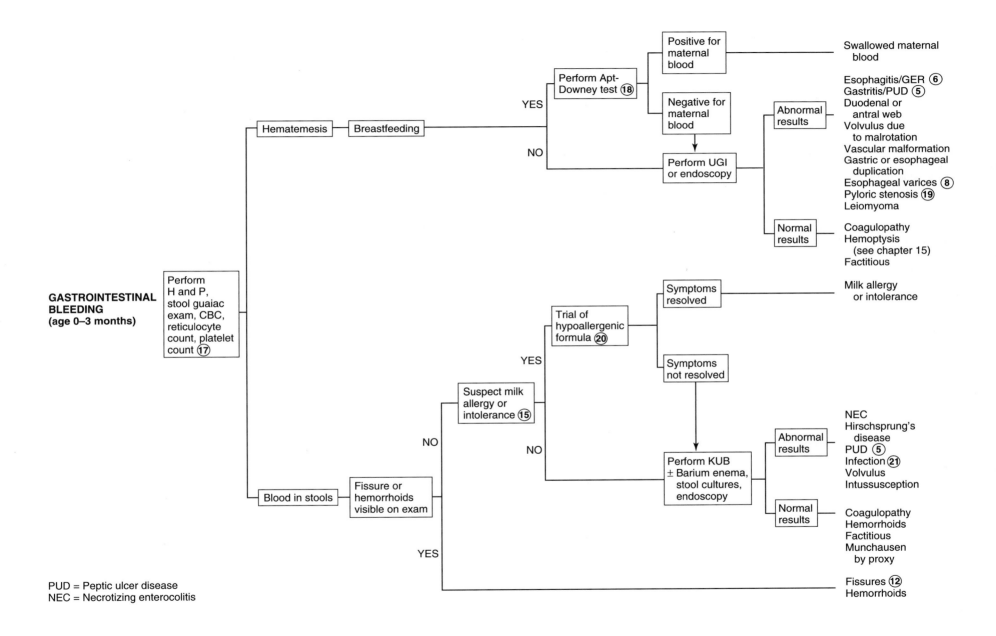

GASTROINTESTINAL BLEEDING (age 0–3 months)

Perform H and P, stool guaiac exam, CBC, reticulocyte count, platelet count ⑰

Hematemesis

Breastfeeding

YES → Perform Apt-Downey test ⑱

Positive for maternal blood → Swallowed maternal blood

Negative for maternal blood → Perform UGI or endoscopy

NO → Perform UGI or endoscopy

Abnormal results →
Esophagitis/GER ⑥
Gastritis/PUD ⑤
Duodenal or antral web
Volvulus due to malrotation
Vascular malformation
Gastric or esophageal duplication
Esophageal varices ⑧
Pyloric stenosis ⑲
Leiomyoma

Normal results →
Coagulopathy
Hemoptysis (see chapter 15)
Factitious

Blood in stools

Fissure or hemorrhoids visible on exam

NO → Suspect milk allergy or intolerance ⑮

YES → Trial of hypoallergenic formula ⑳

Symptoms resolved → Milk allergy or intolerance

Symptoms not resolved → Perform KUB ± Barium enema, stool cultures, endoscopy

NO → Perform KUB ± Barium enema, stool cultures, endoscopy

Abnormal results →
NEC
Hirschsprung's disease
PUD ⑤
Infection ㉑
Volvulus
Intussusception

Normal results →
Coagulopathy
Hemorrhoids
Factitious
Munchausen by proxy

YES →
Fissures ⑫
Hemorrhoids

PUD = Peptic ulcer disease
NEC = Necrotizing enterocolitis

Chapter 26 Jaundice

Jaundice is the yellow discoloration of skin, sclerae, and other tissues caused by the deposition of bilirubin. The degree of jaundice is related to the serum level of bilirubin and the degree of its deposition into the extravascular tissues. The most common source of bilirubin is the breakdown of hemoglobin.

In older infants jaundice should be distinguished from carotenemia, a diffuse yellowish-orange skin discoloration caused by ingestion of large amounts of carotene-containing foods (e.g., carrots, squash).

(1) Although most cases of neonatal jaundice are physiologic, a careful history and physical examination are necessary to rule out more serious disorders. The prenatal and birth history should inquire about delivery complications, maternal infection, diabetes mellitus, and drug use. Oxytocin during labor is associated with an increased risk of jaundice. A history of polyhydramnios suggests an intestinal obstruction. Other conditions resulting in a delayed passage of meconium (Hirschsprung disease, cystic fibrosis) will also contribute to hyperbilirubinemia. Prematurity is a risk factor for hyperbilirubinemia that is often compounded by delayed enteral feeds, parenteral nutrition, and perinatal insults due to hypoxia and acidosis. Vomiting, lethargy, poor feeding, and failure to thrive may suggest an inborn error of metabolism.

Breast-fed infants tend to have higher and more prolonged unconjugated bilirubin levels. A family history of jaundice, anemia, splenectomy, or cholecystectomy suggests a hereditary hemolytic disorder.

(2) Detailed investigation is warranted in children with conjugated hyperbilirubinemia, defined as a conjugated bilirubin level greater than 2.0 mg/dl or a conjugated fraction > 20% of the total bilirubin level. The evaluation should be directed at ruling out infection, metabolic disorders, anatomic abnormalities, and familial cholestatic syndromes.

(3) A congenital infection is suggested by intrauterine growth retardation, microcephaly, and ophthalmologic abnormalities (e.g., cataracts, chorioretinitis, posterior embryotoxon). Characteristic facies may suggest syndromes associated with hyperbilirubinemia.

(4) Nearly all newborns experience some rise in serum bilirubin levels owing to the relative immaturity of their hepatic excretory function. The algorithm lists clinical characteristics and bilirubin values consistent with this benign self-limited hyperbilirubinemia, as well as with breast-feeding jaundice, another benign condition.

(5) The frequent occurrence of hyperbilirubinemia and jaundice—approximately one third of all newborns develop jaundice—has resulted in the term *physiologic jaundice*. Levels higher than those used in the definition may occur (i.e., exaggerated physiologic jaundice), but some evaluation must be done to rule out more serious disorders before making the diagnosis. A well-accepted AAP practice parameter exists for the management of hyperbilirubinemia in the healthy term newborn (see Bibliography).

(6) Breast-fed infants have significantly higher bilirubin levels than formula-fed infants in the first 5 days of life. "Breast-feeding" jaundice describes jaundice occurring in the first week of life in a breast-fed infant and does not require additional workup when the total bilirubin level is < 15 mg/dl.

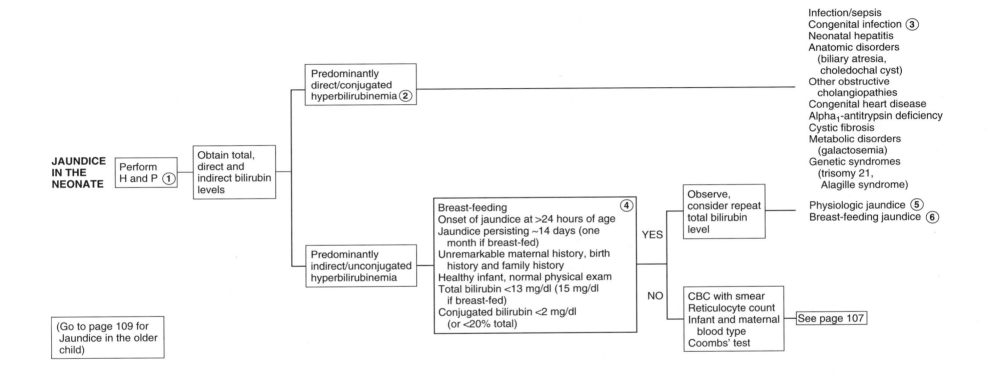

JAUNDICE IN THE NEONATE

Perform H and P ①

Obtain total, direct and indirect bilirubin levels

Predominantly direct/conjugated hyperbilirubinemia ②

Predominantly indirect/unconjugated hyperbilirubinemia

Breast-feeding ④
Onset of jaundice at >24 hours of age
Jaundice persisting ~14 days (one month if breast-fed)
Unremarkable maternal history, birth history and family history
Healthy infant, normal physical exam
Total bilirubin <13 mg/dl (15 mg/dl if breast-fed)
Conjugated bilirubin <2 mg/dl (or <20% total)

YES

NO

Observe, consider repeat total bilirubin level

CBC with smear
Reticulocyte count
Infant and maternal blood type
Coombs' test

Infection/sepsis
Congenital infection ③
Neonatal hepatitis
Anatomic disorders (biliary atresia, choledochal cyst)
Other obstructive cholangiopathies
Congenital heart disease
Alpha₁-antitrypsin deficiency
Cystic fibrosis
Metabolic disorders (galactosemia)
Genetic syndromes (trisomy 21, Alagille syndrome)

Physiologic jaundice ⑤
Breast-feeding jaundice ⑥

See page 107

(Go to page 109 for Jaundice in the older child)

Nelson chapters 98, 355
Practical Strategies chapter 24

Jaundice (continued)

(7) Isoimmune hemolytic disease occurs when maternal antibodies to the erythrocytes of the fetus cross the placenta and cause destruction of the fetal red blood cells. Incompatibility of the Rh factor causes the most severe disease in progressive pregnancies. ABO incompatibility causes less severe hemolysis. On occasion, infants in the latter group will demonstrate a negative or weakly positive direct Coombs test but the indirect Coombs will be positive.

(8) "Breast milk" jaundice is jaundice occurring after the first week of life. A healthy breast-fed infant with unconjugated hyperbilirubinemia, normal hemoglobin, normal reticulocyte count, normal blood smear, negative Coombs test, and no other abnormality on physical examination may be presumed to have breast-feeding jaundice or breast milk jaundice. Approximately one third of healthy breast-fed infants will have jaundice persisting beyond 2 weeks of age.

(9) Any condition causing obstruction or delayed passage of meconium (e.g., Hirschsprung disease, meconium plug syndrome) will increase enterohepatic circulation of bilirubin, contributing to indirect hyperbilirubinemia and jaundice.

(10) Prolonged indirect hyperbilirubinemia may be the earliest clinical manifestation of congenital hypothyroidism. Hypopituitarism is also a cause.

(11) Oxytocin, excess vitamin K in premature infants, some antibiotics, and phenol disinfectants are examples of drugs and toxins that may contribute to unconjugated hyperbilirubinemia.

(12) Red blood cell membrane defects include hereditary spherocytosis, hereditary elliptocytosis, infantile pyknocytosis, hereditary stomatocytosis, and hereditary pyropoikilocytosis.

(13) Review the medical history in the older child who presents with jaundice because certain illnesses are associated with specific liver complications. Examples include AIDS, cystic fibrosis, hemolytic disorders, hemoglobinopathies, and inflammatory bowel disease. Include a travel history, sexual activity, tattoos, drug and alcohol use, and potential exposure to a hepatitis outbreak.

A family history of jaundice, anemia, liver disease, splenectomy, or cholecystectomy suggests a hereditary disorder.

A small liver on examination is consistent with a chronic liver disorder (hepatitis or cirrhosis). A large tender liver suggests acute hepatitis or congestive heart failure. Splenomegaly occurs in hemolytic disorders and in some oncologic disorders.

Neurologic findings such as tremor, fine motor incoordination, clumsy gait, and choreiform movements suggest Wilson disease. Eye examination may reveal Kayser-Fleischer rings (Wilson disease) or posterior embryotoxon (Alagille syndrome).

A workup specifically for jaundice may not be necessary when an underlying diagnosis such as congestive heart failure or sepsis is evident.

(14) Autoimmune hemolytic anemias often demonstrate a direct or indirect positive Coombs test or rouleaux formation on the smear. *Mycoplasma pneumoniae*, Epstein-Barr virus, and lymphoproliferative disorders are associated with cold antibodies. Most cases of hemolytic anemia associated with warm antibodies are idiopathic. Other causes include lymphoproliferative disorders, systemic lupus erythematosus, or immunodeficiency.

(15) Mechanical damage causing fragmentation hemolysis may occur in systemic disorders such as disseminated intravascular coagulation, thrombotic thrombocytopenic purpura, or hemolytic-uremic syndrome. Extracorporeal membrane oxygenation, prosthetic heart valves, and burns may cause hemolysis by a mechanical mechanism.

NEONATAL JAUNDICE
(continued)

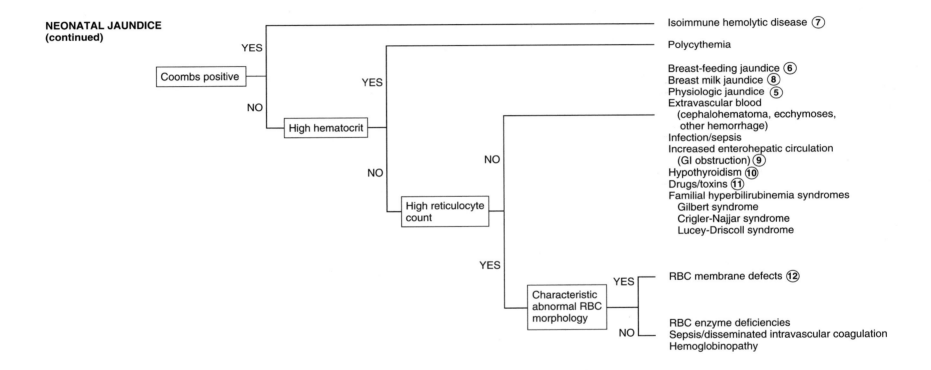

Isoimmune hemolytic disease ⑦

Polycythemia

Breast-feeding jaundice ⑥
Breast milk jaundice ⑧
Physiologic jaundice ⑤
Extravascular blood
    (cephalohematoma, ecchymoses,
    other hemorrhage)
Infection/sepsis
Increased enterohepatic circulation
    (GI obstruction) ⑨
Hypothyroidism ⑩
Drugs/toxins ⑪
Familial hyperbilirubinemia syndromes
    Gilbert syndrome
    Crigler-Najjar syndrome
    Lucey-Driscoll syndrome

RBC membrane defects ⑫

RBC enzyme deficiencies
Sepsis/disseminated intravascular coagulation
Hemoglobinopathy

16 Albumin levels reflect synthetic function of the liver and can aid in distinguishing an acute illness from a chronic liver disorder. The prothrombin time is the best test of liver function and can be abnormal in hepatocellular disorders or cholestatic disorders (malabsorption). In the latter category the prothrombin time will improve after a parenteral dose of vitamin K. Elevated γ-glutamyltransferase is specific for obstructive biliary tract disorders. Hypoglycemia reflects hepatocellular damage; it indicates more severe disease and mandates an urgent workup.

17 Wilson disease, an autosomal recessive disorder of copper metabolism, presents in the preadolescent or adolescent age group. It may present as acute liver disease, neurologic symptoms (e.g., dysarthria, clumsiness, tremor), or both. Kayser-Fleischer rings in the cornea reflect deposited copper and are pathognomonic. Diagnosis is by low serum ceruloplasmin level, high urinary copper excretion, and increased hepatic copper level on liver biopsy.

18 Some drugs that may cause hyperbilirubinemia in older children include antibiotics (erythromycin, tetracycline), anticonvulsants (valproate, phenytoin), acetaminophen, aspirin, alcohol, chlorpromazine, hormones (estrogens, androgens), isoniazid, pemoline, and antineoplastics. Children on total parenteral nutrition are also at risk.

19 Autoimmune hepatitis may occur acutely (malaise, anorexia, nausea, vomiting, jaundice) or with chronic liver disease. Other autoimmune problems (arthritis, thyroiditis, vasculitides, nephritis, diabetes mellitus, or inflammatory bowel disease) may be present. Laboratory evaluation reveals elevated transaminase levels, mild hyperbilirubinemia, hypergammaglobulinemia, and autoantibodies (e.g., antiactin, anti–liver-kidney microsomal, antisoluble liver antigen, antinuclear). Liver biopsy is needed for diagnosis.

BIBLIOGRAPHY

AAP Practice Parameter: Management of hyperbilirubinemia in the healthy term newborn. Pediatrics 94:558, 1994.

Gourley GR: Jaundice. In Wyllie R, Hyams J (eds): Pediatric Gastrointestinal Disease: Pathophysiology, Diagnosis, Management, 2nd ed, p 88. Philadelphia: WB Saunders Company, 1999.

JAUNDICE (continued)

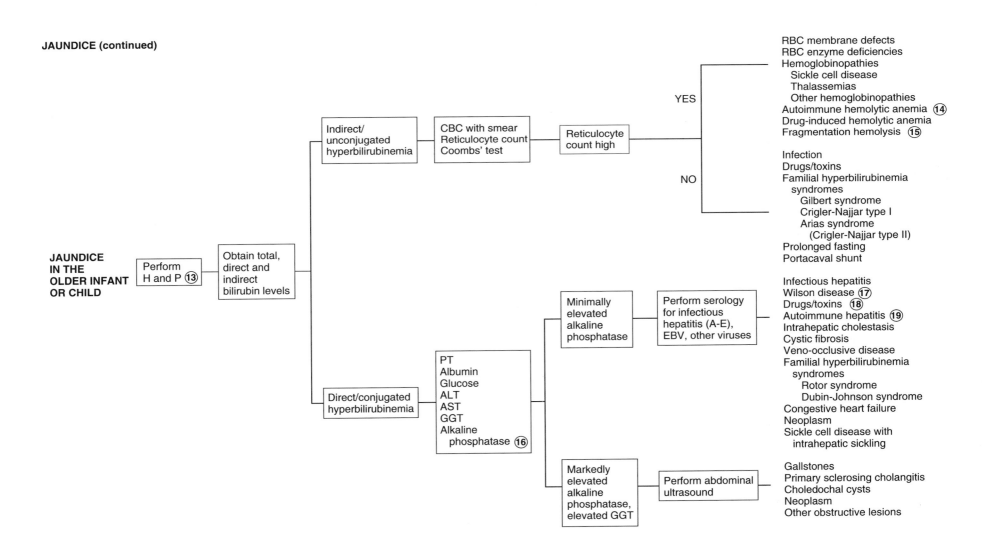

JAUNDICE IN THE OLDER INFANT OR CHILD

Perform H and P ⑬

Obtain total, direct and indirect bilirubin levels

Indirect/ unconjugated hyperbilirubinemia

CBC with smear
Reticulocyte count
Coombs' test

Reticulocyte count high

YES

RBC membrane defects
RBC enzyme deficiencies
Hemoglobinopathies
　Sickle cell disease
　Thalassemias
　Other hemoglobinopathies
Autoimmune hemolytic anemia ⑭
Drug-induced hemolytic anemia
Fragmentation hemolysis ⑮

NO

Infection
Drugs/toxins
Familial hyperbilirubinemia
　syndromes
　　Gilbert syndrome
　　Crigler-Najjar type I
　　Arias syndrome
　　　(Crigler-Najjar type II)
Prolonged fasting
Portacaval shunt

Direct/conjugated hyperbilirubinemia

PT
Albumin
Glucose
ALT
AST
GGT
Alkaline
　phosphatase ⑯

Minimally elevated alkaline phosphatase

Perform serology for infectious hepatitis (A-E), EBV, other viruses

Infectious hepatitis
Wilson disease ⑰
Drugs/toxins ⑱
Autoimmune hepatitis ⑲
Intrahepatic cholestasis
Cystic fibrosis
Veno-occlusive disease
Familial hyperbilirubinemia
　syndromes
　　Rotor syndrome
　　Dubin-Johnson syndrome
Congestive heart failure
Neoplasm
Sickle cell disease with
　intrahepatic sickling

Markedly elevated alkaline phosphatase, elevated GGT

Perform abdominal ultrasound

Gallstones
Primary sclerosing cholangitis
Choledochal cysts
Neoplasm
Other obstructive lesions

Chapter 27 *Hepatomegaly*

1 Inquire about a history of prolonged hyperbilirubinemia as well as underlying conditions that may contribute to liver disease including blood transfusions. Ask about episodic vomiting and associated neurologic changes. The social history should include sexual activity, medication and drug use, and exposure to possible hepatitis outbreaks or jaundiced persons. A family history of hepatic, neurologic, and psychiatric symptoms should be elicited, as well as a history of neonatal deaths.

The normal liver span varies by age, with the average span being 5 to 6.5 cm in healthy term infants, 6 to 7 cm in 1- to 5-year olds, 7 to 9 cm in 5- to 10-year olds, and 8 to 10 cm in 10- to 16-year olds. The span may be about 2 cm less if the lower border is determined by percussion rather than palpation. Cutaneous findings suggestive of liver disease include a prominent abdominal venous pattern, palmar erythema, and spider angiomas. Hepatomegaly is often associated with jaundice. (See Ch. 26 for additional diagnoses to consider.)

2 Elevated transaminase levels provide nonspecific information about hepatocellular injury. Liver function is better assessed by serum albumin and prothrombin time, because they rely on the synthetic function of the liver. Increased levels of alkaline phosphatase and γ-glutamyltransferase usually indicate cholestasis. An abdominal ultrasound will aid in determining whether hepatomegaly is present.

3 Liver involvement of varying severity may occur with multiple systemic disorders.

4 AIDS patients are prone to a variety of hepatobiliary disorders. Other infections that cause hepatosplenomegaly and anicteric hepatitis include cat-scratch disease, typhoid, brucellosis, tularemia, syphilis, Lyme disease, leptospirosis, Rocky Mountain spotted fever, Q fever, tuberculosis, and actinomycosis. Fitz-Hugh-Curtis syndrome is a perihepatitis associated with pelvic inflammatory disease due to *Neisseria gonorrhoeae* or *Chlamydia trachomatis.*

5 Metabolic storage disorders and peroxisomal disorders should be suspected in infants with hepatomegaly, hypotonia, and loss of developmental milestones. Liver biopsy, specific lymphocyte or urine assay, or bone marrow examination may be necessary to diagnose certain metabolic disorders. (See Ch. 22.)

6 Fulminant hepatic failure is the development of advanced liver disease in the absence of previous liver disease. The etiology includes infection, drug reactions, Reye's syndrome, and Wilson disease. Fulminant hepatic failure is unlikely in the absence of jaundice.

HEPATOMEGALY

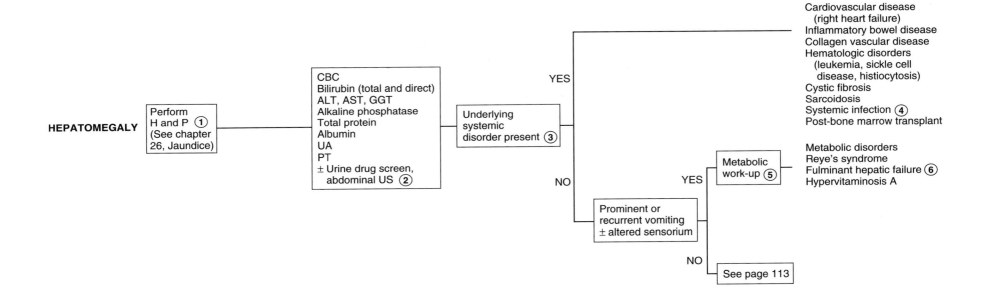

Perform H and P ① (See chapter 26, Jaundice)

CBC
Bilirubin (total and direct)
ALT, AST, GGT
Alkaline phosphatase
Total protein
Albumin
UA
PT
± Urine drug screen, abdominal US ②

Underlying systemic disorder present ③

YES

Cardiovascular disease (right heart failure)
Inflammatory bowel disease
Collagen vascular disease
Hematologic disorders (leukemia, sickle cell disease, histiocytosis)
Cystic fibrosis
Sarcoidosis
Systemic infection ④
Post-bone marrow transplant

NO

Prominent or recurrent vomiting ± altered sensorium

YES

Metabolic work-up ⑤

Metabolic disorders
Reye's syndrome
Fulminant hepatic failure ⑥
Hypervitaminosis A

NO

See page 113

Nelson chapters 81, 355
Practical Strategies chapter 22

PT= Prothrombin time

(7) Zellweger syndrome is the only disorder of peroxisomal metabolism associated with hepatomegaly. Diagnosis is typically made early in life owing to a characteristic phenotype, severe hypotonia, and hepatomegaly.

(8) Wilson disease is in the differential diagnosis of acute hepatitis in all children older than 5 years of age. Kayser-Fleischer rings and neurologic symptoms (e.g., tremor, choreiform movements) are suggestive. Diagnosis is by low serum ceruloplasmin levels, high urinary copper excretion, and increased hepatic copper levels on liver biopsy.

(9) Acute hepatitis may present as a mild or severe illness. Most cases resemble a mild flulike nonicteric illness with only tender hepatomegaly on examination. Mild splenomegaly may also occur. Consider serology for cytomegalovirus and Epstein-Barr virus when a high fever and adenopathy are present. Liver biopsy may occasionally be necessary to diagnose certain forms of chronic hepatitis.

(10) If an ultrasound does not result in a diagnosis, referral for more definitive testing (e.g., biopsy) may be necessary.

(11) A nonspecific fatty infiltration of the liver occurs in response to a variety of disorders (e.g., diabetes, cystic fibrosis, inflammatory bowel disease, metabolic disorders). Chemotherapy, other medication and toxins, malnutrition, and obesity are also risk factors.

(12) Ascites and tender hepatomegaly are common presenting symptoms of hepatic venous outflow obstruction. Serum transaminases and bilirubin levels are minimally affected acutely. Budd-Chiari syndrome is a noncardiogenic hepatic venous outflow obstruction occurring in conditions predisposing to thrombosis.

BIBLIOGRAPHY

Ross H, Hight DW, Weiss RG: Abdominal masses in pediatric patients. In Wyllie R, Hyams J (eds): Pediatric Gastrointestinal Disease: Pathophysiology, Diagnosis, Management, 2nd ed, p 126. Philadelphia: WB Saunders Company, 1999.

HEPATOMEGALY (continued)

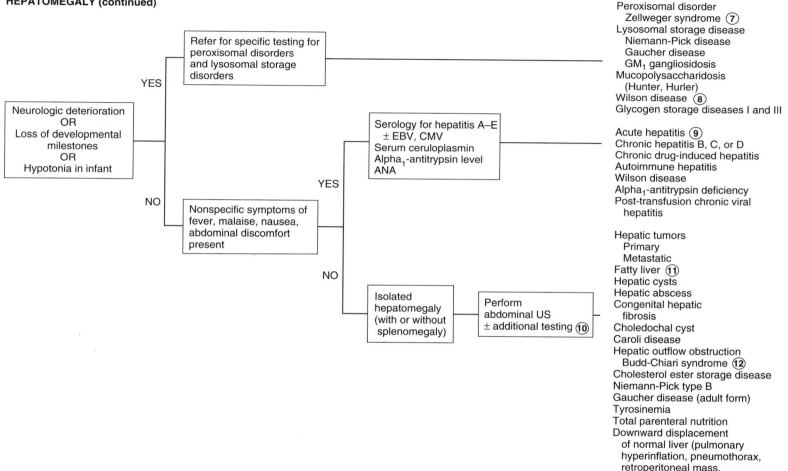

Neurologic deterioration
OR
Loss of developmental milestones
OR
Hypotonia in infant

YES

Refer for specific testing for peroxisomal disorders and lysosomal storage disorders

Peroxisomal disorder
  Zellweger syndrome (7)
Lysosomal storage disease
  Niemann-Pick disease
  Gaucher disease
  GM₁ gangliosidosis
Mucopolysaccharidosis
  (Hunter, Hurler)
Wilson disease (8)
Glycogen storage diseases I and III

NO

Nonspecific symptoms of fever, malaise, nausea, abdominal discomfort present

YES

Serology for hepatitis A–E
± EBV, CMV
Serum ceruloplasmin
Alpha₁-antitrypsin level
ANA

Acute hepatitis (9)
Chronic hepatitis B, C, or D
Chronic drug-induced hepatitis
Autoimmune hepatitis
Wilson disease
Alpha₁-antitrypsin deficiency
Post-transfusion chronic viral
  hepatitis

NO

Isolated hepatomegaly (with or without splenomegaly)

Perform abdominal US ± additional testing (10)

Hepatic tumors
  Primary
  Metastatic
Fatty liver (11)
Hepatic cysts
Hepatic abscess
Congenital hepatic
  fibrosis
Choledochal cyst
Caroli disease
Hepatic outflow obstruction
  Budd-Chiari syndrome (12)
Cholesterol ester storage disease
Niemann-Pick type B
Gaucher disease (adult form)
Tyrosinemia
Total parenteral nutrition
Downward displacement
  of normal liver (pulmonary
  hyperinflation, pneumothorax,
  retroperitoneal mass,
  subdiaphragmatic abscess)

Chapter 28 *Splenomegaly*

In children a palpable spleen may or may not be enlarged because the volume of the spleen may be relatively larger compared with the volume of the abdomen. As a child grows, the absolute and relative size of the spleen decreases. Up to 30% of newborns, 5% to 15% of children, and up to 3% of college freshmen have palpable spleens. A persistently palpable spleen may be normal, but some workup is necessary before making this conclusion. A careful history and physical examination will usually suggest the most likely diagnosis and guide the workup.

(1) A neonatal history of an umbilical catheter is a risk factor for portal vein thrombosis and subsequent venous obstruction. A history of surgery or blood transfusions may be a risk factor for certain bloodborne infections or thrombosis. Hepatic disease of any cause that results in portal hypertension can result in splenomegaly.

Certain ethnic backgrounds suggest a risk of certain disorders, mostly hemolytic or storage disorders. People of Mediterranean or South Asian descent are at risk for thalassemia and glucose-6-phosphate dehydrogenase (G6PD) deficiency. An African ethnicity is a risk factor for sickle cell disease and G6PD deficiency, and an Ashkenazi Jewish ancestry is a risk factor for certain storage disorders, including Gaucher disease. A family history of jaundice, anemia, cholecystectomy, or splenectomy is suggestive of a hemolytic disorder.

A review of systems positive for anemia, failure to thrive or weight loss, night sweats, lethargy, bruising, bony abnormalities, or respiratory symptoms may suggest an underlying systemic disorder. Sudden splenomegaly in a child with sickle cell disease suggests acute splenic sequestration, a life-threatening condition.

The abdominal examination should include attention to the liver and the possibility of ascites and other abdominal masses. Attention to the characteristic notch on the medial or inferior border of the spleen may help identify it, although other nodular masses may be present. Pain occurs secondary to stretching of the splenic capsule and may occur as left upper quadrant pain or referred pain to the left shoulder. Pain on palpation suggests the capsule has been stretched acutely, such as in an acute infection or hemolysis.

(2) Examples of other infections that may cause splenomegaly include spirochetal, rickettsial, parasitic, fungal, mycobacterial, and protozoal (i.e., malaria). Congenital infections (e.g., cytomegalovirus infection, herpes simplex virus infection, toxoplasmosis, rubella) also result in splenomegaly.

(3) Viral infection is the most common cause of splenomegaly in children. In the absence of hemolysis and other worrisome symptoms, a period of observation is acceptable, with additional workup recommended if the splenomegaly persists for 4 to 6 weeks. In the presence of a mononucleosis syndrome, identifying the cause may be reassuring to the physician or family but will not affect the management of the disorder.

(4) Splenomegaly may manifest in multiple collagen vascular disorders (e.g., juvenile rheumatoid arthritis, systemic lupus erythematosus).

SPLENOMEGALY

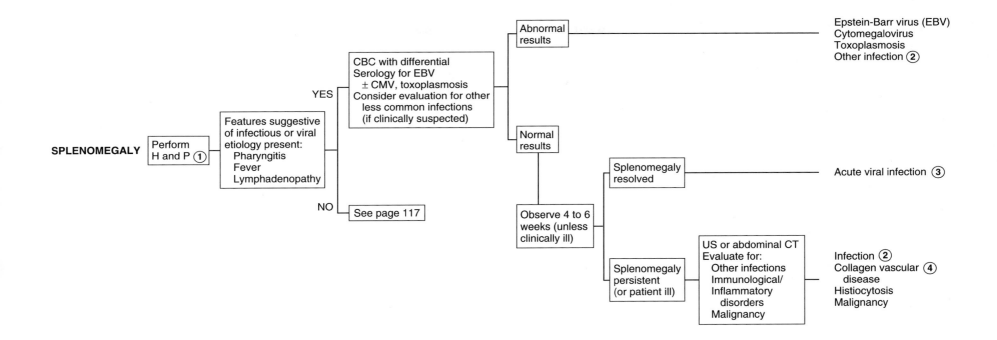

Perform H and P ①

Features suggestive of infectious or viral etiology present:
Pharyngitis
Fever
Lymphadenopathy

YES

CBC with differential
Serology for EBV
± CMV, toxoplasmosis
Consider evaluation for other less common infections (if clinically suspected)

NO

See page 117

Abnormal results

Epstein-Barr virus (EBV)
Cytomegalovirus
Toxoplasmosis
Other infection ②

Normal results

Observe 4 to 6 weeks (unless clinically ill)

Splenomegaly resolved

Acute viral infection ③

Splenomegaly persistent (or patient ill)

US or abdominal CT
Evaluate for:
Other infections
Immunological/
Inflammatory disorders
Malignancy

Infection ②
Collagen vascular ④ disease
Histiocytosis
Malignancy

Nelson chapters 463, 492
Practical Strategies chapter 23

Splenomegaly (continued)

5 A CBC, blood smear, and reticulocyte count may indicate hemolytic disease, chronic anemia, or leukemia.

In a child up to 3 years of age with a normal CBC, a spleen that is palpable 2 cm below the costal margin may be normal.

6 Mechanical damage causing fragmentation hemolysis may occur in systemic disorders such as disseminated intravascular coagulation, thrombotic thrombocytopenic purpura, and hemolytic-uremic syndrome. Extracorporeal membrane oxygenation, prosthetic heart valves, and burns may cause hemolysis by a similar mechanism.

7 Obstruction of venous drainage at a prehepatic or intrahepatic level or in the portal vein can cause a congestive splenomegaly. Congestive heart failure, Budd-Chiari syndrome, and hepatic disorders leading to cirrhosis are causes. Pancytopenia frequently results from excessive pooling (i.e., hypersplenism).

8 Storage disorders (e.g., Gaucher disease, glycogen storage disease, mucopolysaccharidosis) are usually diagnosed early in life with abnormal growth, skeletal abnormalities, and developmental delay.

9 Osteopetrosis refers to disorders of increased skeletal density. Hepatosplenomegaly occurs secondary to extramedullary hematopoiesis in severe forms, Milder variants of the disease may have only a mild anemia and no significant hepatosplenomegaly.

10 Pulmonary hyperinflation due to asthma, bronchiolitis, or a pneumothorax may cause splenic displacement.

BIBLIOGRAPHY

Ross H, Hight DW, Weiss RG: Abdominal masses in pediatric patients. In Wyllie R, Hyams J (eds): Pediatric Gastrointestinal Disease: Pathophysiology, Diagnosis, Management, 2nd ed, p 126. Philadelphia: WB Saunders Company, 1999.

SPLENOMEGALY (continued)

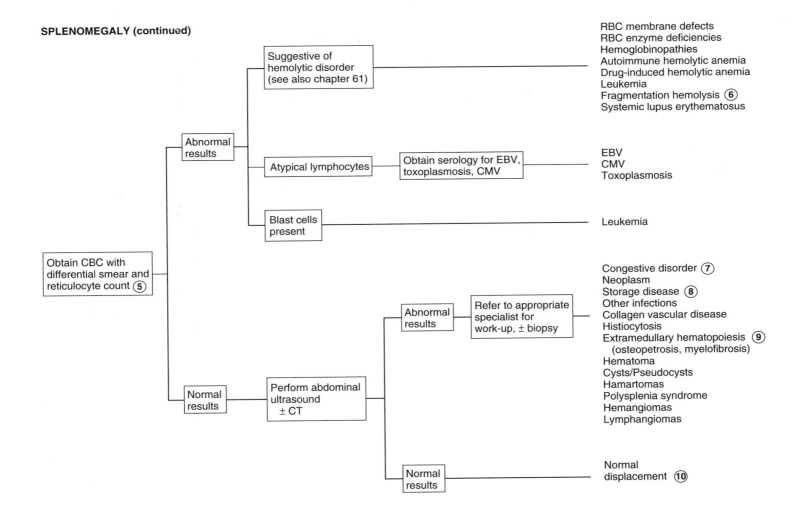

Obtain CBC with differential smear and reticulocyte count ⑤

Abnormal results

Suggestive of hemolytic disorder (see also chapter 61)
- RBC membrane defects
- RBC enzyme deficiencies
- Hemoglobinopathies
- Autoimmune hemolytic anemia
- Drug-induced hemolytic anemia
- Leukemia
- Fragmentation hemolysis ⑥
- Systemic lupus erythematosus

Atypical lymphocytes → Obtain serology for EBV, toxoplasmosis, CMV
- EBV
- CMV
- Toxoplasmosis

Blast cells present
- Leukemia

Normal results

Perform abdominal ultrasound ± CT

Abnormal results → Refer to appropriate specialist for work-up, ± biopsy
- Congestive disorder ⑦
- Neoplasm
- Storage disease ⑧
- Other infections
- Collagen vascular disease
- Histiocytosis
- Extramedullary hematopoiesis ⑨ (osteopetrosis, myelofibrosis)
- Hematoma
- Cysts/Pseudocysts
- Hamartomas
- Polysplenia syndrome
- Hemangiomas
- Lymphangiomas

Normal results
- Normal displacement ⑩

Chapter 29 *Abdominal Masses*

Abdominal masses represent a varied group of entities, many of which are age and gender specific. Because the abdominal cavity allows considerable room for growth, there may be few or nonspecific symptoms.

(1) For infants, a perinatal and birth history may reveal risk factors for certain disorders. Results of a prenatal ultrasound may provide a diagnosis before postnatal imaging. A thorough review of symptoms and social history, including a sexual history, recent travel, and infectious contacts, should be obtained.

The abdominal examination should note the location, size, shape, texture, mobility, and tenderness of the mass. The location will aid in determining which organ is most likely affected. Hepatosplenomegaly is the cause of more than half of childhood abdominal masses. A normal liver is nontender with a sharp edge and is palpated in the right upper quadrant 1 to 2 cm below the right costal margin. The normal spleen is usually nonpalpable, although it may be felt in the left upper quadrant with a round edge. The liver and spleen move with respirations. Renal masses usually extend downward from the kidney location, do not tend to cross the midline, and do not move with respiration.

Abdominal distention due to ascites must be distinguished from abdominal distention due to a mass. Ascites generally causes bulging flanks and dullness to percussion in the flanks. The fluid shifts with movement of the patient and causes a percussion wave or shifting dullness.

In males the external genitalia should be assessed, particularly for a left-sided varicocele, which may be associated with a Wilms tumor. In females with a lower abdominal mass, an assessment should be made to rule out an imperforate hymen.

Although imaging studies have the highest yield in the evaluation of abdominal masses, laboratory evaluation should be considered in certain cases. A urine pregnancy test should be obtained in all adolescent females with a lower abdominal mass. A CBC, serum electrolytes, serum amylase, and urinalysis may screen for other abdominal problems.

(2) An abdominal ultrasound is a safe, noninvasive method for determining whether a mass is cystic or solid. It is the preferred diagnostic test in neonates and may be appropriate in older children.

(3) Hydronephrosis is the most common cause of an abdominal mass in the neonate. It is due to obstruction of the urinary outflow tract. In male infants, posterior urethral valves are the most common cause of hydronephrosis.

(4) In infants, a history of polycythemia, dehydration, diabetic mother, asphyxia, sepsis, or coagulopathy are risk factors for renal vein thrombosis. Hematuria, hypertension, and thrombocytopenia are often present.

(5) Ovarian lesions may appear as a mass or pain due to torsion, adhesions, hemorrhage, or rupture. Some ovarian tumors occur as precocious puberty owing to the production of estrogen.

(6) The etiology of a hepatic mass includes tumors, hemangiomas, cysts, and abscesses. Adenoma, focal nodular hyperplasia, and hamartomas can occur as solitary lesions. Malignant hepatic tumors include hepatoblastoma and hepatocellular carcinoma.

BIBLIOGRAPHY

Ross H, Hight DW, Weiss RG: Abdominal masses in pediatric patients. In Wyllie R, Hyams J (eds): Pediatric Gastrointestinal Disease: Pathophysiology, Diagnosis, Management, 2nd ed, p 126. Philadelphia: WB Saunders Company, 1999.

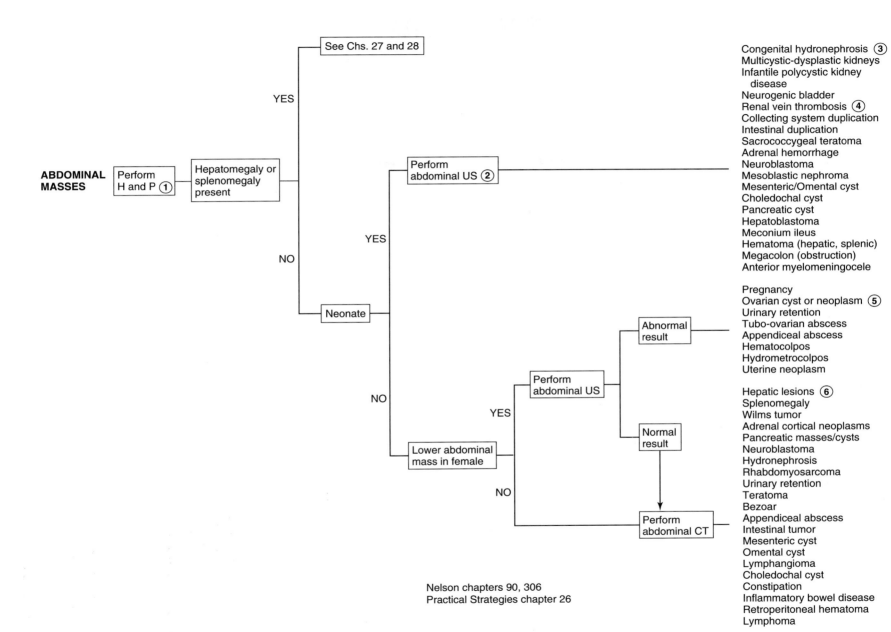

ABDOMINAL MASSES

Perform H and P ①

→ Hepatomegaly or splenomegaly present

YES → See Chs. 27 and 28

NO → Neonate

Neonate — **YES** → Perform abdominal US ②

Congenital hydronephrosis ③
Multicystic-dysplastic kidneys
Infantile polycystic kidney
 disease
Neurogenic bladder
Renal vein thrombosis ④
Collecting system duplication
Intestinal duplication
Sacrococcygeal teratoma
Adrenal hemorrhage
Neuroblastoma
Mesoblastic nephroma
Mesenteric/Omental cyst
Choledochal cyst
Pancreatic cyst
Hepatoblastoma
Meconium ileus
Hematoma (hepatic, splenic)
Megacolon (obstruction)
Anterior myelomeningocele

Neonate — **NO** → Lower abdominal mass in female

Lower abdominal mass in female — **YES** → Perform abdominal US

Perform abdominal US → Abnormal result

Pregnancy
Ovarian cyst or neoplasm ⑤
Urinary retention
Tubo-ovarian abscess
Appendiceal abscess
Hematocolpos
Hydrometrocolpos
Uterine neoplasm

Perform abdominal US → Normal result → Perform abdominal CT

Lower abdominal mass in female — **NO** → Perform abdominal CT

Hepatic lesions ⑥
Splenomegaly
Wilms tumor
Adrenal cortical neoplasms
Pancreatic masses/cysts
Neuroblastoma
Hydronephrosis
Rhabdomyosarcoma
Urinary retention
Teratoma
Bezoar
Appendiceal abscess
Intestinal tumor
Mesenteric cyst
Omental cyst
Lymphangioma
Choledochal cyst
Constipation
Inflammatory bowel disease
Retroperitoneal hematoma
Lymphoma

Nelson chapters 90, 306
Practical Strategies chapter 26

GENITOURINARY SYSTEM

Dysuria is burning or painful urination caused by urethral irritation. It is often associated with urinary symptoms such as frequency, urgency, incontinence, and refusal to void. Dysuria is not specific for urinary tract infections (UTIs) and often occurs in young children.

(1) Toddlers may present with delayed toilet training, secondary enuresis, dribbling, and frequent squatting. Constipation, not being circumcised, female gender, contraceptive diaphragms, and sexual intercourse may predispose to a UTI. Chemical irritants (e.g., detergents, bubble bath) and mechanical irritation (e.g., masturbation, foreign body) may cause dysuria. Dark or tea-colored urine may indicate hematuria. A history of penile or vaginal discharge as well as sexual abuse should be elicited.

Physical examination should include blood pressure, genitalia, abdominal palpation of the kidneys, pelvic when indicated, and neurologic in children with voiding dysfunction to exclude spinal cord pathology.

(2) Urine for urinalysis and culture must be properly obtained. Urinalysis, which includes microscopic examination and dipstick method, correlates with infection, particularly in an older child. Dipstick methods test for leukocyte esterase (an enzyme present in WBC) and nitrites. Microscopic analysis of unspun urine for WBC ($>10/mm^3$) or bacteria is more predictive than spun urine (>5 WBC/high power field). Red blood cells are common with a bacterial UTI. WBC casts, when present, are associated with upper tract infections. Urine culture remains the standard for diagnosis. Any growth in urine collected by suprapubic tap, $> 10,000$ to $50,000$ colonies by catheterization or $> 10^5$ colonies by clean catch, midstream urine indicate infection. "Bagged" specimens may have skin or fecal contaminants and are not recommended. *Escherichia coli* is the most common pathogen; others include *Proteus,*

Klebsiella, Staphylococcus saprophyticus, and enterococcus.

(3) In older children, pyelonephritis may be clinically differentiated from cystitis by the presence of systemic features (fever, vomiting) and signs (flank pain, costovertebral angle tenderness). In infants and young children the clinical picture may be nonspecific, with fever and other symptoms present in upper or lower tract disease. It may be confirmed by renal scan, the most sensitive being ^{99m}Tc-dimercaptosuccinic acid (DMSA). Renal ultrasound may show pyelonephritis but is not as sensitive. The occurrence of the first episode of UTI in a child younger than 3 to 5 years of age may be a marker for congenital anatomic abnormalities, in particular, vesicourethral reflux. Radiologic investigation with a renal ultrasound and voiding cystourethrogram (VCUG) is recommended. For males, a UTI at any age requires evaluation.

(4) The presence of leukocytes on urinalysis may indicate vaginitis due to sexually transmitted diseases (gonorrhea, *Chlamydia*, herpes simplex, *Trichomonas vaginalis*). They may also indicate *Candida albicans*, enteric pathogens, or group A streptococci. Urethritis is caused by *Neisseria gonorrhoeae, Chlamydia, Mycoplasma hominis,* and *Ureaplasma urealyticum.* (See Ch. 41.)

(5) Microscopic hematuria may be seen with UTI. Gross hematuria is seen with hemorrhagic cystitis (adenovirus, cyclophosphamide), renal calculi, and trauma and is rarely tumor related (clots from Wilms tumor). (See Ch. 32.)

(6) Meatal stenosis may occur for a number of reasons. In circumcised boys, it may result from recurrent meatal inflammation from moist diapers. Trauma, hypospadias repair, catheteriza-

tion, and balanitis xerotica obliterans are other causes. It most often appears as an abnormal urine stream, intermittent dysuria, and occasional bleeding. Phimosis is when the foreskin cannot be retracted due to scarring or narrowing of the preputial opening. It must be distinguished from physiologic phimosis when the foreskin has not completed the normal separation from the glans, usually by 3 to 5 years of age. Paraphimosis is the incarceration of the prepuce behind the glans, often after forcible retraction of the foreskin. Balanitis is an inflammation of the prepuce, which is usually due to urine but infection may be involved.

(7) Labial adhesions are common in prepubertal girls and are due to recurrent irritation, trauma, or infection of the hypoestrogenized epithelium of the labia minora. Urethral prolapse is an eversion of the urethral mucosa through the meatus. Bleeding and dysuria are common. Sexual abuse is usually associated with rectal or vaginal bleeding, vaginitis, and abdominal pain. Appropriate cultures should be obtained.

(8) Nonspecific urethritis is often seen in premenarchal girls and is associated with poor hygiene, tight "nonbreathing" clothes, and chemical irritants (bubble bath, harsh soaps). There may be erythema in the periurethral area. Anal pruritus may indicate pinworms, which can cause urethral irritation and can be confirmed by examination with a tape slide test.

BIBLIOGRAPHY

Brown MR, Cartwright PC, Snow BW: Common office problems in pediatric urology and gynecology. Pediatr Clin North Am 44:1091–1116, 1997.
Rushton HG: Urinary tract infections in children: Epidemiology, evaluation, and management. Pediatr Clin North Am 44:1133–1170, 1997.

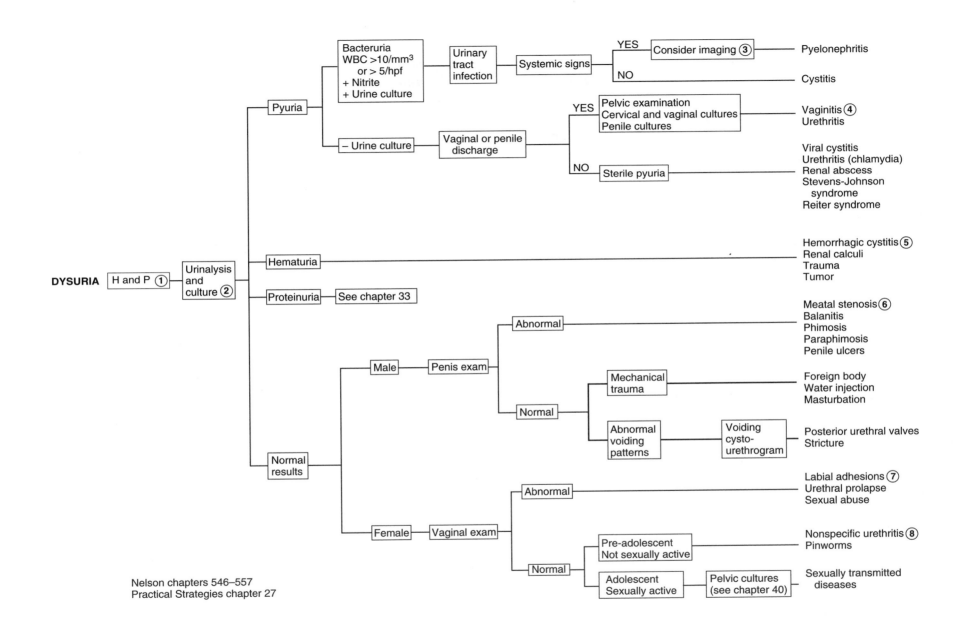

DYSURIA — H and P ①

Urinalysis and culture ②

Pyuria

Bacteruria
WBC >10/mm³
or > 5/hpf
+ Nitrite
+ Urine culture

→ Urinary tract infection → Systemic signs
- YES → Consider imaging ③ — Pyelonephritis
- NO — Cystitis

− Urine culture → Vaginal or penile discharge
- YES → Pelvic examination / Cervical and vaginal cultures / Penile cultures — Vaginitis ④ / Urethritis
- NO → Sterile pyuria — Viral cystitis / Urethritis (chlamydia) / Renal abscess / Stevens-Johnson syndrome / Reiter syndrome

Hematuria — Hemorrhagic cystitis ⑤ / Renal calculi / Trauma / Tumor

Proteinuria — See chapter 33

Normal results

Male → Penis exam
- Abnormal — Meatal stenosis ⑥ / Balanitis / Phimosis / Paraphimosis / Penile ulcers
- Normal
  - Mechanical trauma — Foreign body / Water injection / Masturbation
  - Abnormal voiding patterns → Voiding cysto-urethrogram — Posterior urethral valves / Stricture

Female → Vaginal exam
- Abnormal — Labial adhesions ⑦ / Urethral prolapse / Sexual abuse
- Normal
  - Pre-adolescent / Not sexually active — Nonspecific urethritis ⑧ / Pinworms
  - Adolescent / Sexually active → Pelvic cultures (see chapter 40) — Sexually transmitted diseases

Nelson chapters 546–557
Practical Strategies chapter 27

Enuresis is urinary incontinence at an age when most children are continent. Nocturnal enuresis, the most common form, is the involuntary passage of urine during sleep. Diurnal enuresis is the unintended leakage of urine, when awake, in a child old enough to maintain bladder control. *Primary enuresis* refers to a child who has never been continent at night and is older than 6 years old. *Secondary enuresis* refers to a child who was successfully toilet trained for at least 3 to 6 months and becomes incontinent once again. Most nocturnal enuresis is physiologic and occurs at least monthly in approximately 20% of 5-year olds and in 10% of 6-year olds.

(1) It is most important to distinguish between nocturnal enuresis, which is usually benign, and diurnal enuresis, which may have an organic cause. Urinary tract infection (UTI) is often associated with enuresis, as well as constipation and encopresis. The timing of the wetting should be determined. Children with urge syndrome may have "squatting," urinary frequency, and urgency and may also have symptoms of attention deficit hyperactivity disorder (ADHD). A history of holding urine until the last minute or enuresis associated with giggling, laughing, coughing, straining, or physical activity may indicate the cause. Polyuria and polydipsia may indicate diabetes mellitus or diabetes insipidus. Neurologic symptoms or signs, as well as midline abnormalities, may indicate an underlying neurologic disorder associated with a neurogenic bladder. In children with nocturnal enuresis, a history of snoring and mouth breathing may indicate sleep apnea.

Hypertension or growth failure may indicate chronic renal disease. A careful genitourinary examination should be done to look for meatal stenosis, labial fusion, or other abnormalities. In patients with urethral obstruction the bladder and kidneys may be enlarged.

(2) All children with enuresis should also have a complete urinalysis, with microscopic examination and culture when indicated. (See Ch. 30.)

Children with enuresis due to other causes may be predisposed to UTI. Red blood cells may be seen with urethral obstruction or hydronephrosis, and glucosuria may be due to diabetes mellitus. A first morning urine sample with a specific gravity ≥ 1.015 excludes diabetes insipidus.

(3) Ectopic ureter is a rare congenital anomaly. Incontinence occurs when the ureter is inserted distal to the external sphincter. It is more common in girls, and there is constant dripping of urine.

(4) In children who have leakage of urine after voiding, a careful examination may indicate labial fusion in which there is retention of urine behind the fused labia. In some girls, especially obese or preschool-aged girls who do not open the labia when voiding, there may be "reflux" of the urine into the vagina, which later leaks out. Some girls who have post-void dribble syndrome may feel a sense of wetness after voiding lasting for a few minutes, although there is no evidence of urine. This is believed to be due to detrusor "after contractions."

(5) Giggle incontinence is associated with laughing and is common in girls (up to 8%). The entire bladder empties, in contrast to stress incontinence in which a small amount of urine leaks due to increased intraabdominal pressure. Common causes of stress incontinence are coughing, straining, or physical activity. Another common cause of wetting is micturition deferral. It is common in preschool-aged children who are engrossed in activities. This may increase the risk for UTI as well.

(6) Urge syndrome (i.e., unstable bladder) is a common cause of daytime wetting in girls with ADHD. They may have daytime and nighttime wetting, frequency, and urgency, as well as squatting behavior, which is a characteristic symptom. The squatting is an attempt to suppress detrusor contractions, which can last more than a minute. UTI may be associated with this syndrome.

(7) Hinman syndrome should be considered in children with severe or persistent symptoms of urge syndrome, particularly with associated constipation, encopresis, or UTI. This is a severe manifestation of the same disease process. Imaging shows a trabeculated bladder, significant amount of residual urine after voiding, vesicourethral reflux, upper urinary tract dilation, and renal scarring.

(8) In children with incontinence associated with dysuria, frequency, urgency, and foul-smelling urine, the urinalysis and culture may indicate a UTI. (See Ch. 30.)

(9) Daytime frequency syndrome is more common in boys (mean age 5 years), and they present with sudden onset of urinary frequency. This may occur every 5 to 10 minutes and may be associated with incontinence.

(10) Neurogenic bladder may develop due to a lesion of the central or peripheral nervous system. A careful neurologic examination should be included, assessing strength, tone, sensation and reflexes of the lower extremities, and anal wink. The lumbosacral spine should be examined for hair tufts, dimples, masses, or other skin findings, which might reveal spinal dysraphism. The voiding cystourethrogram demonstrates a trabeculated bladder with a "Christmas tree" or "pine cone" appearance. MRI should be done to look for spinal cord abnormalities when the cause of the neurogenic bladder has not been determined.

(11) Urethral obstruction may appear as an abnormal urinary condition such as dribbling, poor stream, needing to push, or weak thin stream. It may be congenital (e.g., posterior urethral valves, stricture, urethral diverticula) or acquired, owing to development of a stricture due to infection (*Neisseria gonorrhoeae* urethritis) or trauma (traumatic catheterization, urethral foreign body).

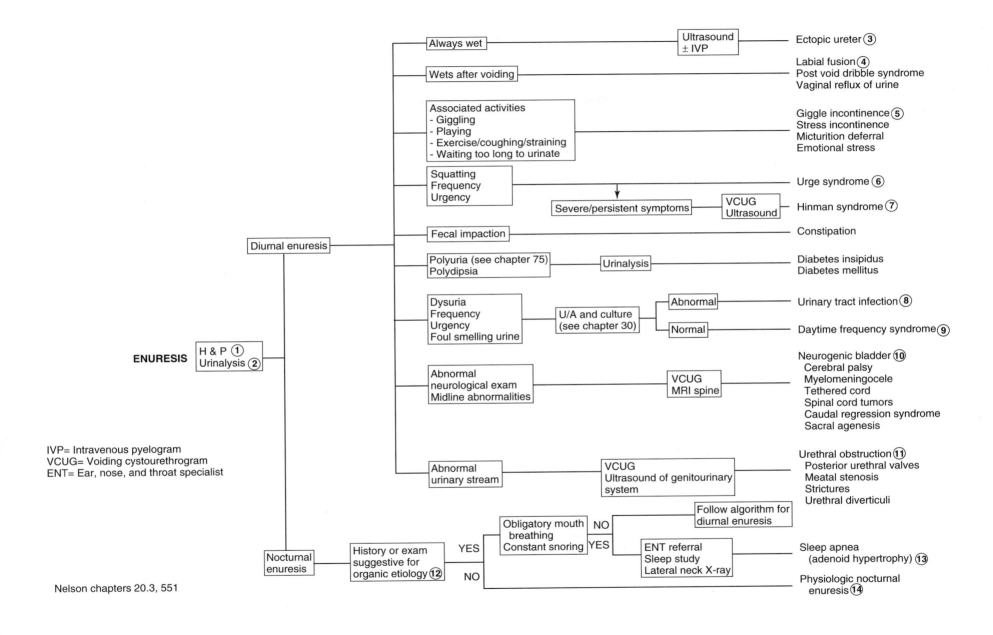

ENURESIS

H & P ①
Urinalysis ②

Diurnal enuresis

Always wet → Ultrasound ± IVP → Ectopic ureter ③

Wets after voiding → Labial fusion ④
Post void dribble syndrome
Vaginal reflux of urine

Associated activities
- Giggling
- Playing
- Exercise/coughing/straining
- Waiting too long to urinate
→ Giggle incontinence ⑤
Stress incontinence
Micturition deferral
Emotional stress

Squatting
Frequency
Urgency
→ Urge syndrome ⑥
→ Severe/persistent symptoms → VCUG Ultrasound → Hinman syndrome ⑦

Fecal impaction → Constipation

Polyuria (see chapter 75)
Polydipsia
→ Urinalysis → Diabetes insipidus
Diabetes mellitus

Dysuria
Frequency
Urgency
Foul smelling urine
→ U/A and culture (see chapter 30) → Abnormal → Urinary tract infection ⑧
→ Normal → Daytime frequency syndrome ⑨

Abnormal
neurological exam
Midline abnormalities
→ VCUG MRI spine → Neurogenic bladder ⑩
Cerebral palsy
Myelomeningocele
Tethered cord
Spinal cord tumors
Caudal regression syndrome
Sacral agenesis

Abnormal
urinary stream
→ VCUG Ultrasound of genitourinary system → Urethral obstruction ⑪
Posterior urethral valves
Meatal stenosis
Strictures
Urethral diverticuli

Nocturnal enuresis → History or exam suggestive for organic etiology ⑫

YES → Obligatory mouth breathing Constant snoring
NO → Follow algorithm for diurnal enuresis
YES → ENT referral Sleep study Lateral neck X-ray → Sleep apnea (adenoid hypertrophy) ⑬

NO → Physiologic nocturnal enuresis ⑭

IVP= Intravenous pyelogram
VCUG= Voiding cystourethrogram
ENT= Ear, nose, and throat specialist

Nelson chapters 20.3, 551

Enuresis *(continued)*

(12) Nocturnal enuresis is rarely due to an organic etiology. A history of dysuria, frequency, urgency, daytime enuresis, polydipsia, polyuria, CNS injury, constipation or encopresis, constant wetness, neurologic signs or symptoms, or abnormal urine stream may indicate an organic cause and prompt further evaluation, as in the case of diurnal enuresis.

(13) In children with sleep apnea, suggested by severe snoring and obligatory mouth breathing, wetting may occur during sleep apnea. Confirmation of the diagnosis is made by lateral neck X-ray and a sleep study. Referral to an ENT specialist should be considered.

(14) Physiologic nocturnal enuresis is a common problem. It is more common in boys and often shows a familial pattern.

BIBLIOGRAPHY

Robson WLM: Diurnal enuresis. Pediatr Rev 18:407–412, 1997.

Schmitt BD: Nocturnal enuresis. Pediatr Rev 18:183–190, 1997.

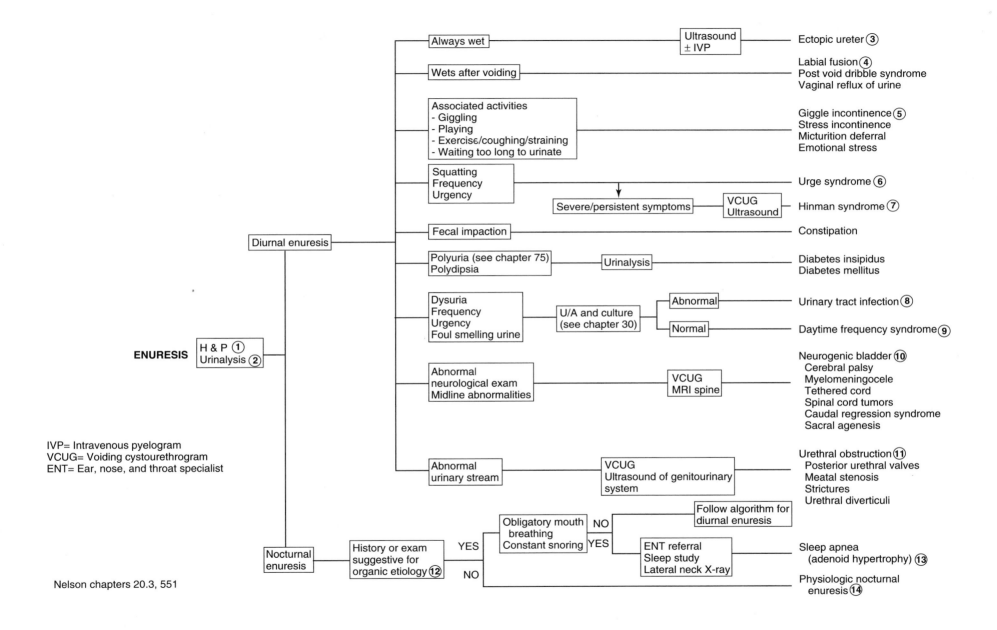

ENURESIS — H & P ①
Urinalysis ②

Diurnal enuresis

- Always wet — Ultrasound ± IVP — Ectopic ureter ③
- Wets after voiding — Labial fusion ④
  Post void dribble syndrome
  Vaginal reflux of urine
- Associated activities
  - Giggling
  - Playing
  - Exercise/coughing/straining
  - Waiting too long to urinate — Giggle incontinence ⑤
  Stress incontinence
  Micturition deferral
  Emotional stress
- Squatting
  Frequency
  Urgency — Urge syndrome ⑥
  → Severe/persistent symptoms — VCUG Ultrasound — Hinman syndrome ⑦
- Fecal impaction — Constipation
- Polyuria (see chapter 75)
  Polydipsia — Urinalysis — Diabetes insipidus
  Diabetes mellitus
- Dysuria
  Frequency
  Urgency
  Foul smelling urine — U/A and culture (see chapter 30) — Abnormal — Urinary tract infection ⑧
  — Normal — Daytime frequency syndrome ⑨
- Abnormal neurological exam
  Midline abnormalities — VCUG MRI spine — Neurogenic bladder ⑩
  Cerebral palsy
  Myelomeningocele
  Tethered cord
  Spinal cord tumors
  Caudal regression syndrome
  Sacral agenesis
- Abnormal urinary stream — VCUG Ultrasound of genitourinary system — Urethral obstruction ⑪
  Posterior urethral valves
  Meatal stenosis
  Strictures
  Urethral diverticuli

Nocturnal enuresis — History or exam suggestive for organic etiology ⑫
- YES — Obligatory mouth breathing / Constant snoring
  - NO — Follow algorithm for diurnal enuresis
  - YES — ENT referral / Sleep study / Lateral neck X-ray — Sleep apnea (adenoid hypertrophy) ⑬
- NO — Physiologic nocturnal enuresis ⑭

IVP= Intravenous pyelogram
VCUG= Voiding cystourethrogram
ENT= Ear, nose, and throat specialist

Nelson chapters 20.3, 551

Red or brown urine may indicate hematuria and possible renal disease. Hematuria is a common finding on urinalysis. Microscopic hematuria is defined as more than 5 red blood cells (RBCs)/high power field in the sediment of freshly voided urine. Gross hematuria is visible to the naked eye. The presence of RBCs in the urine must be confirmed because there are many conditions other than hematuria causing red or brown discoloration of the urine.

(1) History should include urinary symptoms such as dysuria, frequency, and urgency, as well as flank or abdominal pain. A history of exercise or trauma, including a foreign body, catheterization, or sexual/physical abuse, may indicate the cause of the hematuria. A medication, drug, and dietary history should be obtained. The history should include oliguria and hypertension, as well as systemic illnesses often associated with renal disease, such as arthritis and respiratory illness. Family history should include renal abnormalities, hematuria, deafness, renal failure, hypertension, nephrolithiasis, and renal transplant. Blood pressure must be obtained. Physical examination should focus on the genitourinary system and joints and on identifying any abdominal mass or a rash.

(2) A positive reagent strip (dipstick) in the absence of RBCs indicates the presence of hemoglobin or myoglobin. Hemoglobinuria occurs with hemolysis. It may occur in hemolytic anemias, hemolytic-uremic syndrome, mismatched transfusions, fresh water drowning, septicemia, and paroxysmal nocturnal hemoglobinuria. It is also associated with carbon monoxide, fava beans, venoms, mushrooms, naphthalene, quinine, and many other substances. A CBC with smear will often show fragmented cells, and the reticulocyte count may be elevated.

Myoglobinuria occurs with rhabdomyolysis after viral myositis and in children with inborn errors of energy metabolism often after exercise. The clinical picture as well as elevated muscle enzyme levels may aid in distinguishing myoglobinuria from hematuria. If needed, hemoglobin and myoglobin may be measured in the urine.

(3) Microscopic hematuria is often found on routine screening. If the child is asymptomatic, with normal blood pressure and no proteinuria, the urinalysis should be repeated at least two to three times over 2 to 3 months. If follow-up urinalysis is normal, a diagnosis of isolated asymptomatic hematuria is made. If proteinuria is present, the evaluation is the same as for gross hematuria (see algorithm). Loin-pain hematuria syndrome occurs as severe pain and microscopic hematuria and often with proteinuria.

(4) Gross hematuria can be localized to the upper or lower urinary tract. Upper tract bleeding causes brown, smoky, or tea-colored urine. Proteinuria (see Ch. 33) suggests glomerular involvement. Dysmorphic red blood cells due to passage through the glomerular basement membrane also indicate upper tract involvement. Lower tract bleeding is bright red, may have clots, rarely contains significant amounts of protein, and shows isomorphic red blood cell morphology.

(5) Symptomatic gross hematuria may be due to renal disease. Urinary tract infections commonly cause gross hematuria and can be diagnosed by using a positive urine culture when bacterial in origin. Hemorrhagic cystitis is often caused by adenovirus. Nephrolithiasis is associated with renal colic, positive family history, and urinalysis that may show crystals as well as hematuria. Premature infants who received furosemide may have nephrocalcinosis. Stones can be diagnosed by using intravenous pyelography, spiral CT, or ultrasound. X-rays may not detect radiolucent stones. Hypercalciuria, even without the presence of a stone, may cause abdominal or flank pain. Meatal stenosis with ulceration, trauma due to catheterization, and sexual abuse may cause hematuria. Abdominal and renal trauma are also causes and require abdominal CT scan with intravenous contrast medium enhancement. Injury to the bladder and posterior urethra may be associated with pelvic fractures and may be diagnosed by retrograde urethrography.

(6) Henoch-Schönlein purpura (HSP) may appear as abdominal pain, joint pain, and lower extremity rash (palpable purpura). In addition to hematuria, proteinuria may also be present. There is no specific laboratory test for HSP; however, serum IgA levels may be elevated. In tuberous sclerosis, hematuria may be due to associated renal cysts and angiomyolipomas. Systemic infections such as bacterial endocarditis and shunt infections may be associated with hematuria and proteinuria. Nephrotic syndrome may be associated with hematuria, particularly in focal segmental sclerosis and membranoproliferative glomerulonephritis.

(7) Asymptomatic hematuria with proteinuria suggests upper tract involvement. Acute postinfectious glomerulonephritis occurs 4 days to 3 weeks after a febrile illness with hematuria, oliguria, edema, and hypertension. Group A streptococcal infection causing either pharyngitis or impetigo is the most common cause. Laboratory findings include a decrease in C3 and C4 levels and laboratory evidence of a preceding group A streptococcal infection (Streptozyme, antistreptolysin, antihyaluronidase, anti–DNAse B titers). Hematuria from IgA nephropathy appears within 48 hours of an upper respiratory tract infection. Microscopic hematuria may be present between episodes. Alport syndrome is associated with a family history of renal disease, deafness, and hematuria. Tubulointerstitial nephritis is often associated with penicillins, cephalosporins, sulfonamides, rifampin, tetracyclines, nonsteroidal antiinflammatory drugs, furosemide, thiazides, heavy metals, and others. It may also be associated with other diseases, such as systemic lupus erythematosus.

(8) Idiopathic hypercalciuria most often occurs as persistent microscopic hematuria or as recurrent gross hematuria or dysuria. A calcium to creatinine ratio > 0.2 is suggestive. If this is pres-

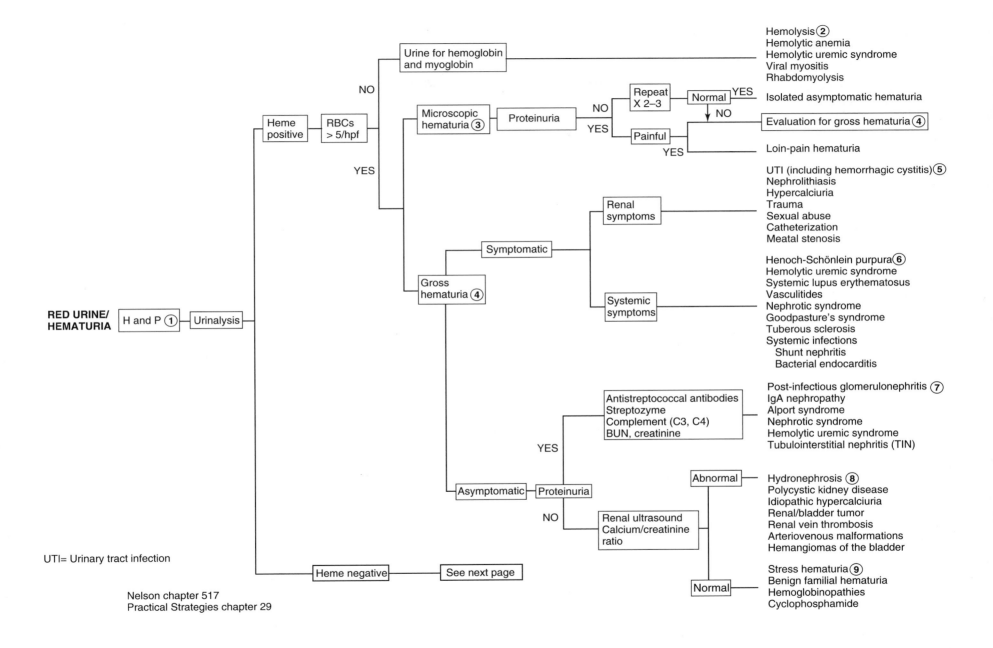

RED URINE/HEMATURIA — H and P ① — Urinalysis

Heme positive → RBCs > 5/hpf

- **NO** → Urine for hemoglobin and myoglobin →
  - Hemolysis ②
  - Hemolytic anemia
  - Hemolytic uremic syndrome
  - Viral myositis
  - Rhabdomyolysis

- **YES** →
  - **Microscopic hematuria** ③ → Proteinuria
    - **NO** → Repeat X 2–3
      - Normal → **YES** → Isolated asymptomatic hematuria
      - Normal → **NO** ↓ → Evaluation for gross hematuria ④
    - **YES** → Painful
      - → Evaluation for gross hematuria ④
      - **YES** → Loin-pain hematuria
  - **Gross hematuria** ④
    - **Symptomatic**
      - **Renal symptoms** →
        - UTI (including hemorrhagic cystitis) ⑤
        - Nephrolithiasis
        - Hypercalciuria
        - Trauma
        - Sexual abuse
        - Catheterization
        - Meatal stenosis
      - **Systemic symptoms** →
        - Henoch-Schönlein purpura ⑥
        - Hemolytic uremic syndrome
        - Systemic lupus erythematosus
        - Vasculitides
        - Nephrotic syndrome
        - Goodpasture's syndrome
        - Tuberous sclerosis
        - Systemic infections
          - Shunt nephritis
          - Bacterial endocarditis
    - **Asymptomatic** → Proteinuria
      - **YES** → Antistreptococcal antibodies / Streptozyme / Complement (C3, C4) / BUN, creatinine →
        - Post-infectious glomerulonephritis ⑦
        - IgA nephropathy
        - Alport syndrome
        - Nephrotic syndrome
        - Hemolytic uremic syndrome
        - Tubulointerstitial nephritis (TIN)
      - **NO** → Renal ultrasound / Calcium/creatinine ratio
        - **Abnormal** →
          - Hydronephrosis ⑧
          - Polycystic kidney disease
          - Idiopathic hypercalciuria
          - Renal/bladder tumor
          - Renal vein thrombosis
          - Arteriovenous malformations
          - Hemangiomas of the bladder
        - **Normal** →
          - Stress hematuria ⑨
          - Benign familial hematuria
          - Hemoglobinopathies
          - Cyclophosphamide

Heme negative → See next page

UTI= Urinary tract infection

Nelson chapter 517
Practical Strategies chapter 29

ent, a 24-hour urine collection for calcium should be obtained. Autosomal dominant polycystic kidney disease often appears as gross hematuria. Symptoms may begin in childhood but more often occur in adulthood. Renal and bladder tumors may rarely occur as hematuria. Arteriovenous malformations of the kidney may present as gross hematuria because of rapid transit of blood down the ureter; localization of bleeding may require cystoscopy or angiography.

(9) Stress hematuria occurs after exercise. It is painless and of short duration; there is no proteinuria. Patients with benign familial hematuria have an excellent prognosis but must be followed. An autosomal dominant inheritance has been proposed. Some patients have thinning of the glomerular basement membrane on electron microscopy.

BIBLIOGRAPHY

Feld LG, Waz WR, Pérez LM, Joseph DB: Hematuria: An integrated medical and surgical approach. Pediatr Clin North Am 44:5, 1997.

RED URINE/HEMATURIA (continued)

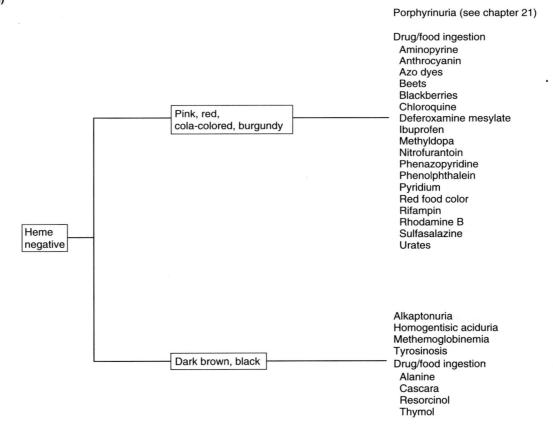

Porphyrinuria (see chapter 21)

Drug/food ingestion
  Aminopyrine
  Anthrocyanin
  Azo dyes
  Beets
  Blackberries
  Chloroquine
  Deferoxamine mesylate
  Ibuprofen
  Methyldopa
  Nitrofurantoin
  Phenazopyridine
  Phenolphthalein
  Pyridium
  Red food color
  Rifampin
  Rhodamine B
  Sulfasalazine
  Urates

Pink, red, cola-colored, burgundy

Heme negative

Alkaptonuria
Homogentisic aciduria
Methemoglobinemia
Tyrosinosis
Drug/food ingestion
  Alanine
  Cascara
  Resorcinol
  Thymol

Dark brown, black

Chapter 33 **Proteinuria**

Proteinuria is a common laboratory finding that is often a symptom of renal disease. It may also be found in normal, healthy children. It is therefore important to distinguish between pathologic and nonpathologic causes of proteinuria. As many as 10% of children will have 1+ proteinuria at some time. Because this is a transient finding in a majority of children, it is important to retest the urine before making a diagnosis.

Proteinuria may be defined qualitatively using a urine dipstick examination. Trace proteinuria is usually not significant; 1+ proteinuria (30 mg/dl) may be significant. This should be repeated and viewed in the context of the urine specific gravity. False-negative results may occur with urine that is too dilute (<1.005), and false-positive results may occur with overlong dipstick immersion, alkaline urine, pyuria, bacteriuria, mucoprotein and quaternary ammonium compounds, and detergents. Quantitative testing for proteinuria is done by a timed 12- to 24-hour urine collection for protein: $< 4 \text{ mg/m}^2\text{/hr}$ is normal; $4\text{–}40 \text{ mg/m}^2\text{/hr}$ is abnormal; and $> 40 \text{ mg/m}^2\text{/hr}$ is in the nephrotic range. An early morning spot testing of urine protein-to-creatinine ratio (in mg/dl) correlates well with 24-hour urine protein excretion. A value of > 0.2 is abnormal in children older than 2 years. This test is not valid in children with decreased muscle mass (i.e., those with nutritional problems).

(1) History should include questions about recent exercise, red or tea-colored urine, and respiratory or other febrile illness. History indicative of edema such as puffiness around the eyes on awakening, increased abdominal girth, and difficulty putting on shoes may indicate nephrotic syndrome and should be investigated. Family history related to renal disease, hematuria, or hypertension should be pursued. Systemic complaints (e.g., arthralgia, rash, fever) may be symptoms of diseases such as systemic lupus erythematosus (SLE) or Henoch-Schönlein purpura (HSP). On physical examination blood pressure must be evaluated as well as evidence of edema. Characteristic rashes may indicate the cause, for example, a malar rash in SLE or purpuric rash with HSP.

(2) Transient proteinuria may occur with fever, which usually resolves within 10 to 14 days of the illness; with strenuous exercise (abates within 48 hours); and with stress, cold exposure, and seizures.

(3) Children who have proteinuria on repeat urinalysis, especially those older than age 4 years, should be tested for orthostatic proteinuria. This is an increased protein excretion in the upright position only and is less common in younger children. It may account for as much as 60% of all proteinuria in children and has a benign clinical course. Testing may be done by ambulatory and recumbent dipstick testing for proteinuria or by quantitative assessment of proteinuria in ambulatory and recumbent urine specimens. The recumbent specimen should have $< 4 \text{ mg/m}^2\text{/hr}$ of protein. The amount in the ambulatory specimen may vary but is usually two to four times that of the recumbent specimen.

(4) In patients who have persistent asymptomatic proteinuria, further evaluation may proceed as in symptomatic patients. It is reasonable to refer even the patient with normal test results to a nephrologist because there are different opinions regarding the need for biopsy.

(5) Patients with proteinuria who are symptomatic (edema, hypertension) or have hematuria, associated systemic complaints (rash, fever, arthralgia), or a significant family history of glomerulonephritis or renal failure should have further evaluation. In most cases, referral to the nephrologist may be necessary. This evaluation includes assessment of renal function with BUN, creatinine, and electrolyte determinations. Nephrotic syndrome consists of proteinuria, hypoalbuminemia, edema, and hyperlipidemia. Total serum protein, albumin, as well as cholesterol and triglycerides are checked. Tests for antistreptococcal antibodies (antistreptolysin, antihyaluronidase, and anti–DNAase B) as well as complement levels (C3, C4) are done to exclude poststreptococcal glomerulonephritis. Antinuclear antibody testing may be considered, especially with hypertension or hematuria, to exclude SLE. Hepatitis B may also be associated with glomerulonephritis. A renal ultrasound should be considered to examine anatomy. A voiding cystourethrogram is indicated if there is a history of febrile urinary tract infections.

(6) Minimal change nephrotic syndrome is more common in boys and usually appears between ages 2 and 6 years. Urinalysis shows +3 to +4 proteinuria, and there may be microscopic hematuria. Renal function may be reduced; cholesterol and triglycerides are elevated; and serum albumin is decreased. The C3 level is normal.

(7) Nephrotic syndrome may develop with any type of glomerulonephritis, especially membranous, membranoproliferative, postinfectious, lupus, chronic infection, and HSP glomerulonephritis. With poststreptococcal glomerulonephritis, antistreptococcal antibody levels are elevated and complement (C3) is decreased. (See Ch. 32 for conditions causing hematuria with proteinuria.)

(8) Nephrotic syndromes may occur with extrarenal neoplasms such as carcinomas and lymphomas (Hodgkin disease).

(9) Drugs or chemicals, such as penicillamine, gold, mercury compounds, probenecid, ethosuximide, methimazole, lithium, phenytoin, and many others, may be associated with nephrotic syndrome.

10 Children younger than age 1 with nephrotic syndrome have a poor prognosis. Congenital nephrotic syndrome (Finnish type) is the most common cause. It is an autosomal recessive condition. It may occur as failure to thrive due to massive proteinuria. Nephrotic syndrome in infants may be occur secondary to infections, such as syphilis, toxoplasmosis, cytomegalovirus, rubella, hepatitis B, HIV, or malaria. Drugs, toxins (e.g., mercury), or SLE may also be causes. Syndromes associated with nephrotic syndrome in infants include nail patella syndrome, Lowe syndrome, congenital brain malformations, and Drash syndrome (Wilms tumor, nephropathy, and genital abnormalities).

BIBLIOGRAPHY

Ettenger RB: The evaluation of the child with proteinuria. Pediatr Ann 23:486–494, 1994.

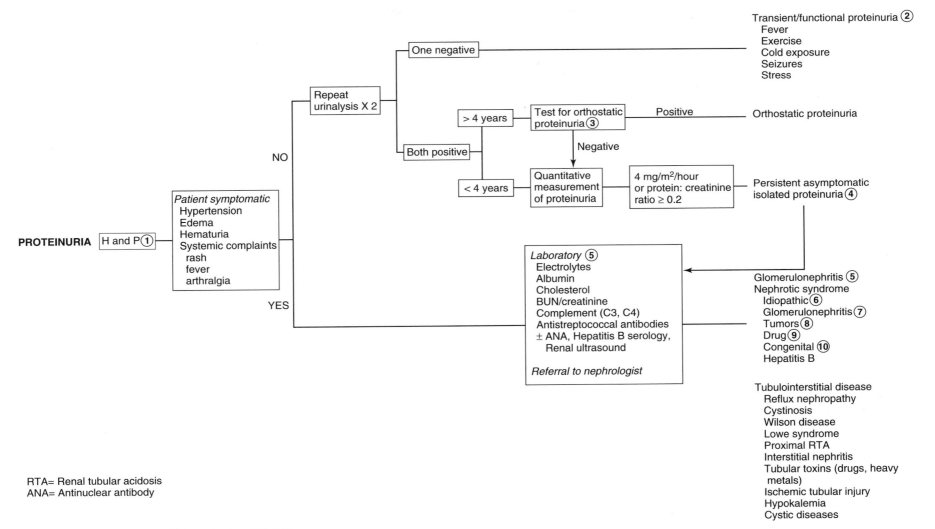

RTA= Renal tubular acidosis
ANA= Antinuclear antibody

Nelson chapters 531–535
Practical Strategies chapters 28, 29

Edema is the excess accumulation of interstitial fluid. It may occur as a result of increased capillary pressure (congestive heart failure [CHF]) or decreased plasma protein concentration. Decreased plasma protein may be due to increased losses (nephrotic syndrome, burns), decreased intake (malnutrition), or impaired lymphatic flow.

(1) The history and physical examination are very important in limiting the differential diagnosis to specific organ systems. Signs and symptoms specific to heart failure, liver failure, and renal disease should be obtained. History of burns and the presence of severe and extensive burns reveal the etiology.

(2) Angioedema is a form of urticaria affecting deeper tissue planes, including the skin and subcutaneous tissues. It often involves the lips, dorsum of the hands and feet, scalp, scrotum, and periorbital tissues. There are many causes, including foods, drugs, contactants (skin products), inhalants (pollen, dander), and infections. A history of recurrent angioedema may indicate episodic angioedema, which is associated with fever and eosinophilia. Hereditary angioedema, which results from a decreased synthesis of C1 esterase inhibitor, occurs as sudden attacks of edema often precipitated by minor trauma, strenuous exercise, or any stressors.

(3) Lymphedema is caused by the obstruction of lymphatic flow. Congenital lymphedema may occur in Turner syndrome, Noonan syndrome, and Milroy disease. Acquired obstruction may be due to tumors, lymphoma, filariasis, postirradiation fibrosis, and postinflammatory or postsurgical scarring. Injury to major lymphatic vessels may result in chylous ascites.

(4) Heart failure occurs when the heart cannot deliver adequate output to meet the metabolic needs of the body. Signs and symptoms include tachycardia, tachypnea, systemic venous congestion (hepatomegaly), and cardiomegaly. Other features may include feeding difficulties, excessive sweating, and failure to thrive in infants. Respiratory symptoms such as wheezing, rales, and cough may be present, owing to pulmonary congestion. Jugular venous distention or a gallop rhythm may be present. An older child may have orthopnea or may experience syncopal symptoms. Poor peripheral perfusion may result in cool extremities, prolonged capillary refill time, and weaker peripheral pulses as compared with central pulses.

(5) Features of hyperthyroidism include goiter and eye findings, including proptosis, exophthalmos, and lid lag. Symptoms due to increased catecholamines include palpitations, tachycardia, hypertension, tremor, and brisk reflexes. A hypermetabolic state results in increased sweating, heat intolerance, and weight loss despite an increased appetite. An associated myopathy may cause weakness, periodic paralysis, and heart failure.

(6) *Kasabach-Merritt* syndrome occurs in children with large cavernous hemangiomas of the trunk, extremities, or abdominal organs, where platelets are trapped in the vascular bed. Thrombocytopenia, a microangiopathic hemolytic anemia, and often a consumptive coagulopathy are present. The severe anemia may cause heart failure. Arteriovenous malformations may also be present within the anomalies, resulting in heart failure.

(7) Chest X-rays, electrocardiography, and echocardiography are useful in identification of an intrinsic cardiac defect. In congestive heart failure the chest X-ray shows cardiac enlargement; evidence of pulmonary edema may be present in severe heart failure. In cardiomyopathies there may be left or right ventricular ischemic changes on the electrocardiogram. In myocarditis and pericarditis there may be low-voltage QRS morphology with ST-T wave abnormalities. Electrocardiography is also useful in determining rhythm abnormalities. Echocardiography is most useful in assessing ventricular function as well as underlying structural causes of the heart failure.

(8) Congenital heart defects are the most common cause of heart failure in infants and children. Cyanotic lesions with CHF include hypoplastic heart syndromes, transposition of the great vessels, and truncus arteriosus. Ventricular septal defects and patent ductus arteriosus are more common causes of CHF.

(9) Cardiomyopathy may occur as a result of a number of diseases. Dilated cardiomyopathy is characterized by massive cardiomegaly and ventricular dilation. The cause is usually unknown (i.e., idiopathic dilated cardiomyopathy). Other causes include genetic (many X-linked), neuromuscular diseases (Friedreich ataxia, Duchenne muscular dystrophy), Kawasaki disease, autoimmune disease (rheumatoid arthritis, systemic lupus erythematosus), hyperthyroidism, and metabolic (mitochondrial disorders) and nutritional disease (beriberi, deficiency of selenium, taurine, and carnitine). Other causes include severe anemia, disorders of coronary arteries (anomalous origin of left coronary), and cardiotoxic drugs (doxorubicin, chronic ipecac abuse). Hypertrophic cardiomyopathy may be secondary to obstructive congenital heart disease, glycogen storage disease, or idiopathic hypertrophic cardiomyopathy. Restrictive cardiomyopathies result in poor ventricular compliance and inadequate ventricular filling; causes include Hurler syndrome and Loeffler hypereosinophilic syndrome.

(10) Viral myocarditis is most commonly caused by adenovirus and coxsackievirus B. It often results in acute or chronic heart failure. Other infectious causes include diphtheria, systemic bacterial infections (sepsis), and Rocky Mountain spotted fever. Parasites and fungal infections are rarely involved.

(11) Arteriovenous malformations may occur within the cranium, as well as in the liver, lungs, extremities, and thoracic wall. Heart failure is more likely with large intracranial arteriovenous fistulas (e.g., vein of Galen malformation) and hepatic malformations. They are less likely with pe-

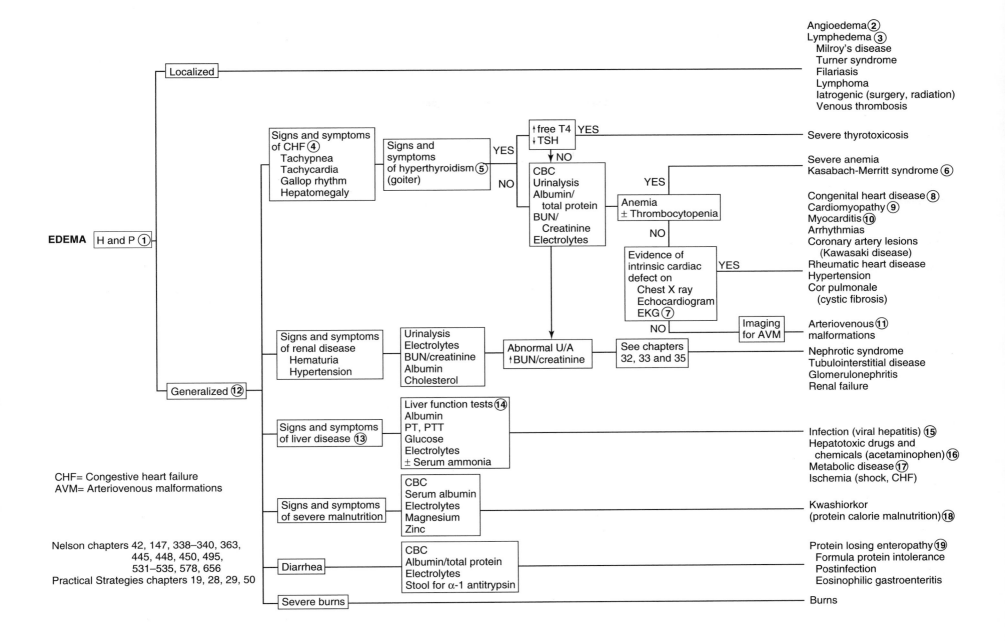

EDEMA | H and P ①

Localized
- Angioedema ②
- Lymphedema ③
  - Milroy's disease
  - Turner syndrome
  - Filariasis
  - Lymphoma
  - Iatrogenic (surgery, radiation)
  - Venous thrombosis

Generalized ⑫

Signs and symptoms of CHF ④
- Tachypnea
- Tachycardia
- Gallop rhythm
- Hepatomegaly

Signs and symptoms of hyperthyroidism (goiter) ⑤ — YES / NO

↑free T4 / ↓TSH — YES → Severe thyrotoxicosis
↓ NO

CBC / Urinalysis / Albumin/total protein / BUN/Creatinine / Electrolytes

Anemia ± Thrombocytopenia — YES → Severe anemia / Kasabach-Merritt syndrome ⑥
NO

Evidence of intrinsic cardiac defect on
- Chest X ray
- Echocardiogram
- EKG ⑦ — YES →
  - Congenital heart disease ⑧
  - Cardiomyopathy ⑨
  - Myocarditis ⑩
  - Arrhythmias
  - Coronary artery lesions (Kawasaki disease)
  - Rheumatic heart disease
  - Hypertension
  - Cor pulmonale (cystic fibrosis)
NO → Imaging for AVM → Arteriovenous ⑪ malformations

Abnormal U/A / ↑BUN/creatinine → See chapters 32, 33 and 35 →
- Nephrotic syndrome
- Tubulointerstitial disease
- Glomerulonephritis
- Renal failure

Signs and symptoms of renal disease
- Hematuria
- Hypertension

Urinalysis / Electrolytes / BUN/creatinine / Albumin / Cholesterol

Signs and symptoms of liver disease ⑬

Liver function tests ⑭ / Albumin / PT, PTT / Glucose / Electrolytes / ± Serum ammonia
- Infection (viral hepatitis) ⑮
- Hepatotoxic drugs and chemicals (acetaminophen) ⑯
- Metabolic disease ⑰
- Ischemia (shock, CHF)

Signs and symptoms of severe malnutrition

CBC / Serum albumin / Electrolytes / Magnesium / Zinc
- Kwashiorkor (protein calorie malnutrition) ⑱

Diarrhea

CBC / Albumin/total protein / Electrolytes / Stool for α-1 antitrypsin
- Protein losing enteropathy ⑲
- Formula protein intolerance
- Postinfection
- Eosinophilic gastroenteritis

Severe burns → Burns

CHF= Congestive heart failure
AVM= Arteriovenous malformations

Nelson chapters 42, 147, 338–340, 363, 445, 448, 450, 495, 531–535, 578, 656
Practical Strategies chapters 19, 28, 29, 50

ripheral arteriovenous fistulas. Physical examination may reveal a bruit, but definitive diagnosis is made by imaging, usually by MRI.

(12) For patients with no clinically obvious etiology, workup should begin by excluding cardiac and renal causes.

(13) Liver failure may be a complication of known liver disease or may be the presenting feature. Features include progressive jaundice, fetor hepaticus, fever, anorexia, vomiting, and abdominal pain. There may be a rapid decrease in liver size without clinical improvement, hemorrhagic diathesis, and ascites. Infants may present with irritability, lethargy, poor feeding, and sleep disturbances. Mental status changes are noted with progression of symptoms. Older children may demonstrate asterixis.

(14) In liver failure, hypoalbuminemia results in edema and bilirubin levels (direct and indirect) are elevated. Serum aminotransferase levels are elevated early but may decrease as the patient's condition deteriorates. Prothrombin time is prolonged and often does not correct with vitamin K administration. The serum ammonia level is usually elevated, and there may be hypoglycemia, hypokalemia, hyponatremia, metabolic acidosis, or respiratory alkalosis.

(15) Viral hepatitis is a common cause of liver failure. It is more likely in children with a combined infection with hepatitis B and D. Other viruses that cause infection may include Epstein-Barr virus, herpes simplex virus, adenovirus, enterovirus, parvovirus B19, and varicella-zoster virus.

(16) Known hepatotoxins include acetaminophen overdose, carbon tetrachloride, and *Amanita phalloides* mushrooms. Idiosyncratic damage may occur with halothane, phenytoin, carbamazepine, or sodium valproate.

(17) Metabolic disorders associated with liver failure include Wilson disease, galactosemia, hereditary tyrosinemia, hereditary fructose intolerance, and urea cycle defects.

(18) Kwashiorkor is a clinical syndrome resulting from severe protein deficiency and inadequate calorie intake (protein calorie malnutrition). Early in the disease, symptoms include anorexia, lethargy, apathy, and irritability. Later there is decreased growth, decreased stamina, muscle loss, increased susceptibility to infections, and edema. The edema may mask poor weight gain. Skin changes may be present, and the hair becomes coarse and discolored, resulting in streaky red or gray hair. Laboratory findings include decreased serum albumin, hypoglycemia, hypophosphatemia, and deficiency of potassium and magnesium. Anemia may be normocytic, microcytic, or macrocytic. Signs of vitamin (especially vitamin A) and mineral (zinc) deficiencies may be present.

(19) Protein-losing enteropathy may result in edema secondary to hypoalbuminemia. α_1-Antitrypsin, unlike albumin, is resistant to digestion. Measurement of levels in the stool is helpful in the diagnosis of protein-losing enteropathy. Causes include intolerance to protein in cow's milk or soy formula and postinfectious enteropathy. Eosinophilic gastroenteritis is another cause; it may be associated with dietary protein hypersensitivity as well as other food allergies. There is often eosinophilia and an elevated serum IgE.

BIBLIOGRAPHY

Hurwitz S (ed): Clinical Pediatric Dermatology, 2nd ed. Philadelphia: WB Saunders Company, 1993.

Gruskin AB: Pediatric nephrology. Pediatr Clin North Am 34(3), 1987.

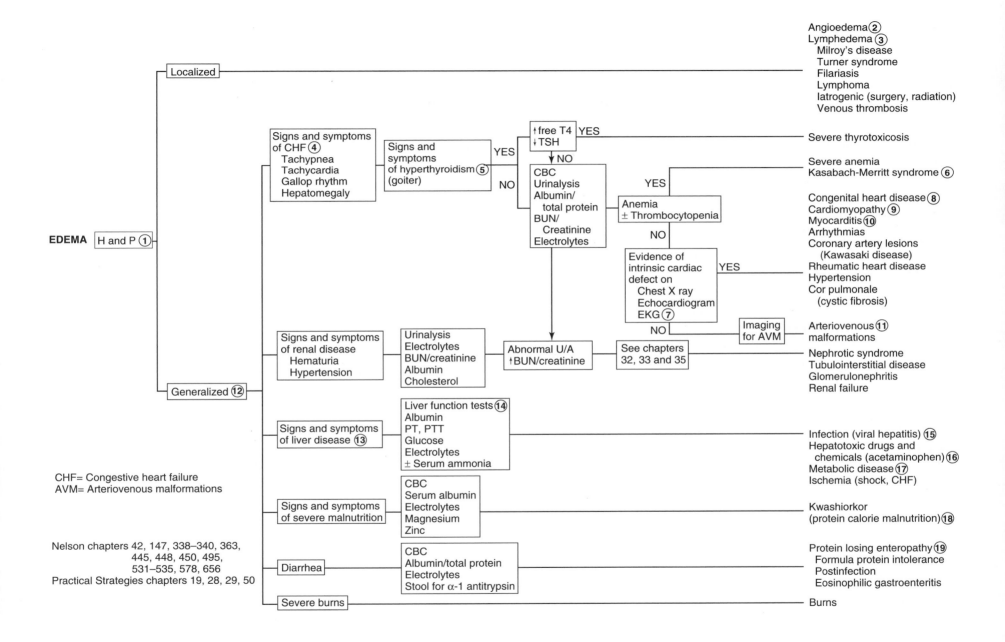

EDEMA H and P ①

Localized

Angioedema ②
Lymphedema ③
  Milroy's disease
  Turner syndrome
  Filariasis
  Lymphoma
  Iatrogenic (surgery, radiation)
  Venous thrombosis

Generalized ⑫

Signs and symptoms of CHF ④
  Tachypnea
  Tachycardia
  Gallop rhythm
  Hepatomegaly

Signs and symptoms of hyperthyroidism ⑤ (goiter)

YES

↑ free T4
↓ TSH   YES

Severe thyrotoxicosis

NO

CBC
Urinalysis
Albumin/
  total protein
BUN/
  Creatinine
Electrolytes

NO

YES

Anemia
± Thrombocytopenia

Severe anemia
Kasabach-Merritt syndrome ⑥

NO

Evidence of intrinsic cardiac defect on
  Chest X ray
  Echocardiogram
  EKG ⑦

YES

Congenital heart disease ⑧
Cardiomyopathy ⑨
Myocarditis ⑩
Arrhythmias
Coronary artery lesions
  (Kawasaki disease)
Rheumatic heart disease
Hypertension
Cor pulmonale
  (cystic fibrosis)

NO

Imaging for AVM

Arteriovenous ⑪
malformations

Signs and symptoms of renal disease
  Hematuria
  Hypertension

Urinalysis
Electrolytes
BUN/creatinine
Albumin
Cholesterol

Abnormal U/A
↑BUN/creatinine

See chapters 32, 33 and 35

Nephrotic syndrome
Tubulointerstitial disease
Glomerulonephritis
Renal failure

Signs and symptoms of liver disease ⑬

Liver function tests ⑭
Albumin
PT, PTT
Glucose
Electrolytes
± Serum ammonia

Infection (viral hepatitis) ⑮
Hepatotoxic drugs and
  chemicals (acetaminophen) ⑯
Metabolic disease ⑰
Ischemia (shock, CHF)

Signs and symptoms of severe malnutrition

CBC
Serum albumin
Electrolytes
Magnesium
Zinc

Kwashiorkor
(protein calorie malnutrition) ⑱

Diarrhea

CBC
Albumin/total protein
Electrolytes
Stool for α-1 antitrypsin

Protein losing enteropathy ⑲
  Formula protein intolerance
  Postinfection
  Eosinophilic gastroenteritis

Severe burns

Burns

CHF= Congestive heart failure
AVM= Arteriovenous malformations

Nelson chapters 42, 147, 338–340, 363,
           445, 448, 450, 495,
           531–535, 578, 656
Practical Strategies chapters 19, 28, 29, 50

Chapter 35 Hypertension

It is currently recommended that all children older than 3 years of age have routine blood pressure screening. It is important to use an appropriate-size cuff that measures 40% of the circumference of the arm or two thirds of the distance between shoulder and elbow. It is also important to use standardized methods of determining systolic (onset of Korotkoff sounds) and diastolic blood pressures (disappearance of sounds) on auscultation. Use of automated devices is acceptable in newborns and infants when auscultation may be difficult and in settings that require continuous monitoring, such as an intensive care unit.

Blood pressure measurement is complicated by the fact that there is wide fluctuation of blood pressure through the day, as well as with activity, stress, and other factors. New blood pressure tables that are adjusted for height should be used to assess for hypertension (see Bibliography). Normal blood pressure is when both systolic and diastolic pressures are less than the 90th percentile for age and sex. A high normal blood pressure is an average systolic or diastolic pressure between the 90th and 95th percentiles. Hypertension is an average systolic or diastolic blood pressure greater than the 95th percentile for age and sex, measured on at least three separate occasions. Although there are ethnic differences in blood pressure, they are not believed to be clinically relevant.

(1) History should include ingestion of medications and toxins, as well as tobacco use. Symptoms such as abdominal pain, dysuria, frequency, nocturia, enuresis, hematuria, and edema may indicate a renal cause. In infants, growth failure, irritability, and feeding problems may be symptoms of hypertension. Joint pain or swelling may be due to collagen vascular diseases. Weight loss, sweating, and pallor may be due to a catecholamine-secreting tumor. Muscle cramps or weakness and constipation may be seen with the hypokalemia associated with hyperaldosteronism. Menstrual disorders, hirsutism, and virilization may indicate forms of congenital adrenal hyperplasia (CAH) associated with hypertension. A neonatal history of umbilical artery line placement can result in renal artery embolization, leading to hypertension.

On physical examination, pallor and edema may indicate a renal cause. A careful skin examination should identify characteristic findings such as café-au-lait spots (neurofibromatosis); tubers, ash leaf spots (tuberous sclerosis); hirsutism (CAH); malar rash (lupus); and purpura (Henoch-Schönlein purpura). Retinal examination may show changes secondary to chronic hypertension. Thyromegaly may be found with hyperthyroidism. There may be a heart murmur with absent or decreased femoral pulses in aortic coarctation and tachyarrhythmias with pheochromocytomas. It is therefore important to always measure blood pressure in all four extremities. Signs of heart failure may be present with chronic or severe hypertension. Bruits may indicate aortic or renal arterial disease. Abdominal examination may identify enlarged kidneys. There may be neurologic deficits or Bell palsy with chronic hypertension. Stigmata of syndromes such as Cushing syndrome (buffalo hump, striae, moon face, truncal obesity, hirsutism), Turner syndrome (short stature, webbed neck, shield chest, low hairline), and William syndrome (elfin facies, poor growth, retardation) should be identified. A complete family history may be helpful in identifying primary or secondary (e.g., polycystic kidney disease) hypertension.

(2) Malignant hypertension is a marked elevation of blood pressure, which may be associated with retinal changes on funduscopy, congestive heart failure, or facial palsy. Hypertensive encephalopathy may occur as nausea, vomiting, altered mental status, visual disturbances, seizures, or stroke. The patient requires emergent diagnosis and management.

(3) Coarctation of the aorta may occur at any point from the arch to the bifurcation. It is more common in males but is also associated with Turner syndrome. The classic features include decreased or absent lower extremity pulses and lower extremity blood pressure less than upper extremity blood pressure; a short systolic murmur may be heard along the left sternal border, as well as an interscapular systolic murmur over the region of the coarctation.

(4) Secondary hypertension is due to an underlying disease process. Seventy-five to 80 percent of secondary hypertension in children is due to renal disease; therefore, initial workup is directed toward detection of renal problems. Urinary tract infections may be associated with an obstructive lesion. Hematuria and/or proteinuria may indicate an underlying renal disease. (See Chs. 32 and 33.) A CBC may reveal anemia, which is often associated with chronic renal disease or a microangiopathic hemolytic anemia associated with hemolytic-uremic syndrome. Determination of BUN and creatinine levels may provide evidence of chronicity of hypertension and renal involvement. Electrolytes may be helpful in the diagnosis of hyperaldosteronism (i.e., low potassium). Renal imaging may also be considered during initial evaluation; renal ultrasound is helpful in determining structural abnormalities; and renal scan may be of value in determining renal scars and ischemic areas secondary to renovascular disease.

(5) In young children with hypertension, renovascular disease is a common cause and further testing may be needed. Renal angiography is the standard. Other tests include captopril-enhanced radionuclide scans, digital subtraction angiography, and MR arteriography. Appropriate referral of children with renal or renovascular disease should be considered for further evaluation. Voiding cystourethrography is used in diagnosis of reflux nephropathy. Computed tomography or MRI is appropriate if a renal tumor is suggested.

(6) Liddle syndrome is an autosomal dominant condition characterized by hypertension and hypokalemia. Renin is suppressed, and aldosterone levels are low.

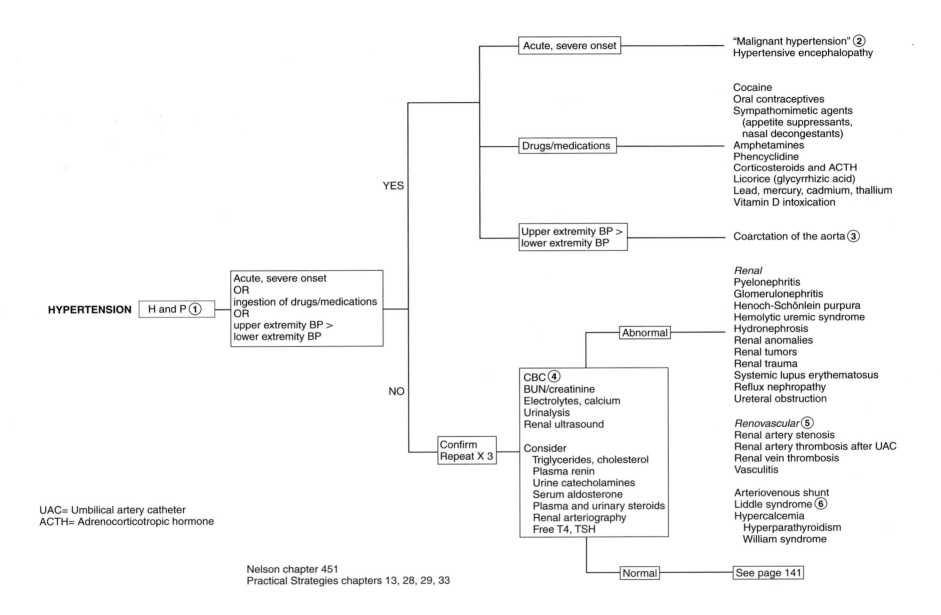

HYPERTENSION H and P ①

Acute, severe onset OR ingestion of drugs/medications OR upper extremity BP > lower extremity BP

YES

Acute, severe onset — "Malignant hypertension" ② Hypertensive encephalopathy

Drugs/medications —
Cocaine
Oral contraceptives
Sympathomimetic agents
   (appetite suppressants,
    nasal decongestants)
Amphetamines
Phencyclidine
Corticosteroids and ACTH
Licorice (glycyrrhizic acid)
Lead, mercury, cadmium, thallium
Vitamin D intoxication

Upper extremity BP > lower extremity BP — Coarctation of the aorta ③

NO

Confirm Repeat X 3

CBC ④
BUN/creatinine
Electrolytes, calcium
Urinalysis
Renal ultrasound

Consider
   Triglycerides, cholesterol
   Plasma renin
   Urine catecholamines
   Serum aldosterone
   Plasma and urinary steroids
   Renal arteriography
   Free T4, TSH

Abnormal —
Renal
Pyelonephritis
Glomerulonephritis
Henoch-Schönlein purpura
Hemolytic uremic syndrome
Hydronephrosis
Renal anomalies
Renal tumors
Renal trauma
Systemic lupus erythematosus
Reflux nephropathy
Ureteral obstruction

Renovascular ⑤
Renal artery stenosis
Renal artery thrombosis after UAC
Renal vein thrombosis
Vasculitis

Arteriovenous shunt
Liddle syndrome ⑥
Hypercalcemia
   Hyperparathyroidism
   William syndrome

Normal — See page 141

UAC= Umbilical artery catheter
ACTH= Adrenocorticotropic hormone

Nelson chapter 451
Practical Strategies chapters 13, 28, 29, 33

Hypertension *(continued)*

(7) Evaluation of hypertension should also include assessment of target organs. This includes funduscopic examination of the retina and echocardiography. Retinal examination may show arteriolar narrowing and arteriovenous nicking. Hemorrhages and exudates are more likely in adults. Echocardiography is used to detect left ventricular hypertrophy.

(8) In older children and adolescents with mild hypertension, normal screening laboratory tests, and no evidence of end organ damage, essential or primary hypertension may be considered. This is especially the case in children with a positive family history. A fasting lipid profile should be considered as part of the assessment, because elevated blood pressure in adults is known to accelerate the development of coronary artery disease.

(9) In children with features of Cushing syndrome, and a negative history of exogenous corticosteroids, further hormonal and imaging studies may be considered. In children with symptoms of hyperthyroidism and systolic hypertension, thyroxine and thyroid-stimulating hormone may be measured. Hypercalcemia, which may be associated with hyperparathyroidism, may cause hypertension.

CAH, due to 11β-hydroxylase deficiency, is characterized by virilization in females and hypertension. There is increased 11-deoxycortisol and 11-deoxycorticosterone (DOC). In 17α-hydroxylase deficiency, there is also increased DOC, leading to hypertension, hypokalemia, and suppression of renin and aldosterone. Affected males are unvirilized and may appear phenotypically female; affected females have failure of pubertal sexual development.

Low plasma renin activity and elevated aldosterone levels may indicate mineralocorticoid excess. It is important to note that random plasma renin activity, which is not profiled against urine sodium ("spot" or 24-hour urinary excretion), may not be specific or sensitive. Primary hyperaldosteronism is characterized by hypertension, hypokalemia, and suppressed plasma renin activity. Elevated plasma renin activity may indicate renovascular disease and should prompt renal referral for further evaluation.

Children with catecholamine-secreting tumors (pheochromocytoma) usually have sustained hypertension. If plasma or urine catecholamine levels are increased, imaging of the adrenal glands should be considered in diagnosis of pheochromocytoma. Neuroblastomas and ganglioneuromas may also produce catecholamines.

(10) Intermittent hypertension may be present in patients with autonomic instability (e.g., Guillain-Barré syndrome, burns, poliomyelitis, Stevens-Johnson syndrome, porphyria). There may be episodic increases in urinary catecholamine excretion.

(11) In children with history or physical examination indicating raised intracranial pressure (e.g., headache, vomiting, papilledema, neurologic changes), cranial imaging should be considered to rule out an intracranial mass. Other conditions associated with raised intracranial pressure are intracranial hemorrhage and brain injury.

BIBLIOGRAPHY

Bartosh SM, Aronson AJ: Childhood hypertension: An update on etiology, diagnosis and treatment. Pediatr Clin North Am 46:235–252, 1999.

Jung FF, Ingelfinger JR: Hypertension in childhood and adolescence. Pediatr Rev 14:169–179, 1993.

Sinaiko AR: Hypertension in children. N Engl J Med 335:1968–1973, 1996.

Task Force on Blood Pressure Control in Children: Report of the Second Task Force on Blood Pressure Control in Children—1987. Pediatrics 79:1–25, 1987.

Update on the Task Force (1987) on High Blood Pressure in Children and Adolescents: A working group from the National High Blood Pressure Education Program. Pediatrics 98:649–658, 1996.

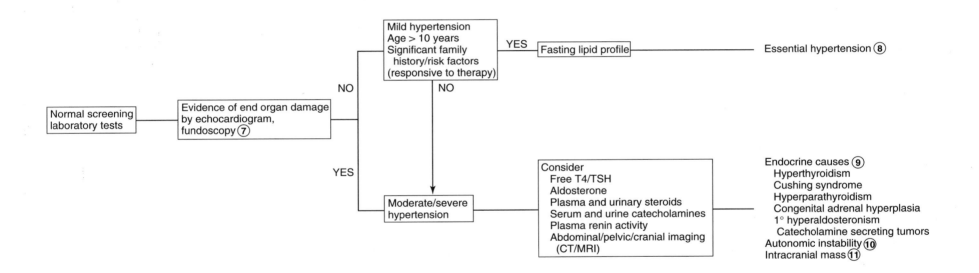

Chapter 36 Scrotal Pain

Painful scrotal swelling requires urgent evaluation to rule out conditions such as testicular torsion or incarcerated inguinal hernias, which require immediate surgical management.

(1) To determine the cause of the painful scrotum, the history should include the duration of pain (acute, chronic, or intermittent), radiation of pain to other areas, any other associated pain symptoms, and whether the pain is associated with exercise or trauma. Genitourinary (dysuria, frequency, hematuria, penile discharge), abdominal, and systemic symptoms may be helpful in diagnosis. Inquire about sexual activity, urinary tract infections, sexually transmitted diseases, and renal stones.

On examination, pubertal development should be assessed. Careful examination of the genitourinary area should include the inguinal canals and spermatic cord, testis and epididymis, and position of testis within the scrotum. Changes in the scrotal skin and presence or absence of the cremasteric reflex should be noted.

(2) Imaging studies are helpful in the diagnosis of painful scrotal swelling. The ^{99mc}Tc-pertechnetate testicular flow scan is used to differentiate ischemia, which appears as a "cold spot," from inflammation of the testis, which causes normal or increased uptake of the radionuclide dye. Color Doppler ultrasound allows differentiation of testicular blood flow from scrotal wall flow. In prepubertal boys Doppler signal may not be demonstrated, owing to small testicular size. Neither test is 100% accurate. Both require clinical correlation and depend on the skill of the radiologist.

(3) Testicular torsion is the cause in one third of cases of painful scrotum. It is a surgical emergency because of risk of gonadal loss. It usually occurs between the ages of 10 and 18 years and is most often associated with a predisposing anatomic abnormality ("bell-clapper" deformity). It also may be associated with trauma. It presents as sudden onset of pain, swelling, and tender enlargement of the testis, which may be high riding with an abnormal transverse lie. The cremasteric reflex is usually absent. There may be referred pain to the groin or abdomen and associated nausea or vomiting. In most cases history and physical examination can help to make the diagnosis. Imaging studies show reduced blood flow.

(4) Epididymitis is most common in sexually active adolescents and is due to retrograde spread of a urethral infection, most often due to *Chlamydia, Mycoplasma,* and *Neisseria gonorrhoeae.* In prepubertal boys, it is usually associated with a urinary tract infection secondary to a structural abnormality of the lower genitourinary tract and involves *Escherichia coli* and other gram-negative organisms. In addition to gradual onset of testicular pain, there may be symptoms of a urinary tract infection and urethral discharge. On examination there is scrotal edema, erythema, warmth, and tenderness. Cremasteric reflex is usually preserved, and there may be a reactive hydrocele. When the inflammation involves the testis it is known as epididymoorchitis. The Prehn sign, which is the relief of pain with elevation of the testis, may be suggestive of epididymitis or orchitis. Urinalysis often shows pyuria or bacteriuria. A urine culture should be obtained and Gram stain and culture of a urethral discharge. If diagnosis is not definitive, imaging may be used to show increased blood flow to the testis and rule out torsion.

(5) Torsion of the testicular appendix is most common between ages 7 and 12 years. There is gradual onset of testicular pain and swelling with a 3- to 5-mm, tender, indurated mass on the upper pole of the testis. If visible, this is the "blue dot" sign. Imaging may show increased flow due to hyperemia of the testis.

(6) Orchitis is rarely an isolated infection. It is usually associated with viral infection: mumps, coxsackievirus, varicella, or dengue.

(7) Incarcerated hernias occur as painful irreducible swellings in the groin or scrotum. Strangulation results from compromised vascular supply.

(8) Henoch-Schönlein purpura is a systemic vasculitis that may present as a purpuric rash or tense edema over the scrotum. There may be swelling and tenderness of the testis.

(9) Idiopathic fat necrosis involves acute painful swelling of the scrotum due to necrosis of intrascrotal fat, the etiology of which is unknown.

(10) Fournier gangrene of the scrotum occurs rarely in children and when present is usually associated with severe diaper rash, insect bites, circumcision, or perianal skin abscess. Organisms involved are *Staphylococcus aureus, Streptococcus, Bacteroides fragilis, Escherichia coli,* and *Clostridium welchii.* There is acute scrotal swelling with redness and tenderness, as well as systemic symptoms of fever, chills, and septicemia.

BIBLIOGRAPHY

Kass EJ, Lundak B: The acute scrotum. Pediatr Clin North Am 44:1251–1266, 1997.

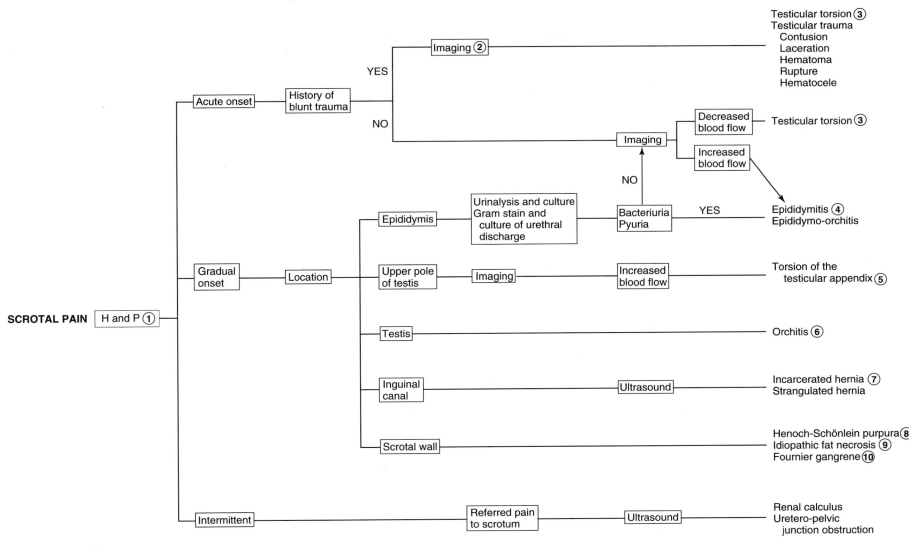

SCROTAL PAIN | H and P ①

- **Acute onset** → History of blunt trauma
  - **YES** → Imaging ② → Testicular torsion ③
    Testicular trauma
    - Contusion
    - Laceration
    - Hematoma
    - Rupture
    - Hematocele
  - **NO** → Imaging
    - Decreased blood flow → Testicular torsion ③
    - Increased blood flow → Epididymitis ④
      Epididymo-orchitis

- **Gradual onset** → Location
  - Epididymis → Urinalysis and culture, Gram stain and culture of urethral discharge → Bacteriuria Pyuria
    - **NO** → Imaging
    - **YES** → Epididymitis ④ / Epididymo-orchitis
  - Upper pole of testis → Imaging → Increased blood flow → Torsion of the testicular appendix ⑤
  - Testis → Orchitis ⑥
  - Inguinal canal → Ultrasound → Incarcerated hernia ⑦ / Strangulated hernia
  - Scrotal wall → Henoch-Schönlein purpura ⑧ / Idiopathic fat necrosis ⑨ / Fournier gangrene ⑩

- **Intermittent** → Referred pain to scrotum → Ultrasound → Renal calculus / Uretero-pelvic junction obstruction

Nelson chapter 553
Practical Strategies chapter 30

Chapter 37 **Scrotal Swelling (Painless)**

Hernias, hydroceles, varicoceles, and spermatoceles are the most common causes of painless scrotal swelling. A testicular mass may be malignant; therefore, the swelling should be carefully localized by examination and, if necessary, by ultrasound.

(1) Physical examination should be done with the patient in the upright and supine positions. Communicating hydroceles, hernias, and varicoceles are accentuated in the upright position and the Valsalva maneuver. Transillumination of the scrotum is used to distinguish solid from cystic lesions. When swelling cannot be adequately assessed on physical examination, or if the testis is not palpable within a cystic mass, an ultrasound evaluation is necessary.

(2) Acute idiopathic scrotal wall edema is a rare cause of acute scrotal swelling in boys between 4 and 7 years old. There may be minimal itching and a waddling gait. There is unilateral or bilateral scrotal wall edema; however, the testicles are not affected. The etiology is unknown but suspected to be allergic.

(3) Solid extratesticular masses may arise from the epididymis, spermatic cord, and scrotal wall. The most common benign lesion is spermatic cord lipoma. Fibromas, leiomyomas, lymphangiomas, adrenal rest tumors, and dermoid cysts are rare. Tumors of the epididymis are usually benign, the most common being the adenomatoid tumor. Paratesticular rhabdomyosarcoma is the most common paratesticular malignancy, with peak incidence between ages 2 and 5 years of age and early metastasis.

(4) Hernias and hydroceles are the most common scrotal/inguinal masses. Hernias are most common in premature infants and low-birthweight infants. A hydrocele is a smooth and nontender collection of fluid in the tunica vaginalis. Transillumination confirms the presence of fluid. Noncommunicating hydroceles are present in 1% to 2% of male neonates. Communicating hydroceles often persist. There is increasing scrotal swelling during the day, with decrease in size overnight. Hernias may be associated. Hydroceles may also be reactive secondary to torsion, epididymitis, or tumor. If the testis is abnormal on palpation or if it is not adequately palpated, ultrasound is needed to rule out an underlying condition. Hematoceles are filled with blood; they are rare and may indicate intraabdominal bleeding. Varicoceles are dilated, elongated veins of the pampiniform plexus, located posterosuperior to the testis, usually on the left side. They resemble a "bag of worms" and are most common in adolescents. They may cause hypotrophy of the testicle and impaired fertility. Spermatoceles and epididymal cysts occur in the rete testis, efferent ductule, or epididymis and contain sperm. On occasion, an ultrasound may be necessary for definitive diagnosis.

(5) Testicular tumors occur as a painless scrotal mass, with secondary hydrocele in 10% to 15%. Pain may occur with torsion or hemorrhage into the tumor. Germ cell tumors are most common. Tumor marker α-fetoprotein is elevated in 80% of yolk sac tumors, whereas β-human chorionic gonadotropin is elevated in teratocarcinomas. Gonadal stromal tumors may produce hormones causing signs and symptoms of precocious puberty and gynecomastia. Lymphomas and leukemia may metastasize to the testis.

(6) Testicular microlithiasis may rarely occur as testicular enlargement. This is diagnosed on ultrasound and may be associated with subsequent development of yolk sac tumors.

BIBLIOGRAPHY

Skoog SJ: Benign and malignant scrotal masses. Pediatr Clin North Am 44(5), 1997.

PAINLESS SCROTAL SWELLING

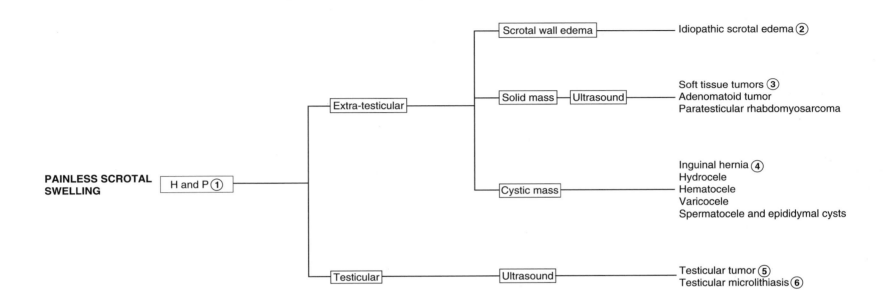

H and P ①

Extra-testicular

Scrotal wall edema —— Idiopathic scrotal edema ②

Solid mass — Ultrasound —— Soft tissue tumors ③
Adenomatoid tumor
Paratesticular rhabdomyosarcoma

Cystic mass —— Inguinal hernia ④
Hydrocele
Hematocele
Varicocele
Spermatocele and epididymal cysts

Testicular —— Ultrasound —— Testicular tumor ⑤
Testicular microlithiasis ⑥

Nelson chapter 553
Practical Strategies chapter 30

Chapter 38 **Dysmenorrhea**

Dysmenorrhea is defined as crampy lower abdominal or low back pain associated with menstruation. It is characterized into primary dysmenorrhea and secondary dysmenorrhea. An increased incidence has been noted in association with sexual abuse and inflammatory bowel disease.

(1) History should include onset of symptoms and whether dysmenorrhea started with menarche. Timing of pain during periods, history of sexual activity, and presence of vaginal discharge should be noted. It is important to obtain a history of disruption of daily activity and response to medications to determine the extent of investigation and treatment required. An abdominopelvic examination may reveal the cause in an older or sexually active adolescent. In a younger virginal adolescent, a rectoabdominal examination or ultrasound may be adequate. A rectal examination should also be done.

(2) Primary dysmenorrhea has no clinically detected pelvic pathology. It is due to uterine contractions caused by prostaglandins produced by the premenstrual secretory endometrium and occurs only with ovulatory cycles. It begins with the onset of the menstrual period and lasts from a few hours to days. Cramping may be associated with nausea, vomiting, diarrhea, and headache. The pelvic examination is normal.

(3) Secondary dysmenorrhea is associated with underlying pathology. New onset of symptoms in a sexually active teen may be due to a complication of pregnancy or pelvic inflammatory disease (PID). (For further discussion on cervicitis and PID, see Ch. 41.) If there is a positive pregnancy test finding, ultrasound evaluation may be needed to exclude an ectopic pregnancy or miscarriage.

(4) Onset of symptoms with menarche when cycles are usually anovulatory may be due to müllerian tract abnormalities with outflow obstruction. Pelvic examination, ultrasound, or laparoscopy may be needed to evaluate outlet obstruction. There may be partial obstruction of menstrual flow causing cyclic dysmenorrhea with accumulation of menstrual fluid resulting in hematocolpos, hematometra, or hematosalpinx depending on the level of the obstruction.

(5) Chronic pelvic pain that is worse during a period may be due to endometriosis and may be diagnosed using laparoscopy. Endometriosis is the presence of endometrial tissue outside the normal intrauterine cavity. Unlike in adults, in adolescents the pelvic examination may be normal or there may be minimal tenderness.

(6) Psychogenic dysmenorrhea may be related to negative sexual experiences, such as child abuse or rape.

BIBLIOGRAPHY
Braverman P, Polaneczky M: Adolescent gynecology: I. Common disorders. Pediatr Clin North Am 46(3), 1999.

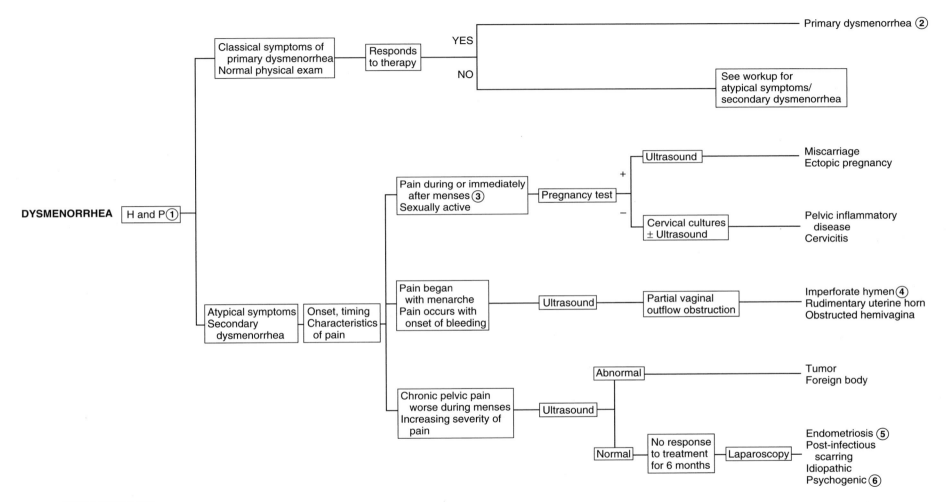

DYSMENORRHEA — H and P ①

- **Classical symptoms of primary dysmenorrhea / Normal physical exam** — Responds to therapy
  - **YES** → Primary dysmenorrhea ②
  - **NO** → See workup for atypical symptoms/ secondary dysmenorrhea

- **Atypical symptoms / Secondary dysmenorrhea** — Onset, timing / Characteristics of pain
  - **Pain during or immediately after menses ③ / Sexually active** — Pregnancy test
    - **+** → Ultrasound → Miscarriage / Ectopic pregnancy
    - **−** → Cervical cultures ± Ultrasound → Pelvic inflammatory disease / Cervicitis
  - **Pain began with menarche / Pain occurs with onset of bleeding** — Ultrasound → Partial vaginal outflow obstruction → Imperforate hymen ④ / Rudimentary uterine horn / Obstructed hemivagina
  - **Chronic pelvic pain worse during menses / Increasing severity of pain** — Ultrasound
    - **Abnormal** → Tumor / Foreign body
    - **Normal** → No response to treatment for 6 months → Laparoscopy → Endometriosis ⑤ / Post-infectious scarring / Idiopathic / Psychogenic ⑥

Nelson chapter 116
Practical Strategies chapter 32

Chapter 39 *Amenorrhea*

Amenorrhea is the absence of menstrual periods. Primary amenorrhea occurs when there is no menstrual period by age 16 years or no signs of puberty with no menses by age 13 years. Secondary amenorrhea occurs when a previously menstruating female has no menstrual bleeding for at least 3 to 6 months.

(1) History should include pubertal development and menstrual patterns in secondary amenorrhea. Pregnancy is the first consideration in an adolescent with secondary amenorrhea, rarely in primary amenorrhea. Information on sexual history including sexual abuse and use of hormonal contraceptives should be carefully elicited. Obtaining a history of weight change, anorexia, stress, athletic participation, and nutrition is important to the diagnosis of amenorrhea. History should also include chronic illness, infections, medications, and substance abuse. Family history should include gynecologic problems and mother's age at the onset of puberty and menses. On physical examination, it is important to assess nutritional status and growth parameters. The presence of congenital anomalies may identify syndromes associated with amenorrhea (e.g., Turner syndrome). Galactorrhea is often associated with amenorrhea; hirsutism and other signs of virilization should be identified. Features suggestive of CNS disease (e.g., headache, visual disturbances) should also be noted. A careful examination of the reproductive tract is useful in identifying anatomic defects and assessing sexual maturity.

(2) Congenital conditions, such as imperforate hymen and transverse vaginal septum, may obstruct menstrual outflow. History of cyclic pain may be present, and a midline lower abdominal mass (hematocolpos/hematometra) may be palpated.

Müllerian agenesis (Mayer-Rokitansky-Küster-Hauser syndrome) is characterized by an absent or a shallow vagina with an absent cervix and uterus. Gonadal function and secondary sexual development are normal, but urinary tract and skeletal anomalies may be present. Androgen insensitivity syndrome (i.e., testicular feminization) occurs in phenotypic females who are chromosomally XY but lack androgen receptors. External genitalia appear female, but the vagina is shallow and testes are intraabdominal. At puberty, breasts develop due to gonadal estrogens; axillary and pubic hair is absent.

(3) Stigmata of Turner syndrome include short stature, pigmented nevi, high arched palate, low hairline, shield chest, ptosis, cutis laxa, pterygium colli, shortened fourth metacarpals, cubitus valgus, heart murmurs, nail changes, and deformed ears.

(4) Pregnancy should always be considered as a possible cause of secondary amenorrhea even in primary amenorrhea. If there is history of contraceptive use (birth control pills or long-acting implantable or injectable progestins), amenorrhea may be attributed to the suppression of ovulation in the progestin-dominated hormonal environment. Menstrual cycles should revert to normal within 6 months of stopping birth control pills and by 12 months after the last injection of medroxyprogesterone (Depo-Provera).

AMENORRHEA

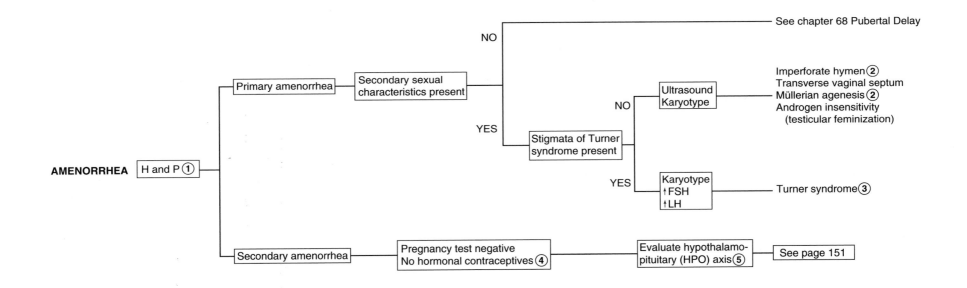

H and P ①

Primary amenorrhea

Secondary sexual characteristics present

NO — See chapter 68 Pubertal Delay

YES

Stigmata of Turner syndrome present

NO

Ultrasound
Karyotype

Imperforate hymen ②
Transverse vaginal septum
Müllerian agenesis ②
Androgen insensitivity
(testicular feminization)

YES

Karyotype
↑FSH
↑LH

Turner syndrome ③

Secondary amenorrhea

Pregnancy test negative
No hormonal contraceptives ④

Evaluate hypothalamo-pituitary (HPO) axis ⑤

See page 151

Nelson Chapter 116
Practical Strategies chapter 32

Amenorrhea (continued)

(5) Evaluation of the hypothalamic-pituitary-ovarian (HPO) axis involves laboratory studies and a progestin challenge. Studies include evaluating thyroid-stimulating hormone and prolactin levels to rule out hypothyroidism and prolactinoma. Estrogen status is evaluated by progestin challenge because blood estrogen levels are unreliable. A 5-day course of oral medroxyprogesterone acetate or a single dose of intramuscular progesterone is given. If bleeding occurs within 2 weeks of treatment, it implies a functional uterus and outflow tract and an endometrium that has been exposed to estrogen. The amount of bleeding is roughly proportional to the amount and duration of prior estrogen exposure. If there is no bleeding, it usually implies a low-estrogen state or hypoestrogenic amenorrhea. Rarely, it may be that the uterus cannot bleed secondary to uterine scarring caused by prior dilatation and curettage or severe uterine infections *(Asherman syndrome)*. This is rare in teenagers. It is important to rule out pregnancy. If there is any question, the pregnancy test must be repeated. Estrogen status may also be confirmed by vaginal smear or the presence of abundant, watery, cervical mucus. In patients with galactorrhea, the sella turcica must be imaged by thin-section coronal CT scan or by MRI, which is the most accurate. Galactorrhea with normal or mildly elevated prolactin levels may be secondary to nipple stimulation.

(6) In chronic anovulation, withdrawal bleeding occurs with a progestin challenge (prolactin and thyroid-stimulating hormone levels are normal). Polycystic ovary syndrome is a common cause. It is characterized by elevated luteinizing hormone, normal follicle-stimulating hormone, and normal or slightly increased free and total testosterone and dehydroepiandrosterone sulfate levels. Patients with premature ovarian failure may have irregular periods and withdrawal bleeding despite elevated follicle-stimulating hormone and luteinizing hormone levels.

(7) Hypothalamic dysfunction leading to amenorrhea is a diagnosis of exclusion. It is caused by suppression of gonadotropin-releasing hormone pulsatile secretion and is most commonly associated with stress, excessive exercise, or weight loss and with anorexia nervosa. Withdrawal bleeding may occur with a progestin challenge.

(8) Elevated levels of gonadotropins imply gonadal failure or dysgenesis. Patients with possible Turner syndrome need a karyotype determination. Autoimmune disease, such as the polyglandular syndrome (hypoparathyroidism, adrenal insufficiency, thyroiditis), may cause premature ovarian failure. Other conditions include myasthenia gravis, idiopathic thrombocytopenic purpura, rheumatoid arthritis, vitiligo, and autoimmune hemolytic anemia. Ovarian failure may result from chemotherapy or from irradiation. Gonadotropin-secreting adenomas are not associated with amenorrhea.

(9) If the gonadotropin levels are low or normal, imaging (CT or MRI) is required to identify a tumor such as a craniopharyngioma or prolactinoma. Symptoms such as headaches or visual disturbances should prompt imaging.

BIBLIOGRAPHY

Emans SJ, Goldstein DP: Delayed puberty and menstrual irregularities. In: Pediatric and Adolescent Gynecology, 4th ed. Boston: Little, Brown & Co, 1990.

Speroff L, Glass RH, Kase NG: Amenorrhea. In Clinical Gynecologic Endocrinology and Infertility, 5th ed. Baltimore: Williams & Wilkins, 1994.

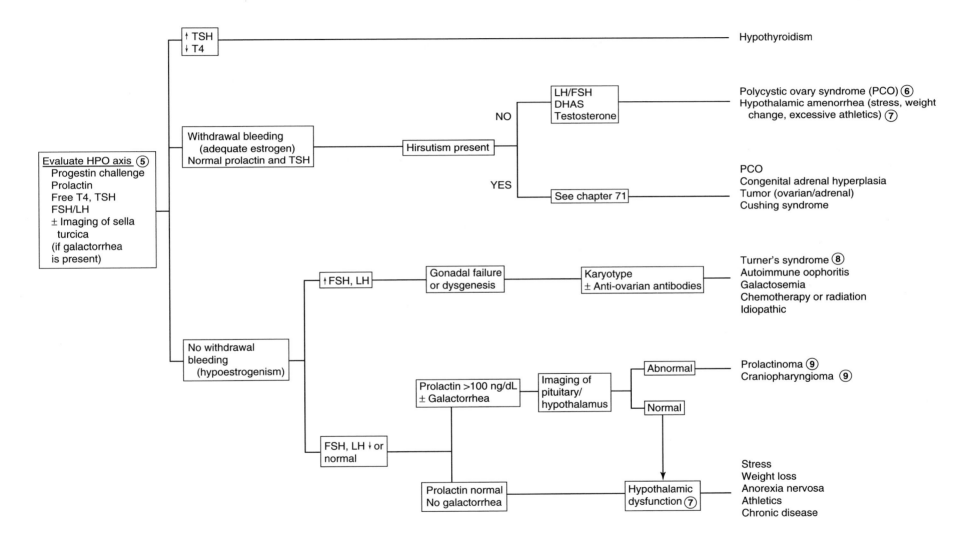

Evaluate HPO axis ⑤
Progestin challenge
Prolactin
Free T4, TSH
FSH/LH
± Imaging of sella
 turcica
(if galactorrhea
is present)

↑ TSH
↓ T4 → Hypothyroidism

Withdrawal bleeding
(adequate estrogen)
Normal prolactin and TSH

Hirsutism present

NO → LH/FSH
DHAS
Testosterone → Polycystic ovary syndrome (PCO) ⑥
Hypothalamic amenorrhea (stress, weight
 change, excessive athletics) ⑦

YES → See chapter 71 → PCO
Congenital adrenal hyperplasia
Tumor (ovarian/adrenal)
Cushing syndrome

No withdrawal
bleeding
(hypoestrogenism)

↑ FSH, LH → Gonadal failure
or dysgenesis → Karyotype
± Anti-ovarian antibodies → Turner's syndrome ⑧
Autoimmune oophoritis
Galactosemia
Chemotherapy or radiation
Idiopathic

FSH, LH ↓ or
normal

Prolactin >100 ng/dL
± Galactorrhea → Imaging of
pituitary/
hypothalamus → Abnormal → Prolactinoma ⑨
Craniopharyngioma ⑨

Normal

Prolactin normal
No galactorrhea → Hypothalamic
dysfunction ⑦ → Stress
Weight loss
Anorexia nervosa
Athletics
Chronic disease

Normal menstrual cycles range from 4 to 6 days, with a normal blood loss of 30 ml. Periodic menstrual bleeding occurring more frequently than every 21 days or greater than every 35 days, lasting longer than 7 days, or with a flow of more than 80 ml/month requires evaluation. With excessive blood loss, iron deficiency anemia may develop.

(1) The age is important, as well as any history of abuse or trauma, including sexual abuse. A history of any foreign body, including intrauterine devices (IUDs) and tampons in older girls, should be elicited. In girls who have reached menarche, a detailed menstrual history should be obtained. Increased clots may signify an abnormality. Variations in menstrual cycles may include menorrhagia (normal intervals, excessive flow and duration of bleeding), metrorrhagia (irregular intervals, excessive flow and duration), polymenorrhea (intervals < 21 days), oligomenorrhea (intervals >35 days), and intermenstrual bleeding. A sexual history is important as well as any use of hormonal contraception. Exposure to medications, including exogenous estrogens, anticoagulants, and platelet inhibitors, may be a cause of bleeding. Abdominal pain or vaginal discharge may indicate infections. On examination, the site of bleeding should be carefully assessed. An examination of external genitalia must be done, and a pelvic examination performed when indicated.

(2) In the newborn a small amount of endometrial bleeding may occur due to withdrawal from relatively high fetal estrogen levels.

(3) In prepubertal-age girls without cyclic bleeding and with no signs of puberty, a vulvovaginal source is most common. Vaginal bleeding is more predictive of a foreign body than a vaginal discharge. The possibility of sexual abuse must be considered. The foreign object may be visualized in the knee-chest position, but, if not, examination using anesthesia may be required.

(4) Infectious vulvovaginitis usually appears as a discharge, but bleeding may be present. The most common organisms obtained on culture are group A streptococci, *Shigella*, and mixed organisms. The presence of gonococci, *Chlamydia,* or *Trichomonas* should prompt evaluation for sexual abuse.

(5) Vulvovaginal trauma is usually caused by straddle injuries and less commonly by vaginal penetration and tearing from forced leg abduction; consider the possibility of sexual abuse.

(6) If a mass is visualized, consider urethral prolapse, which appears as red, friable, often necrotic tissue at the urethra.

(7) In lichen sclerosus, the vulvar skin becomes thin and parchment-like (classically in an hourglass pattern around the introitus and anus) and therefore susceptible to bleeding from minor trauma. The diagnosis may be confirmed by biopsy.

(8) Malignancies are uncommon. A grapelike mass protruding from the vagina is seen in sarcoma botryoides. Adenocarcinoma of the vagina or cervix is rare.

(9) Precocious menarche is a rare form of incomplete precocious puberty, with cyclic menstruation but no other secondary sexual characteristics. There may be a slight increase in serum estrogen levels; gonadotropin levels are prepubertal.

(10) In pubertal-age girls, first exclude pregnancy. Complications of pregnancy such as miscarriage or ectopic pregnancy may appear as abnormal bleeding. If this is suggested, pelvic examination, quantitative serum human chorionic gonadotropin (hCG) levels, and ultrasound are helpful. If the ultrasound shows no ectopic pregnancy, or there is low suspicion of an ectopic pregnancy, serial hCG testing is needed to document complete abortion or to determine if repeat ultrasound or culdocentesis is needed.

(11) If the bleeding site is the vagina, the cause may be injury or laceration, abuse, or foreign body such as a retained tampon or contraceptive sponge. Foul discharge may be present. Cancer is uncommon. Localization of the bleeding site may require anesthesia and possible referral to a gynecologist.

(12) Infections include herpes, chlamydia, gonorrhea, and trichomoniasis. (See Ch. 41.)

(13) Menstrual cycles in adolescents are often "normally" anovulatory in the early years. This is believed to be due to the immaturity of the hypothalamic-pituitary axis. Problems occur when the negative feedback of estrogen does not occur, producing a steady state of estrogen, follicle-stimulating hormone, and luteinizing hormone, as in chronic anovulation. Constant levels of estrogen result in persistent endometrial stimulation and irregular heavy bleeding when the endometrium cannot be sustained (i.e., dysfunctional uterine bleeding).

(14) Coagulopathies often cause abnormal uterine bleeding, especially the more severe bleeding that results in anemias requiring transfusions. Platelet counts, PT, PTT, bleeding time, and von Willebrand factor screening should be obtained to test for idiopathic thrombocytopenic purpura, von Willebrand disease (a common etiology), factor deficiencies, and, rarely, systemic diseases such as leukemia. (See Ch. 62.)

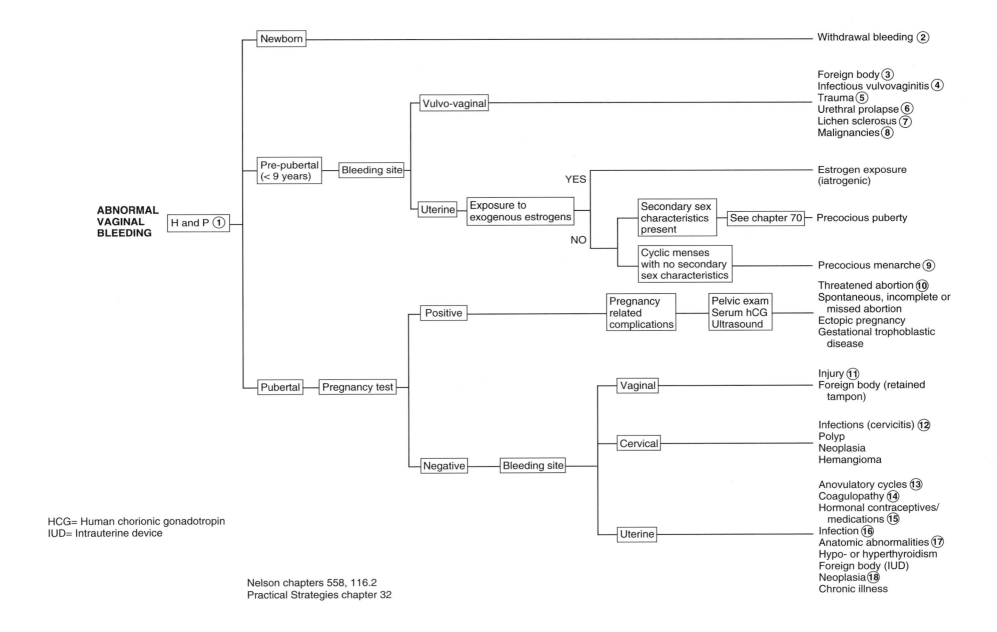

ABNORMAL VAGINAL BLEEDING — H and P ①

- Newborn ——————————————— Withdrawal bleeding ②

- Pre-pubertal (< 9 years) — Bleeding site
  - Vulvo-vaginal ——————————
    - Foreign body ③
    - Infectious vulvovaginitis ④
    - Trauma ⑤
    - Urethral prolapse ⑥
    - Lichen sclerosus ⑦
    - Malignancies ⑧
  - Uterine — Exposure to exogenous estrogens
    - YES ——————————— Estrogen exposure (iatrogenic)
    - NO
      - Secondary sex characteristics present — See chapter 70 — Precocious puberty
      - Cyclic menses with no secondary sex characteristics ——————— Precocious menarche ⑨

- Pubertal — Pregnancy test
  - Positive — Pregnancy related complications — Pelvic exam / Serum hCG / Ultrasound
    - Threatened abortion ⑩
    - Spontaneous, incomplete or missed abortion
    - Ectopic pregnancy
    - Gestational trophoblastic disease
  - Negative — Bleeding site
    - Vaginal ——————————
      - Injury ⑪
      - Foreign body (retained tampon)
    - Cervical ——————————
      - Infections (cervicitis) ⑫
      - Polyp
      - Neoplasia
      - Hemangioma
    - Uterine ——————————
      - Anovulatory cycles ⑬
      - Coagulopathy ⑭
      - Hormonal contraceptives/ medications ⑮
      - Infection ⑯
      - Anatomic abnormalities ⑰
      - Hypo- or hyperthyroidism
      - Foreign body (IUD)
      - Neoplasia ⑱
      - Chronic illness

HCG= Human chorionic gonadotropin
IUD= Intrauterine device

Nelson chapters 558, 116.2
Practical Strategies chapter 32

(15) Oral contraceptive pills and injectable or implantable progestin contraceptives may be associated with abnormal bleeding. Medications include those with hormonal effects (e.g., estrogens, progestins, androgens, prolactin) and those with anticoagulant effects (e.g., warfarin, heparin, aspirin).

(16) Infections such as pelvic inflammatory disease and postpartum or postabortal endometritis may cause uterine bleeding.

(17) Congenital partial obstruction of the hemivagina or uterine horn can result in uterine bleeding.

(18) Neoplasms include fibroids, endometrial polyps, malignant tumors, or estrogen-producing ovarian tumors.

BIBLIOGRAPHY

Speroff L, Glass RH, Kase NG: Dysfunctional uterine bleeding. In Clinical Gynecologic Endocrinology and Infertility, 5th ed. Baltimore: Williams & Wilkins, 1990.

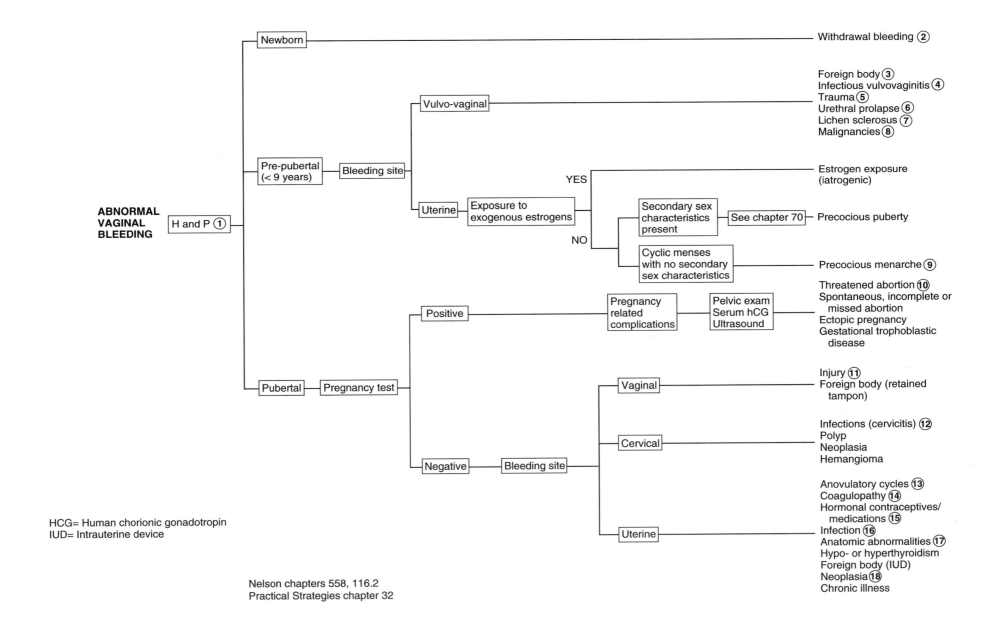

ABNORMAL VAGINAL BLEEDING — H and P ①

- **Newborn** — Withdrawal bleeding ②

- **Pre-pubertal (< 9 years)** — Bleeding site
  - **Vulvo-vaginal**
    - Foreign body ③
    - Infectious vulvovaginitis ④
    - Trauma ⑤
    - Urethral prolapse ⑥
    - Lichen sclerosus ⑦
    - Malignancies ⑧
  - **Uterine** — Exposure to exogenous estrogens
    - YES — Estrogen exposure (iatrogenic)
    - Secondary sex characteristics present — See chapter 70 — Precocious puberty
    - NO — Cyclic menses with no secondary sex characteristics — Precocious menarche ⑨

- **Pubertal** — Pregnancy test
  - **Positive** — Pregnancy related complications — Pelvic exam / Serum hCG / Ultrasound
    - Threatened abortion ⑩
    - Spontaneous, incomplete or missed abortion
    - Ectopic pregnancy
    - Gestational trophoblastic disease
  - **Negative** — Bleeding site
    - **Vaginal**
      - Injury ⑪
      - Foreign body (retained tampon)
    - **Cervical**
      - Infections (cervicitis) ⑫
      - Polyp
      - Neoplasia
      - Hemangioma
    - **Uterine**
      - Anovulatory cycles ⑬
      - Coagulopathy ⑭
      - Hormonal contraceptives/ medications ⑮
      - Infection ⑯
      - Anatomic abnormalities ⑰
      - Hypo- or hyperthyroidism
      - Foreign body (IUD)
      - Neoplasia ⑱
      - Chronic illness

HCG= Human chorionic gonadotropin
IUD= Intrauterine device

Nelson chapters 558, 116.2
Practical Strategies chapter 32

Vaginal discharge is a common but nonspecific sign in female adolescents. It should prompt consideration of sexually transmitted disease in sexually active girls.

(1) Menstrual history including changes in cycle or new onset of dysmenorrhea may be helpful. Sexual history should include recent sexual encounters, number of partners, contraceptive and condom use, dyspareunia, sexually transmitted diseases, and pregnancies if any. Sexual abuse should be considered, particularly in prepubertal girls with vaginal discharge. Most discharge in this age group is not sexually acquired. Examination includes careful inspection of the vulva, vagina, and introitus for any abnormalities, including bruises, lacerations, excoriations, and vesicles, as well as character of the vaginal discharge. Pelvic examination in prepubertal girls may be done using a Huffman speculum. The Pederson speculum is slightly larger and may be used in an adolescent. Rashes may be seen with a sexually transmitted disease (STD), as well as joint and other constitutional symptoms.

(2) Physiologic leukorrhea is a whitish mucoid discharge that occurs in newborns and adolescents. In pubertal adolescents it starts before menarche and may decrease with onset of menses or may continue for a few years. During the middle of the menstrual cycle it is copious and clear; it is scant and sticky during the second half of the cycle. Wet preparation shows epithelial cells and no abnormal findings. If the patient is sexually active an STD must be ruled out.

(3) All cases with suspected sexual abuse require direct cultures for *Neisseria gonorrhoeae* and *Chlamydia,* because results of antigen detection tests are not admissible in court. Referral to persons with expertise in evaluation of sexually abused children is indicated.

(4) In the prepubertal girl the vulvar mucosa is thin and more susceptible to irritation and inflammation. Poor hygiene, use of irritant soaps, bubble baths, and "nonbreathing" underwear may therefore be associated with nonspecific vulvovaginitis. This is caused by an overgrowth of normal flora, including diphtheroids, α-hemolytic streptococci, lactobacilli, and *Escherichia coli*. A bloody vaginal discharge may be seen with *Shigella* or group A streptococcal infections. Bacterial cultures confirm this. If there is possible sexual abuse, vaginal secretions must be cultured to exclude an STD. The presence of gonorrhea or trichomoniasis is consistent with abuse. Chlamydial infection is also highly suspicious. Foreign bodies, often retained toilet tissue, in the vagina cause a foul-smelling discharge, which may be blood tinged. If the foreign body cannot be visualized, examination using anesthesia may be needed. Anal pruritus may indicate pinworms and can be diagnosed by using a tape test. Pinworms are more common in younger children. Neoplasms may also cause discharge—rhabdomyosarcoma; adenosis and adenocarcinoma in girls whose mothers were exposed to diethylstilbestrol during pregnancy.

(5) The appearance of secretions may help in diagnosis; *Candida* causes a thick, whitish, curdy discharge and *Trichomonas* has a yellow frothy discharge. A mucopurulent discharge with evidence of cervicitis may be seen with *Chlamydia trachomatis, N. gonorrhoeae,* and herpes. Microscopic examination of secretions may help to provide the diagnosis. Trichomonads are motile flagellated organisms. Clue cells (i.e., epithelial cells coated with refractile bacteria) are seen with bacterial vaginosis. Potassium hydroxide (KOH) reveals pseudohyphae in *Candida*. A positive "whiff" test due to release of amine odor is present with bacterial vaginosis and sometimes with *Trichomonas*. Staining may reveal gram-variable coccobacilli and curved, gram-negative rods in bacterial vaginosis; gram-negative intracellular diplococci are seen in *N. gonorrhoeae*. Specific methods for detection of *C. trachomatis* include enzyme immunoassay, ligase chain reaction, polymerase chain reaction, and culture. Papanicolaou (Pap) smear may also indicate the diagnosis: intranuclear inclusions and multinucleate giant cells with herpes simplex and cytoplasmic inclusions with *Chlamydia*. Gonorrheal infections may also involve the pharynx, rectum, and joints; disseminated infection may occur. *Candida albicans* is the most common fungal infection of the vagina; other *Candida* species may be involved. Diabetes mellitus, pregnancy, and use of antibiotics are predisposing factors. Chlamydial infections usually cause vaginal discharge, dysuria, or frequency. Endometritis with menorrhagia or metrorrhagia may be present. Perihepatitis (Fitz-Hugh-Curtis syndrome) may occur with gonorrhea or chlamydial infection; these are also responsible for most pelvic inflammatory disease. HIV testing should be considered in all girls diagnosed with an STD.

(6) In primary syphilis, there is initially a papule that develops into an ulcer with a clean base with rounded borders that is usually painless. There may be painless inguinal lymphadenopathy. Diagnosis can be made by direct fluorescent antibody or darkfield microscopy of exudate or tissue. Diagnosis is usually made using serology, which may be negative in the early stages. Serologic tests include rapid plasma reagin (RPR) and Venereal Disease Research Laboratory (VDRL) tests. Nontreponemal tests are sensitive but can be falsely positive and so need confirmation by specific treponemal tests, such as fluorescent treponemal antibody absorption test (FTA-ABS) and the microhemagglutination assay for antibodies to *Treponema pallidum* (MHA-TP).

(7) Herpes appears initially as vesicles and pustules, associated with vaginal discharge and dysuria, followed by ulceration of the lesions with associated constitutional symptoms. Tender inguinal lymphadenopathy may be present. Tzanck preparation, herpes cultures, and direct fluorescent antibody testing may be done.

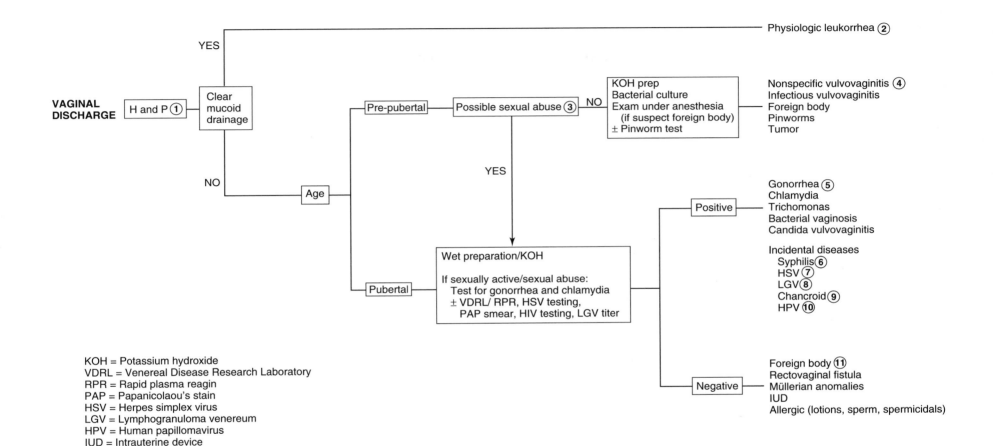

VAGINAL DISCHARGE — H and P ①

YES → Physiologic leukorrhea ②

Clear mucoid drainage

NO → Age

Pre-pubertal → Possible sexual abuse ③

NO →
KOH prep
Bacterial culture
Exam under anesthesia
 (if suspect foreign body)
± Pinworm test

Nonspecific vulvovaginitis ④
Infectious vulvovaginitis
Foreign body
Pinworms
Tumor

YES ↓

Pubertal →
Wet preparation/KOH

If sexually active/sexual abuse:
 Test for gonorrhea and chlamydia
 ± VDRL/ RPR, HSV testing,
  PAP smear, HIV testing, LGV titer

Positive →
Gonorrhea ⑤
Chlamydia
Trichomonas
Bacterial vaginosis
Candida vulvovaginitis

Incidental diseases
 Syphilis ⑥
 HSV ⑦
 LGV ⑧
 Chancroid ⑨
 HPV ⑩

Negative →
Foreign body ⑪
Rectovaginal fistula
Müllerian anomalies
IUD
Allergic (lotions, sperm, spermicidals)

KOH = Potassium hydroxide
VDRL = Venereal Disease Research Laboratory
RPR = Rapid plasma reagin
PAP = Papanicolaou's stain
HSV = Herpes simplex virus
LGV = Lymphogranuloma venereum
HPV = Human papillomavirus
IUD = Intrauterine device

Nelson chapters 192, 557, 583
Practical Strategies chapter 31

8 Lymphogranuloma venereum (LGV) is rare and is caused by three serotypes of *C. trachomatis*. The ulcer is transient; there is tender inguinal adenopathy that may suppurate. Rectal strictures may also occur. Diagnosis is by LGV titer.

9 Chancroid is also rare; it occurs as multiple, deep, purulent ulcerations and tender, fluctuant, inguinal lymphadenopathy, which may suppurate. Diagnosis is often by exclusion. Gram stain of smear obtained from the ulcer base may be done. Culture of the ulcer base for *Haemophilus ducreyi* is difficult.

10 Human papillomavirus (HPV) infection usually occurs as exophytic warts in the anogenital area. Vulvar lesions cause local burning; vaginal lesions cause discharge, pruritus, and postcoital bleeding.

11 Foreign bodies may also cause discharge in pubertal-age girls. Often it is a retained tampon. Other causes of vaginitis include allergic vulvovaginitis caused by soaps, douches, contraceptive gels or creams, and, rarely, sperm. Chronic discharge may be due to the intrauterine device string. Rectovaginal fistulas may be seen with Crohn disease. Müllerian anomalies may also be present with vaginal discharge.

BIBLIOGRAPHY

Emans SJ, Goldstein DP: Vulvovaginal complaints in the adolescent. In Pediatric and Adolescent Gynecology, 3rd ed. Boston: Little, Brown & Co, 1990.

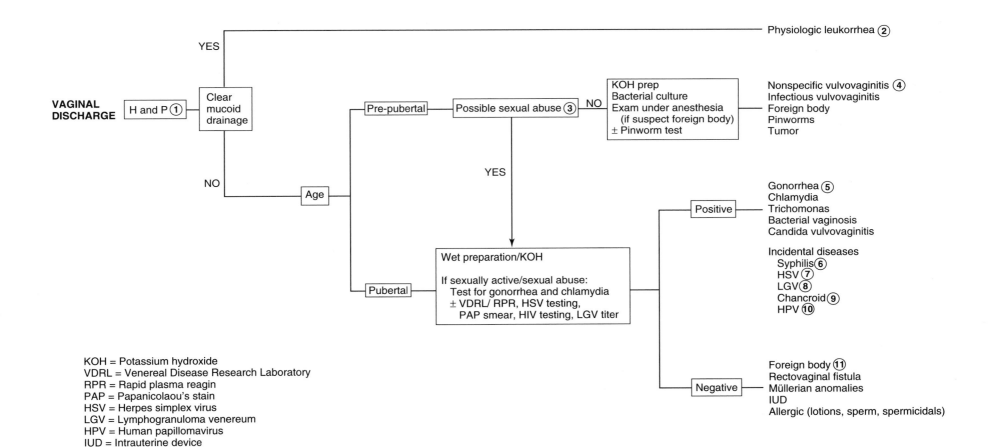

VAGINAL DISCHARGE — H and P ①

Clear mucoid drainage
- YES → Physiologic leukorrhea ②
- NO → Age

Age:
- Pre-pubertal → Possible sexual abuse ③
  - NO → KOH prep / Bacterial culture / Exam under anesthesia (if suspect foreign body) / ± Pinworm test → Nonspecific vulvovaginitis ④ / Infectious vulvovaginitis / Foreign body / Pinworms / Tumor
  - YES → Wet preparation/KOH
- Pubertal → Wet preparation/KOH

Wet preparation/KOH
If sexually active/sexual abuse:
  Test for gonorrhea and chlamydia
  ± VDRL/ RPR, HSV testing,
    PAP smear, HIV testing, LGV titer

- Positive → Gonorrhea ⑤ / Chlamydia / Trichomonas / Bacterial vaginosis / Candida vulvovaginitis

  Incidental diseases
    Syphilis ⑥
    HSV ⑦
    LGV ⑧
    Chancroid ⑨
    HPV ⑩

- Negative → Foreign body ⑪ / Rectovaginal fistula / Müllerian anomalies / IUD / Allergic (lotions, sperm, spermicidals)

KOH = Potassium hydroxide
VDRL = Venereal Disease Research Laboratory
RPR = Rapid plasma reagin
PAP = Papanicolaou's stain
HSV = Herpes simplex virus
LGV = Lymphogranuloma venereum
HPV = Human papillomavirus
IUD = Intrauterine device

Nelson chapters 192, 557, 583
Practical Strategies chapter 31

MUSCULOSKELETAL SYSTEM

Chapter 42 Limp

An abnormal gait in a child may be due to pain, torsional deformity, or musculoskeletal disorder.

(1) A birth history and developmental history are particularly important for problems noticed early or around the time a child begins walking. Prematurity and birth complications are risk factors for hypoxic brain damage (i.e., cerebral palsy). For older children, systemic signs and symptoms (e.g., fever, rash, generalized weakness, weight loss) may suggest infections or rheumatic disorders.

The musculoskeletal examination should include careful attention to all the joints and the spine. Hip pathology may occur as pain in the knee. Careful observation of the gait, ideally over a distance such as a long hallway, is critical. Having the child adequately undressed is necessary for a good evaluation. In a painful gait the child's stance phase on the affected limb is shortened. A nonpainful or Trendelenburg gait indicates proximal muscle weakness or hip instability; stance phase is equal from side to side, but the child shifts the weight over the involved side for balance. Bilateral involvement produces a waddling gait.

(2) Children are more at risk for epiphyseal fractures than ligamentous sprains because their ligaments are generally stronger than the adjacent growth plates. Because X-rays may be normal or show only physeal widening, the diagnosis is often clinical. Consultation should always be considered when in doubt.

(3) Slipped capital femoral epiphysis (SCFE) is the most common hip disorder in adolescents presenting with pain or an abnormal gait. In many cases an undiagnosed chronic slip appears when it is acutely worsened by trauma. A careful history may elicit chronic complaints of pain, subtle limp, or self-imposed activity restrictions. Examination reveals limited internal rotation of the affected hip and an out-toed, painful gait. Anteroposterior and "frog leg" lateral X-rays are usually adequate to make the diagnosis. When SCFEs occur before puberty, an underlying hormonal ab-

normality (i.e., hypothyroidism or pituitary disorders) should be ruled out.

(4) When infection or inflammation is suspected, laboratory tests (CBC, ESR, CRP) may be helpful. Blood cultures yield a positive result in 50% to 60% of cases of osteomyelitis. If the X-ray is negative, consider a bone scan. Ultrasound may aid in detecting joint effusions, especially of the hip.

(5) Infection confined to the capsule of a joint is termed *septic arthritis*. Infection within the bone, even with secondary spread to involve the joint, is osteomyelitis. Both disorders may present with localized pain and tenderness in an acutely ill child. Osteomyelitis may also occur subacutely with prolonged pain and limp but without fevers or systemic complaints. Bone changes on X-ray may not become evident for 7 to 10 days; soft tissue changes may be evident earlier. Ultrasound-guided aspiration of the suspected site may be diagnostic if pus is obtained. Bone scans are a sensitive and specific diagnostic modality early in the clinical course. MRI is sensitive but is costly and usually requires sedation.

(6) Septic arthritis is a medical emergency requiring prompt diagnosis and treatment. Patients typically present with fever, malaise, refusal to walk, and localized joint pain, most commonly knee or hip. Examination reveals erythema, warmth, swelling, and pain with passive motion. An ultrasound evaluation may suggest the diagnosis by demonstrating an effusion, but joint aspiration is mandated.

(7) Acute transient synovitis (toxic synovitis or hip monoarticular synovitis) is one of the most common causes of hip pain and limping in children usually between 3 and 8 years of age. It occurs as unilateral hip pain, painful limp, and slightly restricted abduction and internal rotation. Fevers may be present, but rarely do patients present with the acute toxicity suggestive of septic arthritis. The diagnosis is one of exclusion. An

evaluation to rule out more serious causes is always indicated. Laboratory results are usually normal or suggest a mild inflammatory process. X-rays are also usually normal or may show a lightly widened medial joint space or accentuated pericapsular shadow. In acute cases when fever is present, ultrasound and aspiration to evaluate the effusion may be necessary to rule out septic arthritis.

(8) Avascular necrosis (AVN or Legg-Calvé-Perthes disease) is an ischemic necrosis and bony collapse of the femoral head followed by subsequent repair. Children between 2 and 12 years of age are most commonly affected and typically present with a history of mild or intermittent groin, knee, or thigh pain that is aggravated by activity. Common physical findings include a leg-length discrepancy and slightly restricted abduction and internal rotation. Anteroposterior and "frog leg" lateral X-rays will confirm the diagnosis.

(9) Night pain is characteristic of both benign and malignant primary or metastatic tumors. Characteristic X-ray findings usually suggest the diagnosis of benign bone tumors, but excisional biopsy is usually recommended to confirm the diagnosis. A bone scan or MRI is indicated if nerve or spinal cord involvement is suggested.

(10) A child whose gait abnormality was noted shortly after beginning to walk is likely to have a congenital neurologic or musculoskeletal disorder, such as developmental dysplasia of the hip (DDH). Ultrasound can be used to diagnose DDH in the newborn; however, interpretation by a radiologist experienced in the examination is recommended.

(11) Spastic diplegia is the most common type of cerebral palsy. The condition is characterized by toe-walking and a painless limp. Examination reveals increased muscle tone, spasticity, hyperactive deep tendon reflexes, tight heel cords, and persistent pathologic reflexes.

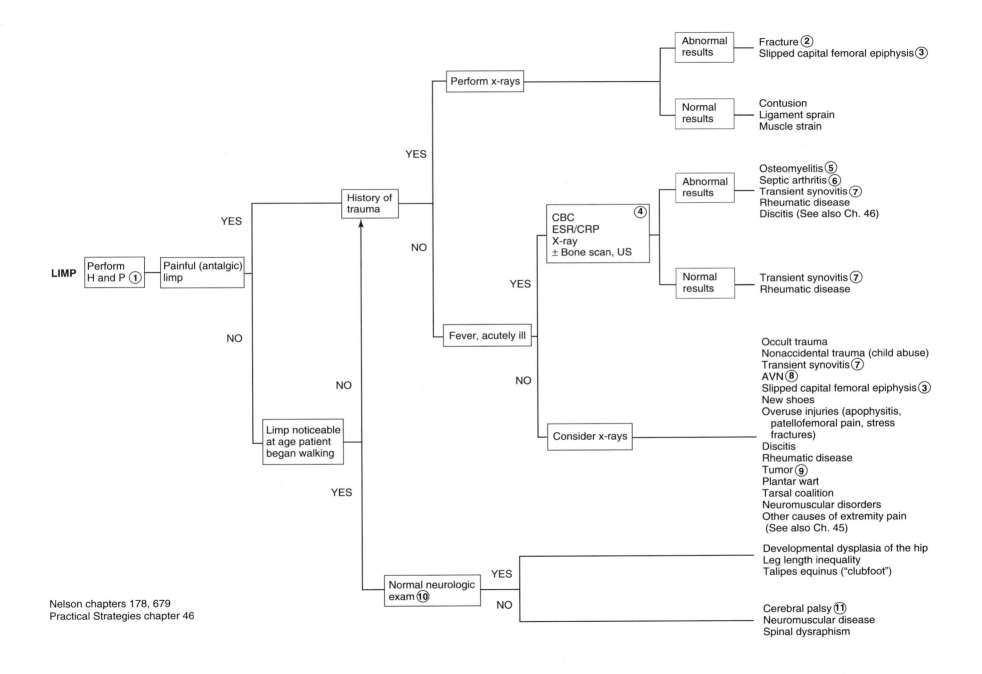

LIMP

Perform H and P ①

Painful (antalgic) limp

YES → History of trauma

NO → Limp noticeable at age patient began walking

History of trauma **YES** → Perform x-rays

Perform x-rays:
- **Abnormal results** → Fracture ② / Slipped capital femoral epiphysis ③
- **Normal results** → Contusion / Ligament sprain / Muscle strain

History of trauma **NO** → Fever, acutely ill

Fever, acutely ill **YES** → CBC / ESR/CRP / X-ray / ± Bone scan, US ④
- **Abnormal results** → Osteomyelitis ⑤ / Septic arthritis ⑥ / Transient synovitis ⑦ / Rheumatic disease / Discitis (See also Ch. 46)
- **Normal results** → Transient synovitis ⑦ / Rheumatic disease

Fever, acutely ill **NO** → Consider x-rays → Occult trauma / Nonaccidental trauma (child abuse) / Transient synovitis ⑦ / AVN ⑧ / Slipped capital femoral epiphysis ③ / New shoes / Overuse injuries (apophysitis, patellofemoral pain, stress fractures) / Discitis / Rheumatic disease / Tumor ⑨ / Plantar wart / Tarsal coalition / Neuromuscular disorders / Other causes of extremity pain (See also Ch. 45)

Limp noticeable at age patient began walking **YES** → Normal neurologic exam ⑩
- **YES** → Developmental dysplasia of the hip / Leg length inequality / Talipes equinus ("clubfoot")
- **NO** → Cerebral palsy ⑪ / Neuromuscular disease / Spinal dysraphism

Nelson chapters 178, 679
Practical Strategies chapter 46

BIBLIOGRAPHY

AAP Committee on Quality Improvement and Subcommittee on Developmental Dysplasia of the Hip: Clinical practice guideline: Early detection of developmental dysplasia of the hip. Pediatrics 105:896, 2000.

Greene W (section ed): Pediatric orthopaedics. In Snider RK (ed): Essentials of Musculoskeletal Care, p 549. Rosemont, IL: American Academy of Orthopaedic Surgeons, 1997.

Koop S, Quanbeck D: Three common causes of childhood hip pain. Pediatr Clin North Am 43:1053–1066, 1996.

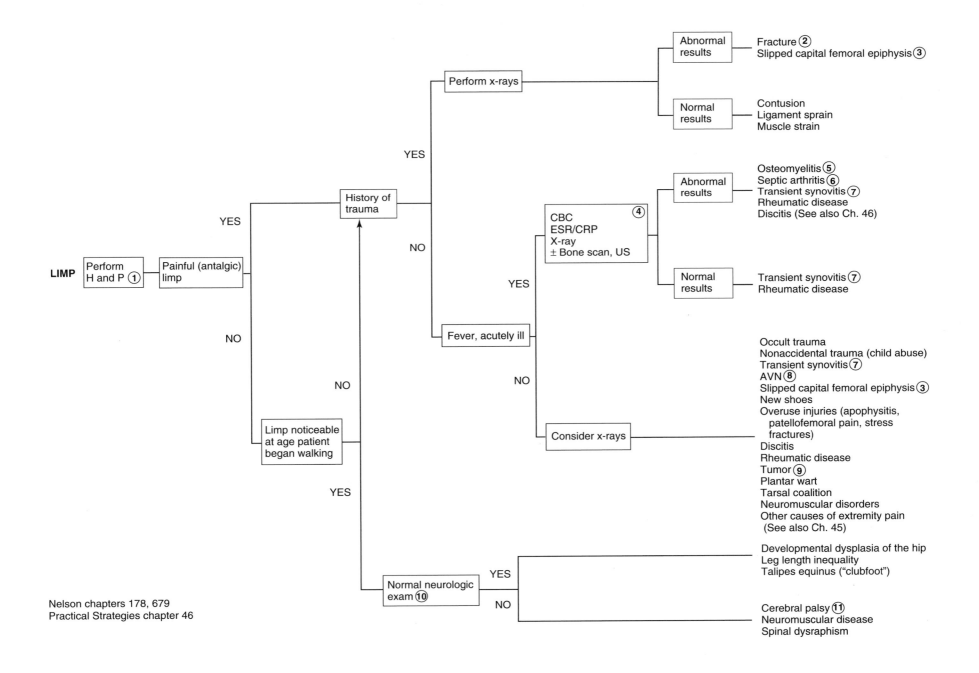

LIMP

Perform H and P ①

Painful (antalgic) limp

YES → History of trauma

History of trauma → **YES** → Perform x-rays

Perform x-rays →
- Abnormal results → Fracture ②
  Slipped capital femoral epiphysis ③
- Normal results → Contusion
  Ligament sprain
  Muscle strain

History of trauma → **NO** → Fever, acutely ill

Fever, acutely ill → **YES** → CBC / ESR/CRP / X-ray / ± Bone scan, US ④

CBC ESR/CRP X-ray ± Bone scan, US →
- Abnormal results → Osteomyelitis ⑤
  Septic arthritis ⑥
  Transient synovitis ⑦
  Rheumatic disease
  Discitis (See also Ch. 46)
- Normal results → Transient synovitis ⑦
  Rheumatic disease

Fever, acutely ill → **NO** → Consider x-rays →
Occult trauma
Nonaccidental trauma (child abuse)
Transient synovitis ⑦
AVN ⑧
Slipped capital femoral epiphysis ③
New shoes
Overuse injuries (apophysitis, patellofemoral pain, stress fractures)
Discitis
Rheumatic disease
Tumor ⑨
Plantar wart
Tarsal coalition
Neuromuscular disorders
Other causes of extremity pain (See also Ch. 45)

Perform H and P → **NO** → Limp noticeable at age patient began walking

Limp noticeable at age patient began walking → **NO** → History of trauma

Limp noticeable at age patient began walking → **YES** → Normal neurologic exam ⑩

Normal neurologic exam ⑩ → **YES** →
Developmental dysplasia of the hip
Leg length inequality
Talipes equinus ("clubfoot")

Normal neurologic exam ⑩ → **NO** →
Cerebral palsy ⑪
Neuromuscular disease
Spinal dysraphism

Nelson chapters 178, 679
Practical Strategies chapter 46

Arthralgia is joint pain; arthritis is joint swelling or the presence of both pain and limitation of motion in at least one joint. The degree of joint pain and diminished function accompanying arthritis is variable.

(1) Arthritis may occur as warmth or swelling of a joint without any evidence of pain or obviously restricted motion. Clinical manifestations of arthritis are nonspecific in the neonate and include poor feeding, irritability, and pseudoparalysis of an extremity. Morning stiffness or stiffness after prolonged periods of inactivity are more common than pain. Children may also experience referred pain. Hip disease may be referred to the knees, and pelvic pain may be referred to the back, hip, or anterior thigh. Arthritis may also occur as a limp. (See Ch. 42.)

A thorough review of systems is important because rheumatic disorders (also called connective tissue disorders) can include virtually all organ systems. Findings consistent with a viral syndrome may also aid in the diagnosis. Bone pain, especially at night, accompanied by signs of systemic illness (e.g., fever, weight loss) should prompt a workup to rule out malignancy.

In addition to a careful examination of each joint, the physical examination should assess for any back or neck stiffness. Muscle atrophy could indicate significant involvement of adjacent joints. Additional laboratory and radiographic testing should be obtained based on the suspected cause.

(2) An acutely inflamed joint needs to be aspirated. Imaging may or may not be obtained before referring for aspiration, depending on the preference of the consultant performing the aspiration.

(3) The most common agent of septic arthritis is *Staphylococcus aureus* in all age groups. *Haemophilus influenzae* type B is now uncommon due to immunization. Other streptococci and *Pseudomonas aeruginosa*, as a sequela to a puncture wound through a tennis shoe, are also causes. Tuberculosis is a rare cause. Group B *Streptococcus* and gram-negative enteric rods can be causative in neonates. Gonococcal disease should be considered in sexually active adolescents, although a monoarticular arthritis is a less common presentation of this disease. It more commonly appears as a migratory tenosynovitis involving the wrists, hands, and fingers, plus fever and rash. The genitourinary tract, rectum, or pharynx is also usually infected.

Acute toxic synovitis (see Ch. 42) usually occurs with a less fulminant onset than a septic arthritis. Joint aspiration may be necessary to distinguish between the two conditions.

(4) Lyme disease titers should be obtained in patients with risk factors, including exposure in an endemic area. When clinically suspicious, obtain an enzyme-linked immunosorbent assay (ELISA) followed by a confirmatory Western blot test if the ELISA is positive.

(5) Juvenile rheumatoid arthritis (JRA) is defined as the persistence of a nonmigratory arthritis for 6 weeks or longer in a child younger than 16 years. It is subclassified as systemic onset, pauciarticular, or polyarticular. In systemic-onset JRA the systemic symptoms are predominant (e.g., high spiking fevers, evanescent rash). The arthritis is usually polyarticular when it develops. There are no specific diagnostic laboratory criteria.

In pauciarticular JRA, four or fewer joints are involved. Iridocyclitis is a frequent complication in this subgroup. Test results for antinuclear antibodies may be positive, although those for rheumatoid factor are always negative. A subgroup of children develops spondyloarthropathy.

(6) The spondyloarthropathies (ankylosing spondylitis [AS], arthritis of inflammatory bowel disease, psoriasis, Reiter syndrome) are seronegative arthritides characterized by arthritis that is usually spinal and enthesopathies (i.e., pain at the site of tendon or ligament insertions). Sacroiliitis and an association with HLA-B27 are also common. Reiter syndrome is characterized by urethritis and uveitis and is often misdiagnosed as pauciarticular JRA. AS may appear with arthritis, usually of large joint and lower extremity. Heel pain and enthesopathies are common in both Reiter syndrome and AS. In AS, characteristic sacroiliac (SI) and lumbosacral spine involvement may occur at the onset of symptoms or months to years later. Lower back, hip, and thigh pain is also characteristic of AS.

(7) Arthritis precedes psoriasis in approximately one half of the cases of psoriatic arthritis. Arthritis may be pauciarticular or polyarticular and frequently includes the distal interphalangeal joints.

(8) Lyme disease arthritis may be mild or severe. Erythema chronicum migrans (an expanding annular rash) is the characteristic skin finding for Lyme disease when it occurs. Arthritis is typically a late manifestation. It usually involves large joints, although any joint can be affected, and may be migratory. Joint swelling and tenderness are common, although the tenderness is not as severe as with pyogenic-septic joints.

(9) Arthritis and arthralgias have been associated with many viral infections, including rubella, parvovirus, Epstein-Barr virus, cytomegalovirus, varicella, and influenza. The joint symptoms may occur during the course of the infection or as a postinfectious reaction. Symptoms usually resolve within 6 weeks.

(10) Arthralgias and arthritis in the peripheral small joints may occur 1 to 3 weeks after immunization with rubella vaccine. This reaction occurs most commonly in postpubertal females. An associated rash may occur.

(11) Arthritis is a frequent component of vasculitis syndromes, including Henoch-Schönlein purpura, polyarteritis nodosa, Wegener's granulomatosis, and Takayasu arteritis. Characteristic skin findings occur with many of the disorders.

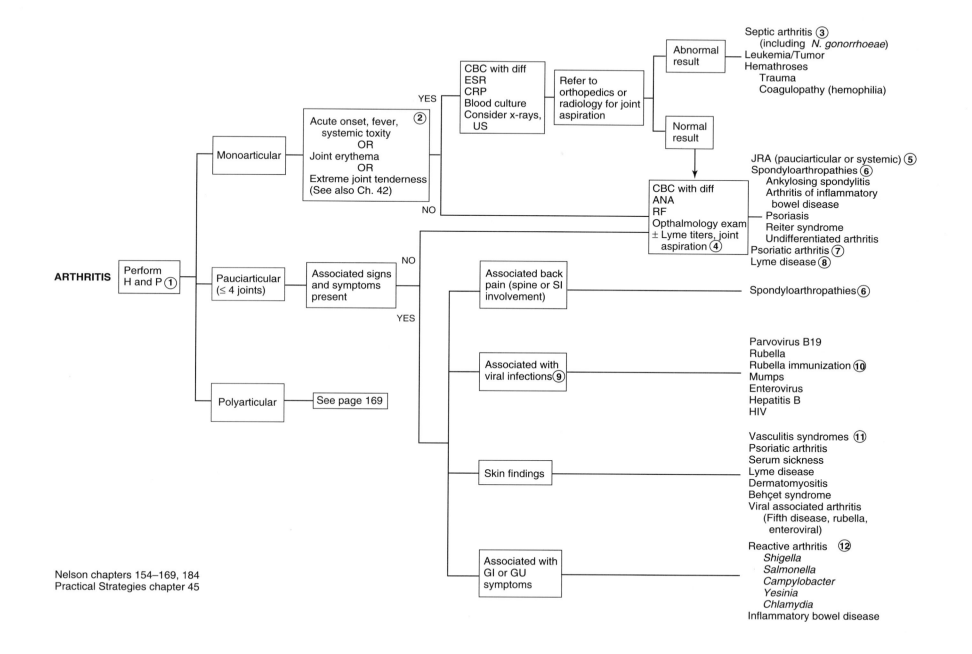

ARTHRITIS — Perform H and P ①

Monoarticular

Acute onset, fever, systemic toxicity OR Joint erythema OR Extreme joint tenderness (See also Ch. 42) ②

YES →
CBC with diff
ESR
CRP
Blood culture
Consider x-rays, US

→ Refer to orthopedics or radiology for joint aspiration

Abnormal result →
Septic arthritis ③ (including *N. gonorrhoeae*)
Leukemia/Tumor
Hemathroses
Trauma
Coagulopathy (hemophilia)

Normal result →

CBC with diff
ANA
RF
Opthalmology exam
± Lyme titers, joint aspiration ④

JRA (pauciarticular or systemic) ⑤
Spondyloarthropathies ⑥
Ankylosing spondylitis
Arthritis of inflammatory bowel disease
Psoriasis
Reiter syndrome
Undifferentiated arthritis
Psoriatic arthritis ⑦
Lyme disease ⑧

Pauciarticular (≤ 4 joints) — Associated signs and symptoms present

NO → (to CBC with diff / ANA / RF ④)

YES ↓

Associated back pain (spine or SI involvement) → Spondyloarthropathies ⑥

Associated with viral infections ⑨ →
Parvovirus B19
Rubella
Rubella immunization ⑩
Mumps
Enterovirus
Hepatitis B
HIV

Skin findings →
Vasculitis syndromes ⑪
Psoriatic arthritis
Serum sickness
Lyme disease
Dermatomyositis
Behçet syndrome
Viral associated arthritis (Fifth disease, rubella, enteroviral)

Associated with GI or GU symptoms →
Reactive arthritis ⑫
Shigella
Salmonella
Campylobacter
Yesinia
Chlamydia
Inflammatory bowel disease

Polyarticular — See page 169

Nelson chapters 154–169, 184
Practical Strategies chapter 45

Arthritis *(continued)*

(12) A reactive arthritis is believed to be an auto-immune reaction occurring after an infection outside the joint, usually the gastrointestinal or genitourinary tract. A reactive arthritis may progress to a chronic spondyloarthropathy.

(13) The polyarthritis that constitutes one of the Jones criteria for the diagnosis of rheumatic fever is migratory and characterized by extreme tenderness, redness, and swelling of affected joints. It may affect several joints but rarely the fingers, toes, or spine. This arthritis classically responds very quickly to treatment with aspirin. Arthralgias constitute a minor criterion for the diagnosis of rheumatic fever. In contrast to those cases fulfilling the Jones criteria, poststreptococcal arthritis has also been described as a pauciarticular nonmigratory arthritis affecting both small and large joints after infection with group A *Streptococcus*. Controversy exists over whether poststreptococcal arthritis is a distinct entity or an incomplete form of acute rheumatic fever.

(14) All collagen vascular diseases may cause arthralgias and arthritis. Arthralgias and arthritis are frequently early manifestations of systemic lupus erythematosus (SLE). The subjective complaint of pain in SLE-related arthritis is typically greater than expected for the clinical signs. Diagnosis is based on evidence of multisystem involvement and supportive laboratory studies, including specific antinuclear antibody tests and complement levels. Arthritis is also associated with chronic fatigue syndrome and fibromyalgia.

(15) In polyarticular JRA, involvement of large joints is frequently followed by involvement of the small joints of the hands. A positive rheumatoid factor, which only occurs in 5% to 10% of JRA patients overall, may occur in this subtype.

(16) Of the disorders occurring as pauciarticular arthritis, only the spondyloarthropathies are unlikely to appear as polyarticular.

BIBLIOGRAPHY

Aronoff SC, Scoles PV: Musculoskeletal infection. In Scoles PV (ed): Pediatric Orthopedics in Clinical Practice, 2nd ed, p 269. Chicago: Year Book Medical Publishers, 1988.

Jacobs JC: Pediatric Rheumatology for the Practitioner, 2nd ed. New York: Springer-Verlag, 1993.

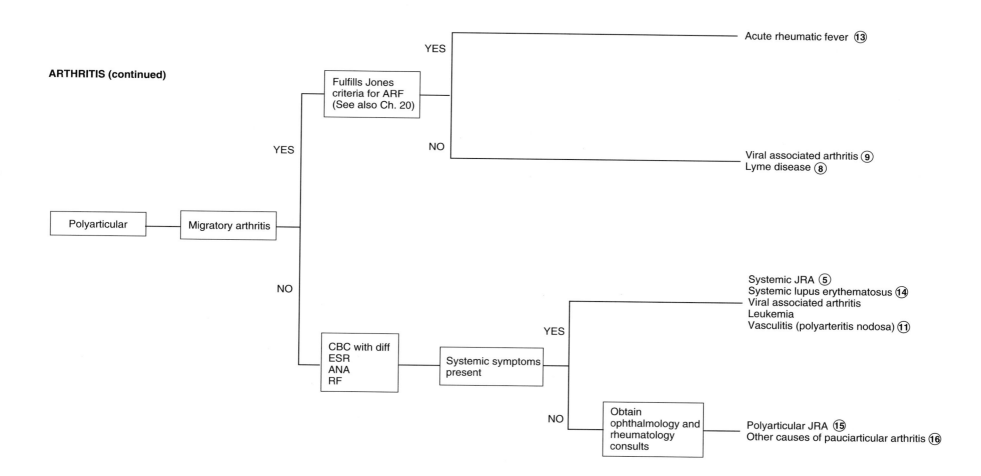

Chapter 44 Knee Pain

Knee pain can be an indicator of problems related to the distal femur, proximal tibia, hip, or the knee itself.

(1) Knee pain in children may occur secondary to acute or chronic processes. A thorough history and examination, including patient age, pain location, duration of the complaint, and relationship to trauma, narrow the differential diagnosis. The disorder suspected should aid in the selection of radiographic aids.

True locking occurs when the knee is stuck in approximately 45 degrees of flexion and requires some type of manipulation by the patient to release it.

Range of motion may be affected simply by pain or by intraarticular damage. Forced range of motion should never be attempted. Bilateral knee evaluation allows comparison for symmetry and better detection of subtle findings. A careful examination of the hips is critical in the evaluation of knee pain, especially nontraumatic. Knee pain, especially if poorly localized and without knee tenderness, accompanied by an abnormal hip examination suggests a primary hip disorder such as avascular necrosis or a slipped capital femoral epiphysis.

Effusions are most likely to occur in association with a traumatic injury. Immediate development of an effusion after an injury usually indicates hemarthrosis. Effusions may develop slowly (2 to 3 days) after an injury or may occur intermittently owing to an intracapsular injury (e.g., meniscal tear), overuse, or a rheumatoid process. Septic arthritis should be considered when a knee is acutely painful, warm, and swollen, and if the patient is febrile or toxic. Aspiration is essential when septic arthritis is suspected. It may be helpful in the diagnosis of chronic or recurrent knee effusions. Asymmetric thigh girth suggests a chronic problem with resultant muscular atrophy.

(2) Children are at greater risk for fractures than ligament sprains because the physes (i.e., growth plates) are weaker than ligaments.

(3) The Lachman test can assess the integrity of the anterior cruciate ligament (ACL). To perform this test, the patient should be supine with the knee flexed approximately 20 degrees, and the examiner should first stabilize the thigh. This can be done by grasping the distal thigh (positioning the hand so the thumb wraps over the thigh just above the patella). The examiner could also stabilize the patient's knee by placing his or her own knee under the patient's knee. The proximal tibia should then be grasped with the other hand and pulled forward. The nonpainful knee should be examined first and then compared with the painful knee. A normal examination reveals a small amount of anterior displacement and a fixed endpoint. Significant displacement and lack of a distinct endpoint indicate injury to the ACL. Mild injuries may be characterized by pain on ligamentous testing and absence of laxity or instability. Evaluation of a suspected ACL injury should include X-rays to rule out a physeal or avulsion fracture of the tibial eminence. Because ACL tears are often associated with meniscal injury in children, referral for further evaluation (arthroscopy or MRI) is recommended.

(4) Patellofemoral pain comprises a spectrum of disorders due to patellar malalignment that causes inflammation of the patellofemoral articulation. The term most commonly refers to a pain syndrome typically experienced by adolescents after a growth spurt, minor injury, or change in activity level. Pain is vaguely described as located around the knee or behind the patella. It is exacerbated by climbing stairs and after sitting with the knee flexed for extended periods and is relieved by rest. Patients may complain of occasional buckling or stiffness, but true locking does not occur. The pain is frequently bilateral, and examination may be normal or reveal peripatellar tenderness with mild patellar compression. Contraction of the quadriceps while the examiner pushes down on the upper pole of the patella frequently causes pain. Diagnosis is usually clinical. X-rays may be indicated in atypical or prolonged symptoms not responding to therapy. Significant pain or guarding with attempted lateral or medial displacement of the patella (i.e., positive apprehension test) suggests a more serious disorder of chronic or recurrent subluxation or dislocation. These disorders should be classified as distinct entities rather than simply as patellofemoral pain syndrome.

The term chondromalacia patellae has frequently been used to describe patellofemoral pain syndrome. By definition, the term implies a histologic or an arthroscopic diagnosis of articular softening or fissuring. These changes do not generally occur in children and adolescents with this patellofemoral pain syndrome, although they may be at risk for articular changes as adults.

(5) Certain congenital conditions (e.g., high-riding patella, shallow intercondylar notch, genu valgum deformity) may predispose children to patellar malalignment significant enough to produce recurrent subluxation or dislocation. Significant pain or guarding with attempted lateral or medial displacement (i.e., positive apprehension sign) suggests subluxation. In patellar dislocation the knee is usually locked in approximately 45 degrees of flexion.

(6) A bipartite patella occurs when secondary ossification centers in the patella fail to fuse to the primary ossification center. Most are asymptomatic, but occasionally pain may occur with sports, especially with jumping, or climbing stairs or after nonunion of a fracture between the ossification centers. Symptoms are usually unilateral, and the examination typically reveals pain at the superolateral pole of the patella. X-rays are diagnostic.

(7) Sinding-Larsen-Johansson syndrome is an overuse syndrome similar to Osgood-Schlatter disease, except that the apophysitis occurs at the insertion of the patellar tendon on the inferior pole of the patella. Pain is localized to the inferior pole of the patella and is aggravated by activity. As in Osgood-Schlatter disease, diagnosis is frequently clinical. Patients with similar complaints

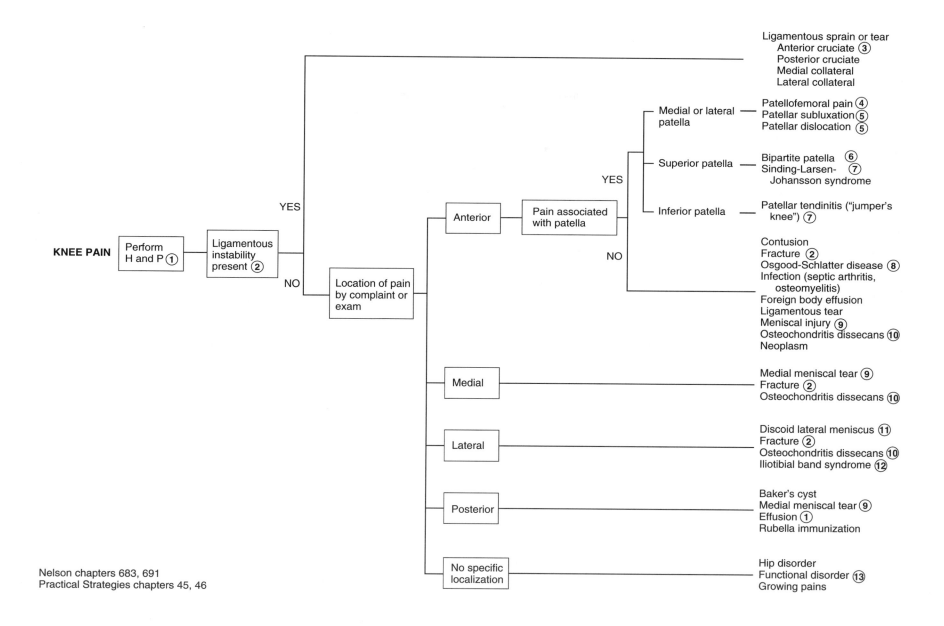

KNEE PAIN

Perform H and P ①

Ligamentous instability present ②

YES

Ligamentous sprain or tear
Anterior cruciate ③
Posterior cruciate
Medial collateral
Lateral collateral

NO

Location of pain by complaint or exam

Anterior

Pain associated with patella

YES

Medial or lateral patella — Patellofemoral pain ④
Patellar subluxation ⑤
Patellar dislocation ⑤

Superior patella — Bipartite patella ⑥
Sinding-Larsen-Johansson syndrome ⑦

Inferior patella — Patellar tendinitis ("jumper's knee") ⑦

NO

Contusion
Fracture ②
Osgood-Schlatter disease ⑧
Infection (septic arthritis, osteomyelitis)
Foreign body effusion
Ligamentous tear
Meniscal injury ⑨
Osteochondritis dissecans ⑩
Neoplasm

Medial

Medial meniscal tear ⑨
Fracture ②
Osteochondritis dissecans ⑩

Lateral

Discoid lateral meniscus ⑪
Fracture ②
Osteochondritis dissecans ⑩
Iliotibial band syndrome ⑫

Posterior

Baker's cyst
Medial meniscal tear ⑨
Effusion ①
Rubella immunization

No specific localization

Hip disorder
Functional disorder ⑬
Growing pains

Nelson chapters 683, 691
Practical Strategies chapters 45, 46

Knee Pain (continued)

and tenderness over the patellar ligament near but not involving the bony attachments are most likely to have patellar tendinitis (i.e., "jumper's knee").

8 Osgood-Schlatter disease is an apophysitis at the site of insertion of the patellar tendon into the tibial tuberosity. It is most common in adolescent athletes who are undergoing a growth spurt. Examination reveals tenderness and swelling at the tibial tubercle and exacerbation of pain with resisted knee extension. Symptoms are commonly bilateral, although one side may be more symptomatic than the other. Patients complain of worsening pain with flexion activities (e.g., running, jumping, kneeling, climbing stairs). Typical X-ray findings are soft tissue swelling and possibly avulsed bony spicules over the tibial tuberosity, although X-rays are not usually indicated when the condition is bilateral. X-rays should be obtained when the pain is unilateral, not located directly over the tibial tuberosity, and in cases unresponsive to treatment.

9 Meniscal injuries are more common in adolescents than in younger age groups. They are most commonly sports injuries due to a twisting motion that occurs when the knee is flexed and the foot is firmly planted on the ground. Medial meniscal tears are more common than lateral tears. Patients complain of vague pain, recurrent effusions, stiffness, giving way, clicking, and sometimes locking. Examination reveals joint line tenderness and occasionally a small effusion. X-rays are not helpful. Arthroscopy is a better diagnostic modality than MRI, which is not very specific for meniscal tears in adolescents.

10 Osteochondritis dissecans is a condition of primary necrosis of the bone with subsequent involvement of the underlying cartilage. The lateral aspect of the medial femoral condyle is the most common site of this lesion. Patients complain of nonspecific pain usually associated with activity and sometimes effusion. Locking may occur if a bony fragment has become dislodged into the joint. X-rays with a notch view may be helpful in diagnosing this condition. The MRI will yield the most accurate assessment.

11 Discoid lateral meniscus is a congenital abnormality in which a plump disc of cartilage replaces the normal semilunar shape. It is usually unstable in the joint, which makes it prone to injury. Patients typically present in late childhood or adolescence with vague, inconsistent complaints of pain and an audible click or clunk with flexion. Examination reveals a palpable, visible "clunk" at the lateral joint line when the knee is flexed. Standing X-rays may show a widened lateral joint space. MRI may be necessary for definitive diagnosis.

12 Iliotibial band tendonitis is a common cause of lateral knee pain in runners.

13 Functional knee pain should be considered a diagnosis of exclusion for persistent knee pain in the presence of a normal examination and evaluation. Environmental stress and anxiety and parental pressure about athletic performance are often contributors.

BIBLIOGRAPHY

Davids JR: Pediatric knee: Clinical assessment and common disorders. Pediatr Clin North Am 43:1067–1090, 1996.

Kelley SS(section ed): Knee and lower leg. In Snider RK (ed): Essentials of Musculoskeletal Care, p 304. Rosemont, IL: American Academy of Orthopaedic Surgeons, 1997.

Smith AD, Scoles PV: The knee. In Scoles PV (ed): Pediatric Orthopedics in Clinical Practice, 2nd ed, p 122. Chicago, Year Book Medical Publishers, 1988.

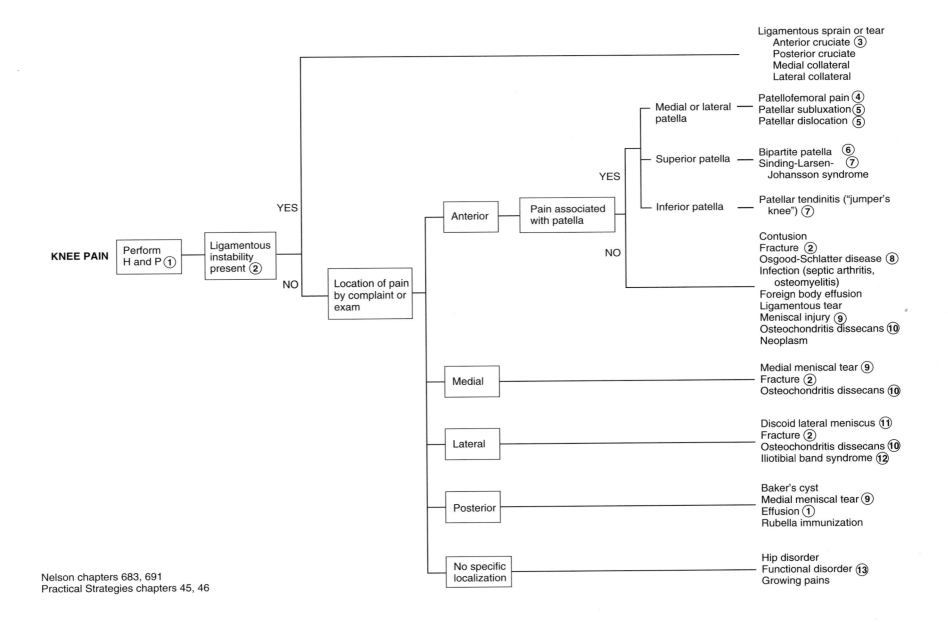

KNEE PAIN

Perform H and P ①

Ligamentous instability present ②

YES

Ligamentous sprain or tear
Anterior cruciate ③
Posterior cruciate
Medial collateral
Lateral collateral

NO

Location of pain by complaint or exam

Anterior

Pain associated with patella

YES

Medial or lateral patella —
Patellofemoral pain ④
Patellar subluxation ⑤
Patellar dislocation ⑤

Superior patella —
Bipartite patella ⑥
Sinding-Larsen-Johansson syndrome ⑦

Inferior patella —
Patellar tendinitis ("jumper's knee") ⑦

NO

Contusion
Fracture ②
Osgood-Schlatter disease ⑧
Infection (septic arthritis, osteomyelitis)
Foreign body effusion
Ligamentous tear
Meniscal injury ⑨
Osteochondritis dissecans ⑩
Neoplasm

Medial

Medial meniscal tear ⑨
Fracture ②
Osteochondritis dissecans ⑩

Lateral

Discoid lateral meniscus ⑪
Fracture ②
Osteochondritis dissecans ⑩
Iliotibial band syndrome ⑫

Posterior

Baker's cyst
Medial meniscal tear ⑨
Effusion ①
Rubella immunization

No specific localization

Hip disorder
Functional disorder ⑬
Growing pains

Nelson chapters 683, 691
Practical Strategies chapters 45, 46

Chapter 45 *Extremity Pain*

Extremity pain only is covered in this chapter. Joint problems, including knee pain, are covered in other chapters. (See Chs. 43 and 44.) Associated symptoms or circumstances should be used to narrow the differential diagnosis.

(1) Be aware of the possibility of unobserved trauma as well as intentional trauma (i.e., child abuse). Inquire specifically about the lifting of a child by the child's extended arm, resulting in a radial head subluxation or "nursemaid's elbow."

(2) Nursemaid's elbow or radial head subluxation commonly occurs when a preschool-aged child is lifted up by the extended pronated forearm. The injury is only mildly painful, but the child is reluctant to use the arm. The child may prefer holding the arm splinted close to the body, often giving the impression of wrist pain. X-rays are nonspecific but should be considered if the history is unclear to rule out other injuries.

(3) "Burners" or "stingers" due to traumatic stretching of the brachial plexus manifest as severe transient pain extending from the shoulder to the fingertips. Accompanying weakness and numbness may occur. These injuries occur most commonly in football players and wrestlers.

(4) Children and adolescents are more susceptible to physeal (growth plate) injury than ligament sprains or diaphyseal (shaft) fractures, because physes in growing children are weaker than ligaments. Injury may be due to physeal fractures (separations) or repetitive microtrauma.

Be aware of the possibility of child abuse when unsuspected fractures are detected.

(5) Night pain is especially characteristic of both benign and malignant primary bone or metastatic tumors. Pain in the absence of local tenderness is another clue.

(6) A contusion of the quadriceps muscle may be complicated by ossification of the hematoma (i.e., myositis ossificans) causing pain and stiffness for several months after the injury.

(7) If symptoms persist, further radiographic investigation (MRI) or repeat studies may be indicated.

(8) Shin splints (i.e., medial tibial stress syndrome) occur as diffuse tenderness along the posteromedial border of the tibia. Imaging is not necessary for diagnosis. Consider X-rays only if a stress fracture is suspected. Bone scans if performed will be abnormal, although the uptake will be less dense than with stress fractures.

(9) Stress fractures occur owing to repetitive overuse. Pain and tenderness are localized with a gradual onset and exacerbation by activity. Swelling may or may not be associated. X-rays may be normal until 3 to 4 weeks after symptom onset when subperiosteal new bone formation may be visible. A bone scan aids in early diagnosis.

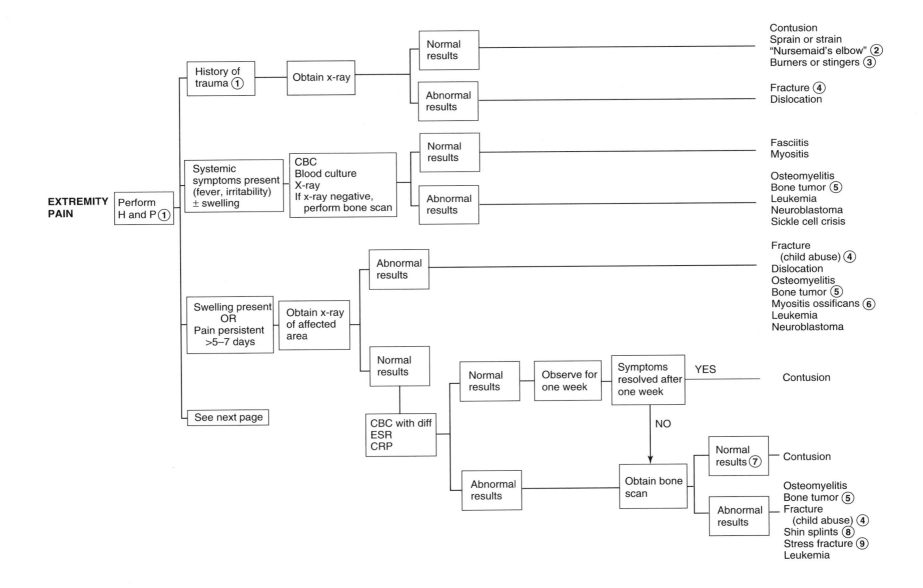

EXTREMITY PAIN — Perform H and P ①

History of trauma ① → Obtain x-ray

- Normal results → Contusion / Sprain or strain / "Nursemaid's elbow" ② / Burners or stingers ③
- Abnormal results → Fracture ④ / Dislocation

Systemic symptoms present (fever, irritability) ± swelling → CBC / Blood culture / X-ray / If x-ray negative, perform bone scan

- Normal results → Fasciitis / Myositis
- Abnormal results → Osteomyelitis / Bone tumor ⑤ / Leukemia / Neuroblastoma / Sickle cell crisis

Swelling present OR Pain persistent >5–7 days → Obtain x-ray of affected area

- Abnormal results → Fracture (child abuse) ④ / Dislocation / Osteomyelitis / Bone tumor ⑤ / Myositis ossificans ⑥ / Leukemia / Neuroblastoma
- Normal results → CBC with diff / ESR / CRP
  - Normal results → Observe for one week → Symptoms resolved after one week
    - YES → Contusion
    - NO → Obtain bone scan
  - Abnormal results → Obtain bone scan
    - Normal results ⑦ → Contusion
    - Abnormal results → Osteomyelitis / Bone tumor ⑤ / Fracture (child abuse) ④ / Shin splints ⑧ / Stress fracture ⑨ / Leukemia

See next page

Extremity Pain (continued)

(10) Reflex sympathetic dystrophy is a rare condition occurring with an acute, severe complaint of intense extremity pain. There is either no history or one of a very minor injury followed by acute pain, swelling, and color and temperature change of the affected area. Erythema and warmth occur initially; chronically, disuse atrophy and cool, clammy skin develop. Laboratory studies and X-ray findings are normal. Bone scan shows a decreased uptake of radioactive material on the affected side. The syndrome occurs most commonly in preteenaged and teenaged girls.

(11) Growing pains (i.e., idiopathic limb pains of childhood) are common. Pain that is unilateral or persists during the day should never be assumed to be growing pains. Children with growing pains complain of diffuse extremity pain, usually in the legs, typically at night that does not affect daytime activity. The physical examination is normal. Massaging characteristically produces relief in these children; it aggravates pain in many other conditions.

(12) Nerve compression manifests by tingling, numbness, and paresthesias ("pins and needles") in addition to pain. Carpal tunnel syndrome classically occurs as numbness on the radial side of the hand, and ulnar nerve entrapment occurs as numbness on the ulnar side of the hand (4th and 5th fingers). Although rare in children, cervical nerve compression should be considered, especially if there is a history of neck trauma or symptoms are worse with the arm in an overhead position (i.e., thoracic outlet syndrome). MRI or an electromyogram should be considered when arm or shoulder pain accompanies numbness and tingling to rule out cervical nerve compression.

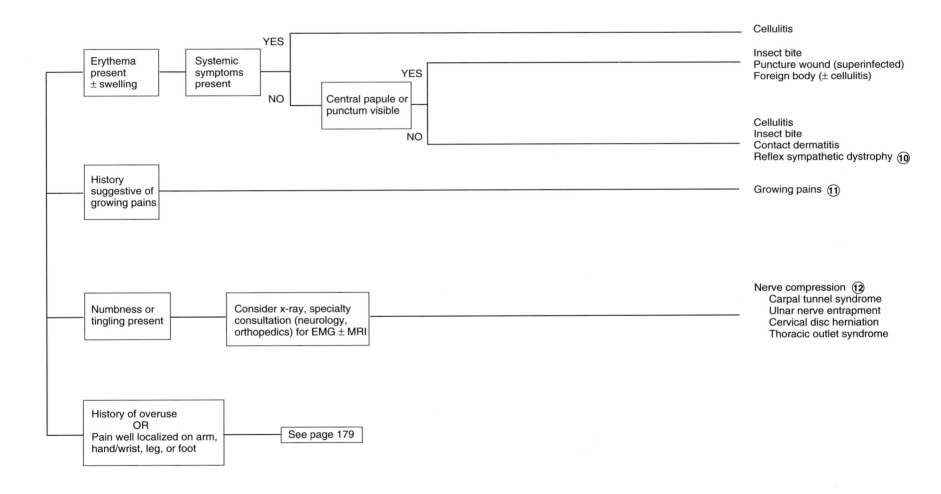

EMG = Electromyography

(13) Overuse syndromes do not require X-rays for diagnosis. X-rays or consultation with a sports medicine physician should be considered if symptoms do not improve in response to an appropriate course of treatment. X-rays may also aid in the diagnosis of those conditions listed here that are not evident by history or physical examination and those that are not consistent with overuse syndromes.

(14) Carpal tunnel syndrome is caused by entrapment of the median nerve at the wrist and occurs as vague pain and numbness in the thenar region and proximal forearm.

(15) Tenosynovitis of the wrist occurs as pain and swelling of the lateral aspect of the wrist. A locking or sticking sensation may occur as the patient moves the thumb.

(16) Ulnar nerve irritation or ulnar nerve entrapment appears as tingling, numbness, and weakness of the fourth and fifth fingers.

(17) Tarsal coalitions may develop in late childhood or adolescence as stiff and painful flat feet.

(18) Plantar fasciitis is heel pain that may radiate over the entire plantar fascial surface and is typically worse in the morning but improves over the course of the day.

(19) Sever disease is an apophysitis at the site of the heel cord (Achilles tendon) insertion into the calcaneus due to overuse. Children 6 to 10 years of age are affected and complain of posterior heel pain. A limp is often present.

(20) Accessory navicular bones may become symptomatic in late childhood or early adolescence with pain and tenderness along the medial aspect of the navicular bone.

(21) Freiberg infraction (i.e., osteonecrosis of the head of the metatarsal bone) causes pain in the forefoot that worsens with activity. The condition is usually related to trauma and occurs most commonly in adolescent females.

Köhler disease (i.e., osteonecrosis of the tarsal navicular) occurs in children 4 to 8 years of age. Patients complain of pain in the medial arch.

(22) The term "Little League elbow" encompasses a variety of disorders in and around the elbow, the most common of which is a traction apophysitis (i.e., inflammation at the site of tendon insertion into the bone) of the medial epicondyle.

(23) Panner disease, an osteochondrosis of the lateral epicondyle of the distal humeral epiphysis, occurs acutely with lateral elbow pain in the young (<10 years old) athlete. In older athletes, the condition is called osteochondritis dissecans. Its onset is more insidious and more likely to be associated with a loose body.

(24) Slipped capital femoral epiphysis (SCFE) and avascular necrosis of the hip (AVN or Legg-Calvé-Perthes disease) occur as a limp and hip pain or poorly localized medial thigh or knee pain. If either condition is suspected, X-rays should be obtained. (See Ch. 42.)

(25) Localized tenderness over the anterior iliac crest characterizes iliac apophysitis. It is seen most commonly in adolescent runners, especially during a growth spurt and when they are increasing their mileage.

BIBLIOGRAPHY

Greene W (section ed): Pediatric orthopaedics. In Snider RK (ed): Essentials of Musculoskeletal Care, p 549. Rosemont, IL: American Academy of Orthopaedic Surgeons, 1997.

Hoffinger SA: Evaluation and management of pediatric foot deformities. Pediatr Clin North Am 43:1091–1111, 1996.

Saperstein AL, Nicolas SJ: Pediatric and adolescent sports medicine. Pediatr Clin North Am 43:1013–1033, 1996.

Schaller JG: Pain syndromes. In Behrman RE, Kliegman RM, Arvin AM (eds): Nelson Textbook of Pediatrics, 15th ed, p 686. Philadelphia: WB Saunders Company, 1996.

Smith AD: Children and sports. In Scoles PV (ed): Pediatric Orthopedics in Clinical Practice, 2nd ed, p 269. Chicago: Year Book Medical Publishers, 1988.

EXTREMITY PAIN (continued)

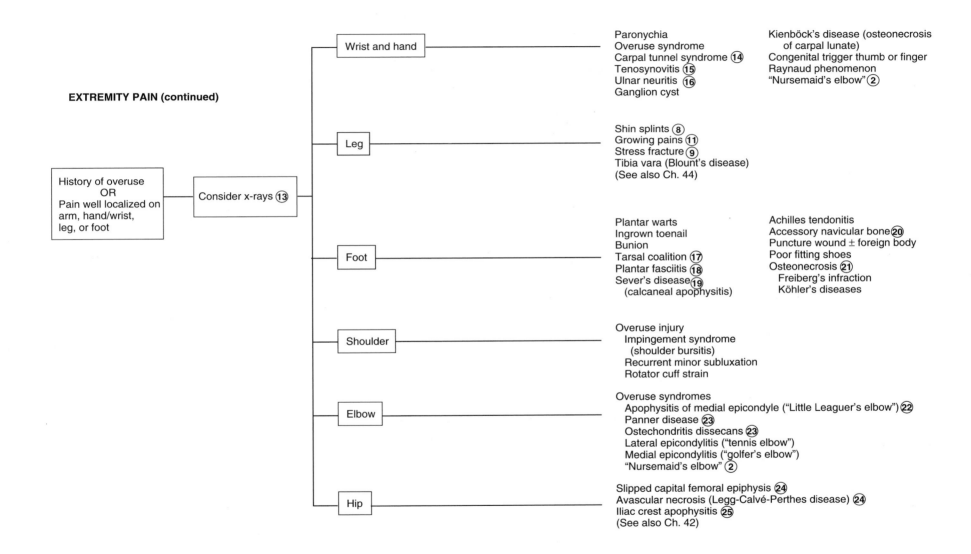

History of overuse
OR
Pain well localized on arm, hand/wrist, leg, or foot → Consider x-rays ⑬

Wrist and hand

Paronychia
Overuse syndrome
Carpal tunnel syndrome ⑭
Tenosynovitis ⑮
Ulnar neuritis ⑯
Ganglion cyst

Kienböck's disease (osteonecrosis of carpal lunate)
Congenital trigger thumb or finger
Raynaud phenomenon
"Nursemaid's elbow" ②

Leg

Shin splints ⑧
Growing pains ⑪
Stress fracture ⑨
Tibia vara (Blount's disease)
(See also Ch. 44)

Foot

Plantar warts
Ingrown toenail
Bunion
Tarsal coalition ⑰
Plantar fasciitis ⑱
Sever's disease ⑲
   (calcaneal apophysitis)

Achilles tendonitis
Accessory navicular bone ⑳
Puncture wound ± foreign body
Poor fitting shoes
Osteonecrosis ㉑
   Freiberg's infraction
   Köhler's diseases

Shoulder

Overuse injury
   Impingement syndrome
      (shoulder bursitis)
   Recurrent minor subluxation
   Rotator cuff strain

Elbow

Overuse syndromes
   Apophysitis of medial epicondyle ("Little Leaguer's elbow") ㉒
   Panner disease ㉓
   Ostechondritis dissecans ㉓
   Lateral epicondylitis ("tennis elbow")
   Medial epicondylitis ("golfer's elbow")
   "Nursemaid's elbow" ②

Hip

Slipped capital femoral epiphysis ㉔
Avascular necrosis (Legg-Calvé-Perthes disease) ㉔
Iliac crest apophysitis ㉕
(See also Ch. 42)

Chapter 46 Back Pain

Back pain is rare in children, especially severe or persistent back pain. Most children who complain of back pain have mild self-resolving symptoms of limited duration. Symptoms of severe or persistent back pain, as well as any abnormal finding on physical examination, mandate a thorough evaluation.

(1) The history should include trauma, associated leg pain, gait abnormalities, enuresis or incontinence, and any systemic signs or symptoms (e.g., fever, malaise, rashes, gastrointestinal symptoms). The physical should include a careful neurologic examination.

(2) Discitis is an infection or inflammation of an intervertebral disc space. The most common pathogen is *Staphylococcus aureus*. Common clinical findings are back pain, stiff straight posture due to loss of normal lumbar lordosis, and pain with flexion of the hips and/or lumbar spine. The degree of systemic illness is variable with younger children (i.e., younger than 3 years old), more likely to present with a toxic picture of fever, refusal to walk, irritability, and decreased appetite. Older children and adolescents may also complain of leg pain and may be afebrile. Bone scan or MRI may be necessary for early diagnosis; typical X-ray changes within 2 to 4 weeks are narrowing of the involved disc space and irregularities of adjacent vertebral endplates.

(3) X-ray or bone scan may not be as reliable for detecting leukemic involvement of the spine as it is for other sites. MRI may be more useful to assess spinal and intraspinal involvement.

(4) Primary vertebral osteomyelitis is rare in young children. It typically occurs in children older than 8 years of age as a result of hematogenous infection. It may present as a constant dull backache or as an acute febrile illness after a more chronic complaint of back pain. Pott disease is tuberculosis spondylitis, the most common bone manifestation of untreated tuberculosis.

(5) Intraabdominal or retroperitoneal processes can cause referred back pain. More specific signs and symptoms should aid in the diagnosis of problems such as pyelonephritis, pancreatitis, nephrolithiasis, and perinephric or muscle (e.g., paraspinal, psoas) abscesses.

(6) If pain persists, a bone scan should be performed to rule out a fracture not detected by X-ray.

(7) Contusions and abrasions are the most common back injuries sustained in routine play and sports in young children. If no associated injuries are present, and the physical examination is normal with no abnormalities of trunk configuration or lower extremities, no additional workup is needed.

(8) Back pain associated with bowel or bladder deficits, gait abnormalities, lower extremity pain, weakness, or reflex or sensation deficits is suggestive of space-occupying lesions (e.g., spinal cord tumors, metastatic lesions). Prompt diagnosis and treatment is critical to minimize morbidity.

(9) Spondylolysis is a defect of the bony connection between a vertebral body and its arch (i.e., pars interarticularis). Spondylolisthesis is the forward slippage or displacement of one vertebra in relation to another. Classic spondylolisthesis in children and adolescents involves the fifth lumbar and first sacral units. In these cases fatigue or stress fractures of the pars interarticularis bilaterally allow the posterior articulation of L5 and S1 to persist while the body of L5 slips forward. Children participating in sports involving repetitive flexion and hyperextension are at increased risk for spondylolysis. Symptoms (poorly localized lumbar and lumbosacral pain, hamstring tightness) often do not occur until the adolescent growth spurt. Defects often remain asymptomatic indefinitely. When symptoms do occur, they are not always consistent with the severity of the spondylolytic defect or the degree of slippage. In contrast to adults, nerve root signs and symptoms are rare in children and adolescents.

(10) Kyphosis is an exaggeration of the normal thoracic or thoracolumbar curve in the sagittal plane. X-rays should be taken in severe cases and when back pain is present to rule out Scheuermann disease. In Scheuermann disease, vertebral endplate irregularities and vertebral body wedging are associated with the kyphosis. Most cases of scoliosis, regardless of the age at onset, are idiopathic. Idiopathic scoliosis is not painful during childhood and adolescence. If pain is noted with a scoliotic curve, rule out infectious, inflammatory, and neoplastic causes.

(11) Benign tumors of the spine are rare. The most common ones are osteoid osteoma, osteoblastoma, and eosinophilic granuloma. Presentation is typically a prolonged period of back pain (especially at night) that eventually evolves to stiffness and a painful scoliosis. Aneurysmal bone cysts are also considered benign tumors.

(12) Overuse syndromes are more common in athletic adolescents than younger children. The stress of normal physiologic activity results in microtrauma, which typically resolves. Overuse injuries result when repetitive activity without adequate conditioning or rest prohibits this resolution. Both bone and soft tissues (muscles, ligaments, bursae) are susceptible to overuse injuries. Gymnasts and dancers are particularly prone to overuse injuries of the back. Carrying a heavy book bag or backpack may cause back pain.

BIBLIOGRAPHY

Scoles PV: The spine. In Scoles PV (ed): Pediatric Orthopedics in Clinical Practice, 2nd ed, p 179. Chicago: Year Book Medical Publishers, 1988.

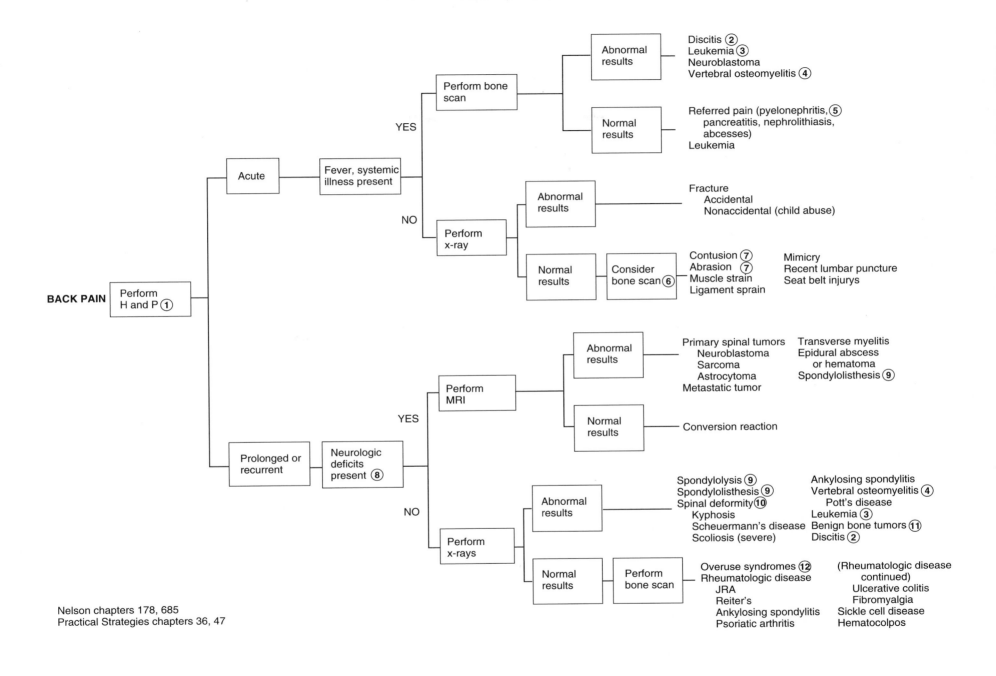

BACK PAIN — Perform H and P ①

Acute → Fever, systemic illness present

YES → Perform bone scan
- Abnormal results:
  - Discitis ②
  - Leukemia ③
  - Neuroblastoma
  - Vertebral osteomyelitis ④
- Normal results:
  - Referred pain (pyelonephritis, ⑤ pancreatitis, nephrolithiasis, abcesses)
  - Leukemia

NO → Perform x-ray
- Abnormal results:
  - Fracture
    - Accidental
    - Nonaccidental (child abuse)
- Normal results → Consider bone scan ⑥
  - Contusion ⑦
  - Abrasion ⑦
  - Muscle strain
  - Ligament sprain
  - Mimicry
  - Recent lumbar puncture
  - Seat belt injurys

Prolonged or recurrent → Neurologic deficits present ⑧

YES → Perform MRI
- Abnormal results:
  - Primary spinal tumors
    - Neuroblastoma
    - Sarcoma
    - Astrocytoma
  - Metastatic tumor
  - Transverse myelitis
  - Epidural abscess or hematoma
  - Spondylolisthesis ⑨
- Normal results:
  - Conversion reaction

NO → Perform x-rays
- Abnormal results:
  - Spondylolysis ⑨
  - Spondylolisthesis ⑨
  - Spinal deformity ⑩
    - Kyphosis
    - Scheuermann's disease
    - Scoliosis (severe)
  - Ankylosing spondylitis
  - Vertebral osteomyelitis ④
    - Pott's disease
  - Leukemia ③
  - Benign bone tumors ⑪
  - Discitis ②
- Normal results → Perform bone scan
  - Overuse syndromes ⑫
  - Rheumatologic disease
    - JRA
    - Reiter's
    - Ankylosing spondylitis
    - Psoriatic arthritis
  - (Rheumatologic disease continued)
    - Ulcerative colitis
    - Fibromyalgia
    - Sickle cell disease
    - Hematocolpos

Nelson chapters 178, 685
Practical Strategies chapters 36, 47

Chapter 47 Stiff or Painful Neck

Most causes of neck pain and stiffness in children are benign; however, potentially life-threatening conditions (e.g., meningitis, cervical spine fracture) must always be ruled out.

(1) The history should clarify the nature and duration of the complaint, as well as a comprehensive review of systems. The physical examination should assess stiffness (nuchal rigidity) and range of motion of the neck (lateral movement and flexion-extension) and attempt to localize the pain (muscle spasm, muscle or bone tenderness). The differential diagnosis for a child whose neck can be moved, even if painful, is different from that of a child whose range of motion is limited.

Torticollis or "wry neck" describes a condition in which the infant or child holds the neck in a rotated, tilted condition. It may be the sole manifestation of a disorder (congenital torticollis) or be an accompanying symptom of numerous disorders (infectious, CNS neoplasia, structural, inflammatory, neurologic).

A thorough neurologic examination including mental status, cranial nerve involvement, upper extremity pain or weakness, and cerebellar function is important.

(2) Congenital muscular torticollis appears in the first several weeks of life. The head is tilted toward a shortened sternocleidomastoid muscle; a fibrous mass is frequently palpable in the muscle belly. X-rays should be performed to rule out congenital bony abnormalities.

(3) A suspected cervical spine injury should be treated in the acute setting with cervical spine immobilization until appropriate X-rays can be taken. Anteroposterior, lateral, and open mouth odontoid views should be taken with good visualization of the vertebral bodies from the occiput to the top of the first thoracic vertebrae.

(4) Cervical spine subluxation that is usually atlantoaxial may occur as a result of mild as well as severe trauma. Torticollis occurs with neck pain and sternocleidomastoid muscle tenderness on the same side the as the head rotation. Spinal cord compromise and neurologic symptoms generally do not occur.

(5) The ligamentous laxity and hypermobility of the cervical spine and a potentially narrow spinal canal in young children place them at risk for spinal cord injury in the absence of radiographic abnormalities. The injury due to hyperflexion, hyperextension, or ischemia may occur as a progressive paralysis within 48 hours of injury. Sometimes transient neurologic symptoms occur and then resolve and recur in a more severe form within a day.

(6) In meningitis, meningeal signs (e.g., nuchal rigidity, Kernig and Brudzinski signs) are usually accompanied by systemic signs of illness, including fever, altered consciousness, and possibly seizures. The neck stiffness is due to inflammation of the cervical dura and spasm of the neck extensor muscles. Meningeal signs may not be present with meningitis in children younger than 18 to 24 months of age.

With bacterial meningitis, CSF analysis usually reveals a low glucose level of usually less than 40 mg/dl, a high protein level, a neutrophilic leukocytosis, and a positive Gram stain.

(7) Postinfectious encephalitis mimics meningitis with signs and symptoms of fever, headache, stiff neck, and occasionally mental status changes, coma, and seizures. The condition occurs 1 to 3 weeks after common viral or bacterial infections in children. The CSF may be normal, show elevated pressure only, or show increased white cells or protein. Culture is always sterile.

(8) Tumor of any origin (nerve, muscle, bone) may occur acutely with a stiff neck, owing to swelling or nerve compression. Nocturnal pain may indicate an osteoid osteoma. Diagnosis is by X-ray or bone scan.

(9) Approximately 15% of children with Down syndrome have atlantoaxial instability or subluxation (i.e., increased mobility at the atlantoaxial joint), which may be a risk factor for catastrophic spinal cord injury. Patients may be asymptomatic or have slowly progressive neurologic symptoms ranging from neck pain to clumsiness, sensory deficits, spasticity, or, rarely, paralysis. Currently, lateral neck films of patients with Down syndrome are required for participation in the Special Olympics, although their value is limited. Careful longitudinal assessment of these patients is critical. The families must be carefully educated regarding the patient's risks and presenting symptoms.

Occasionally, a mild atlantoaxial subluxation may occur in children without risk factors (Down syndrome, rheumatoid arthritis, skeletal dysplasias) and in the absence of trauma. The cause is presumed to be inflammation related to pharyngitis or an upper respiratory tract infection causing increased laxity of spinal ligaments. Children between 6 and 12 years of age are most commonly affected and present with a painful torticollis with the head rotation and neck pain localized to the side opposite the site of inflammation. If routine X-rays are not diagnostic, high-resolution CT with three-dimensional reconstruction may be necessary to make the diagnosis. Neurologic symptoms are rare.

(10) Abnormal eye movements (e.g., nystagmus, superior oblique muscle weakness) or strabismus may result in compensatory neck stiffness and torticollis in infants.

(11) Neuroimaging may not be indicated if a drug effect is suspected. Certain drugs, including neuroleptic agents and anticonvulsants, can produce dystonic reactions. Ingestion of phenothiazines will occasionally result in an "oculogyric crisis" with torticollis, involuntary deviation and fixation of the gaze, usually upward, and associated "cogwheeling" neck stiffness.

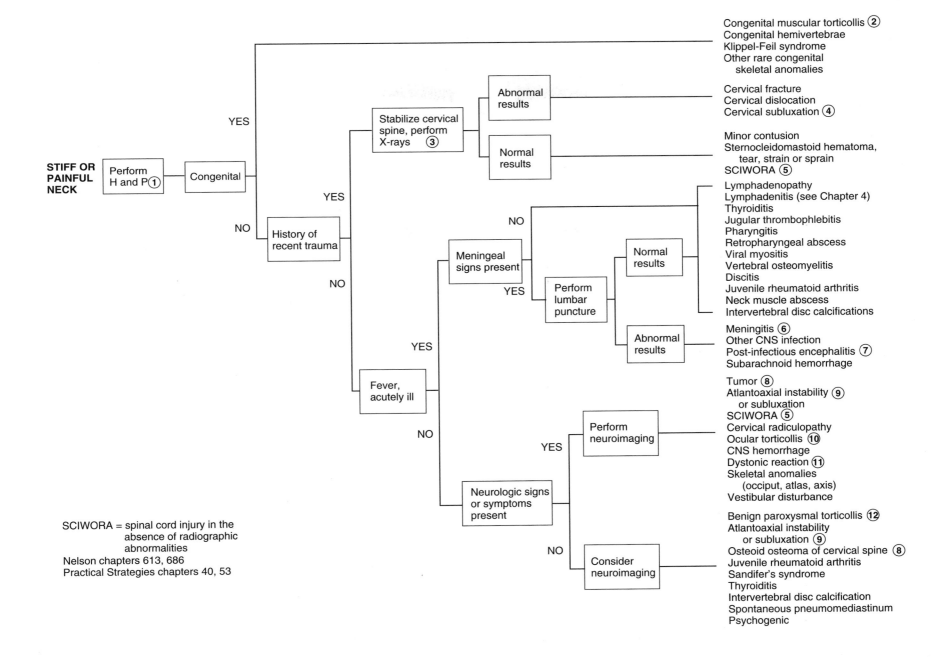

STIFF OR PAINFUL NECK → Perform H and P ①

Congenital — **YES** →
Congenital muscular torticollis ②
Congenital hemivertebrae
Klippel-Feil syndrome
Other rare congenital skeletal anomalies

— **NO** → History of recent trauma — **YES** → Stabilize cervical spine, perform X-rays ③

Abnormal results →
Cervical fracture
Cervical dislocation
Cervical subluxation ④

Normal results →
Minor contusion
Sternocleidomastoid hematoma, tear, strain or sprain
SCIWORA ⑤

— **NO** → Fever, acutely ill — **YES** → Meningeal signs present

NO →
Lymphadenopathy
Lymphadenitis (see Chapter 4)
Thyroiditis
Jugular thrombophlebitis
Pharyngitis
Retropharyngeal abscess
Viral myositis
Vertebral osteomyelitis
Discitis
Juvenile rheumatoid arthritis
Neck muscle abscess
Intervertebral disc calcifications

YES → Perform lumbar puncture

Normal results →
(above list)

Abnormal results →
Meningitis ⑥
Other CNS infection
Post-infectious encephalitis ⑦
Subarachnoid hemorrhage

— **NO** → Neurologic signs or symptoms present — **YES** → Perform neuroimaging →
Tumor ⑧
Atlantoaxial instability ⑨ or subluxation
SCIWORA ⑤
Cervical radiculopathy
Ocular torticollis ⑩
CNS hemorrhage
Dystonic reaction ⑪
Skeletal anomalies (occiput, atlas, axis)
Vestibular disturbance

— **NO** → Consider neuroimaging →
Benign paroxysmal torticollis ⑫
Atlantoaxial instability or subluxation ⑨
Osteoid osteoma of cervical spine ⑧
Juvenile rheumatoid arthritis
Sandifer's syndrome
Thyroiditis
Intervertebral disc calcification
Spontaneous pneumomediastinum
Psychogenic

SCIWORA = spinal cord injury in the absence of radiographic abnormalities
Nelson chapters 613, 686
Practical Strategies chapters 40, 53

12 Benign paroxysmal torticollis is characterized by torticollis of variable duration that may or may not be accompanied by symptoms of pallor, agitation, or vomiting. The onset is in the first year of life, and consciousness is not impaired.

BIBLIOGRAPHY

American Academy of Pediatrics, Committee on Sports Medicine and Fitness: Atlantoaxial instability in Down syndrome: Subject review. Pediatrics 96:151, 1995.

Epps HR, Salter RB: Orthopedic conditions of the cervical spine and shoulder. Pediatr Clin North Am 43:919–931, 1996.

Kuppermann N: Neck stiffness. In Fleisher G, Ludwig S: Textbook of Pediatric Emergency Medicine, 4th ed, p 391. Baltimore: Williams and Wilkins, 2000.

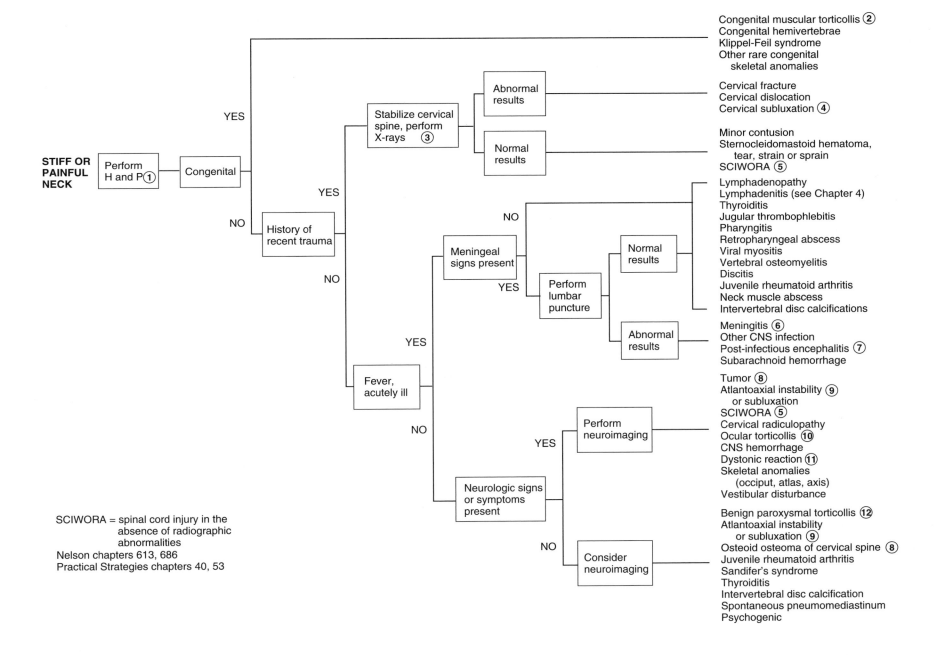

STIFF OR PAINFUL NECK → Perform H and P ① → Congenital

YES → Congenital muscular torticollis ②
Congenital hemivertebrae
Klippel-Feil syndrome
Other rare congenital
    skeletal anomalies

NO → History of recent trauma

YES → Stabilize cervical spine, perform X-rays ③

Abnormal results → Cervical fracture
Cervical dislocation
Cervical subluxation ④

Normal results → Minor contusion
Sternocleidomastoid hematoma,
    tear, strain or sprain
SCIWORA ⑤

NO → Fever, acutely ill

YES → Meningeal signs present

NO → Lymphadenopathy
Lymphadenitis (see Chapter 4)
Thyroiditis
Jugular thrombophlebitis
Pharyngitis
Retropharyngeal abscess
Viral myositis
Vertebral osteomyelitis
Discitis
Juvenile rheumatoid arthritis
Neck muscle abscess
Intervertebral disc calcifications

YES → Perform lumbar puncture

Normal results →

Abnormal results → Meningitis ⑥
Other CNS infection
Post-infectious encephalitis ⑦
Subarachnoid hemorrhage

NO → Neurologic signs or symptoms present

YES → Perform neuroimaging → Tumor ⑧
Atlantoaxial instability ⑨
    or subluxation
SCIWORA ⑤
Cervical radiculopathy
Ocular torticollis ⑩
CNS hemorrhage
Dystonic reaction ⑪
Skeletal anomalies
    (occiput, atlas, axis)
Vestibular disturbance

NO → Consider neuroimaging → Benign paroxysmal torticollis ⑫
Atlantoaxial instability
    or subluxation ⑨
Osteoid osteoma of cervical spine ⑧
Juvenile rheumatoid arthritis
Sandifer's syndrome
Thyroiditis
Intervertebral disc calcification
Spontaneous pneumomediastinum
Psychogenic

SCIWORA = spinal cord injury in the
    absence of radiographic
    abnormalities
Nelson chapters 613, 686
Practical Strategies chapters 40, 53

Chapter 48 *In-Toeing, Out-Toeing, and Toe-Walking*

In-toeing and out-toeing are the most common gait disturbances and can be due to disorders occurring anywhere between the hip and foot. Torsional deformities are most common.

Version is the normal degree of rotation or twisting of a limb segment. Femoral anteversion is normal. The distal aspect of the femur (femoral condyles) is rotated medially or twisted anteriorly, relative to the proximal aspect (i.e., femoral head and neck). Torsion, also called rotational malalignment, is the term used to describe version that is in excess of 2 standard deviations of the norm. It frequently results in an in-toed (or out-toed if the rotation is lateral) gait but rarely in functional disability. Femoral anteversion is greatest at birth, although its impact is compensated by normally tight hip contractures, resulting in some degree of lateral hip rotation. Remodeling slowly normalizes femoral anteversion by 8 or 9 years of age.

The distal aspect of the tibia is normally rotated medially relative to the proximal aspect (tibial torsion), resulting in a bowed or in-toed appearance of the lower extremity. This appearance is usually exaggerated in the infant due to *in utero* positioning.

(1) The history for a child presenting with a gait problem should include the age at onset, a birth and developmental history, and any exacerbating factors (e.g., fatigue, running). In addition to a careful spine, lower extremity, and neurologic examination, a rotational profile (see the algorithm) is very helpful in the evaluation of torsional deformities.

(2) Internal (medial) tibial torsion is the most common cause of in-toeing in children younger than 2 years of age. Remodeling typically decreases the degree of tibial torsion to normal by 2 to 3 years of age.

(3) Internal (medial) femoral torsion is the most common cause of in-toeing in children older than 2 years of age. Females are affected more often than males. In addition to "W" sitting, affected children frequently exhibit generalized ligamentous laxity and exaggeration of their in-toeing when fatigued.

(4) An atavistic great toe "searches" or "wanders" and gives the impression of an active or dynamic in-toeing process. The abnormality is not evident at rest.

(5) Metatarsus adductus occurs as an effect of *in utero* molding (compression) on the developing foot. The forefoot is adducted and occasionally supinated relative to the normal midfoot and hindfoot. The lateral border of the foot is not straight but convex or "C" shaped. Assessment of the mobility of the deformity is very important; feet that correct to neutral or overcorrect are mild cases and may be observed. If the deformity is fixed and does not actively or passively correct, referral for orthopedic consultation is indicated. In 10% of metatarsus adductus cases, developmental dysplasia of the hip is associated.

(6) External (lateral) femoral torsion is an occasional cause of bilateral out-toeing. It is more commonly unilateral if it occurs with a slipped capital femoral epiphysis.

(7) External (lateral) tibial torsion usually occurs in conjunction with a calcaneovalgus foot. The *in utero* foot is forced into a hyperdorsiflexed position, resulting in a dorsiflexed foot with varying degrees of eversion, forefoot abduction, and an abnormally high degree of tibial external rotation. When associated with a calcaneovalgus foot, X-rays may be necessary to rule out a posteromedial bow of the tibia or vertical talus. Neuromuscular assessment should rule out a paralyzed gastrocnemius muscle.

(8) Flat feet ("pes planus") may give the impression of out-toeing when the patient is standing.

(9) Habitual toe-walking may be a normal finding until 3 years of age. Neurologic examination and range of motion (i.e., passive dorsiflexion beyond 15 degrees) are normal. Beyond 3 years of age, or if acquired after the patient has been walking normally for a period of time, assessment to rule out other causes is indicated. Referral for electromyography or gait analysis may be necessary to distinguish between mild cerebral palsy and congenital contracture of the Achilles tendon.

(10) A small amount of length-leg discrepancy is normal. Most children easily compensate for a 1- to 2-cm discrepancy. Acquired toe-walking with a leg-length asymmetry should be evaluated by a pediatric orthopedist.

(11) Torsion dystonia, previously called idiopathic dystonia musculorum deformans, is a movement disorder that appears late in the first or second decade of life. It typically begins with unilateral foot or leg involvement presenting as toe-walking and progresses to generalized involvement.

BIBLIOGRAPHY

Bruce RW: Torsional and angular deformities. Pediatr Clin North Am 43:867–881, 1996.

Hoffinger SA: Evaluation and management of pediatric foot deformities. Pediatr Clin North Am 43:1091–1111, 1996.

Scoles PV: Lower extremity development. In Scoles PV (ed): Pediatric Orthopedics in Clinical Practice, 2nd ed, p 82. Chicago: Year Book Medical Publishers, 1988.

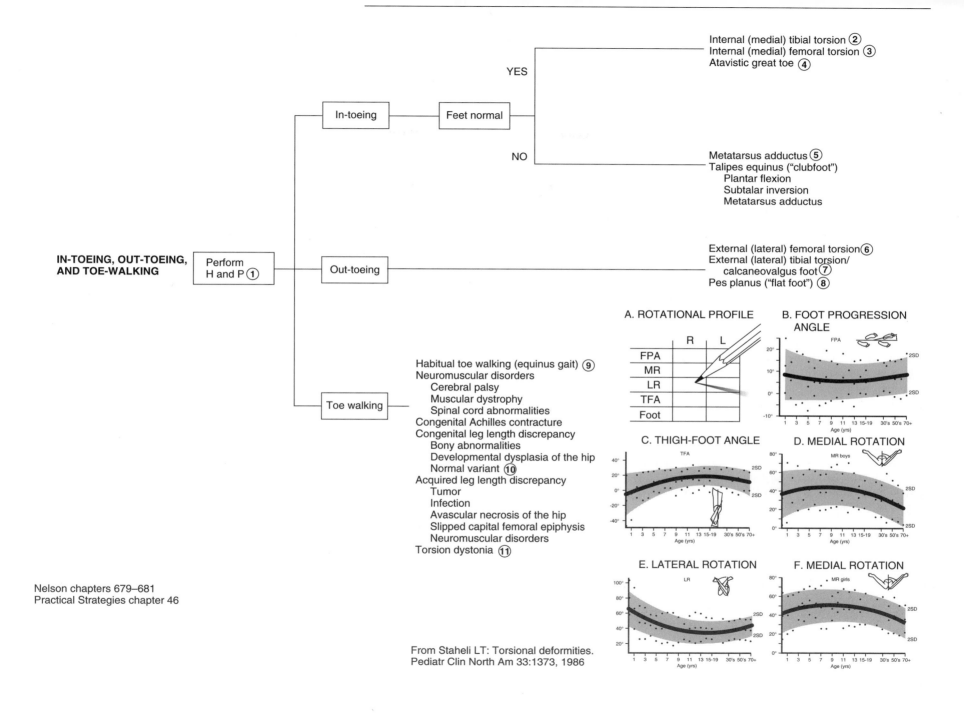

IN-TOEING, OUT-TOEING, AND TOE-WALKING

Perform H and P ①

In-toeing → Feet normal

YES
- Internal (medial) tibial torsion ②
- Internal (medial) femoral torsion ③
- Atavistic great toe ④

NO
- Metatarsus adductus ⑤
- Talipes equinus ("clubfoot")
  - Plantar flexion
  - Subtalar inversion
  - Metatarsus adductus

Out-toeing
- External (lateral) femoral torsion ⑥
- External (lateral) tibial torsion/ calcaneovalgus foot ⑦
- Pes planus ("flat foot") ⑧

Toe walking
- Habitual toe walking (equinus gait) ⑨
- Neuromuscular disorders
  - Cerebral palsy
  - Muscular dystrophy
  - Spinal cord abnormalities
- Congenital Achilles contracture
- Congenital leg length discrepancy
  - Bony abnormalities
  - Developmental dysplasia of the hip
  - Normal variant ⑩
- Acquired leg length discrepancy
  - Tumor
  - Infection
  - Avascular necrosis of the hip
  - Slipped capital femoral epiphysis
  - Neuromuscular disorders
- Torsion dystonia ⑪

Nelson chapters 679–681
Practical Strategies chapter 46

From Staheli LT: Torsional deformities.
Pediatr Clin North Am 33:1373, 1986

A. ROTATIONAL PROFILE

	R	L
FPA		
MR		
LR		
TFA		
Foot		

B. FOOT PROGRESSION ANGLE

C. THIGH-FOOT ANGLE

D. MEDIAL ROTATION

E. LATERAL ROTATION

F. MEDIAL ROTATION

Chapter 49 **Bowlegs and Knock-Knees**

Angular deformities such as bowlegs and knock-knees are common complaints. Spontaneous resolution is the rule for most cases. It is important to know when to be concerned about a potentially pathologic diagnosis when treating an angular deformity.

Angular alignment of the lower extremities at birth is typically varus at the knee (bowlegged), although most of this impression is due to lateral hip external rotation and tibial torsion rather than an angular problem. Normal bony remodeling occurs over the first 2 years of life with typical resolution of this physiologic genu varum or bowlegs to a near-neutral position. Subsequent development over the second and third year of life normally results in a valgus alignment at the knees (i.e., genu valgum or knock-knees), which slowly neutralizes to the normal adult alignment of slight valgus by age 7 or 8 years.

(1) The history should clearly elucidate the nature of the complaint, age at onset, progression, and previous treatment. It may also be helpful to ask the parents to clarify their exact concerns and fears about the child's appearance and future prognosis. A complete medical, developmental, and family history should be part of the evaluation. A birth history and history of breast-feeding or unusual diet may also be helpful.

The physical assessment should include careful measurements and observation of the gait. A rotational profile should be done because rotational malalignment may contribute to the appearance of genu varum or valgum. (See Ch. 48.) Joints should be assessed for laxity and swelling suggesting arthritis. Extremities should be assessed for asymmetry suggesting bony abnormalities (congenital absence, hypoplasia). Café-au-lait spots or neurofibromas may indicate neurofibromatosis.

(2) Gentle reassurance of parental concerns and education about the expected course of these conditions are often all that is necessary. Certain indicators, such as short stature and significant asymmetry, do indicate further workup for a cause other than physiologic. A preliminary X-ray (standing anteroposterior) evaluation of the lower extremities should be done if any worrisome conditions are present to localize the deformity and identify any obvious bony abnormalities. Failure to follow a normal developmental sequence, rapid progression of the deformity, family history of a pathologic condition, and physical findings suggestive of an underlying abnormality (e.g., neurofibromatosis, arthritis, infection) warrant further evaluation.

(3) Genu varum (i.e., physiologic bowlegs) is usually a combination of a normal varus angulation of the knee and internal tibial torsion that is normal in the infant and toddler. Neutralization by 2 to 3 years of age is the norm. Persistence beyond age 3 years or a severe case (>4–5 inches intercondylar distance, 20-degree tibial femoral angle) warrants investigation to rule out a pathologic cause.

(4) Physiologic genu valgum (i.e., knock-knees) develops as the natural overcorrection of physiologic genu varus and occurs between the second and third years of life. Resolution generally occurs between 5 and 8 years of age.

(5) Asymmetric growth of the tibial growth plate results in tibia vara (Blount disease), characterized by severe, progressive bowing. Infantile onset (age 1 to 3 years) is most common and is characterized by a female and black predominance, marked obesity, and mostly (80%) bilateral involvement. Late onset (age 4 years or older) is characterized by a male and black predominance, marked obesity, bilateral involvement in approximately 50% of patients, and pain rather than deformity as the primary complaint. X-rays show medial metaphyseal irregularity, beaking of the proximal tibia, and wedging of the proximal epiphysis.

(6) Congenital pseudoarthrosis of the tibia appears early in infancy as an anterolateral bowing of the tibia. It occurs in 50% of children with neurofibromatosis.

(7) Bony dysplasias may be characterized by metaphyseal, diaphyseal, epiphyseal, or physeal plate abnormalities.

(8) Neuromuscular disorders generally occur as knock-knee (valgus) deformities.

BIBLIOGRAPHY

Bruce RW: Torsional and angular deformities. Pediatr Clin North Am 43:867–881, 1996.

Mankin KP, Zimbler S: Gait and leg alignment: What's normal and what's not. Contemp Pediatr 14:41, 1997.

Scoles PV: Lower extremity development. In Scoles PV (ed): Pediatric Orthopedics in Clinical Practice, 2nd ed, p 82. Chicago: Year Book Medical Publishers, 1988.

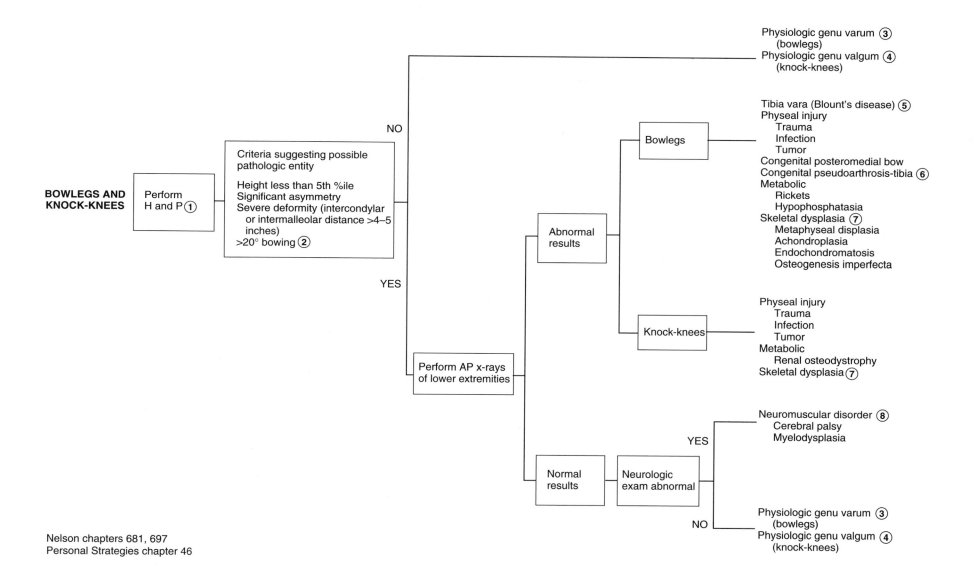

BOWLEGS AND KNOCK-KNEES

Perform H and P ①

Criteria suggesting possible pathologic entity

Height less than 5th %ile
Significant asymmetry
Severe deformity (intercondylar or intermalleolar distance >4–5 inches)
>20° bowing ②

NO → Physiologic genu varum ③ (bowlegs)
Physiologic genu valgum ④ (knock-knees)

YES → Perform AP x-rays of lower extremities

Abnormal results

Bowlegs → Tibia vara (Blount's disease) ⑤
Physeal injury
　Trauma
　Infection
　Tumor
Congenital posteromedial bow
Congenital pseudoarthrosis-tibia ⑥
Metabolic
　Rickets
　Hypophosphatasia
Skeletal dysplasia ⑦
　Metaphyseal displasia
　Achondroplasia
　Endochondromatosis
　Osteogenesis imperfecta

Knock-knees → Physeal injury
　Trauma
　Infection
　Tumor
Metabolic
　Renal osteodystrophy
Skeletal dysplasia ⑦

Normal results → Neurologic exam abnormal

YES → Neuromuscular disorder ⑧
　Cerebral palsy
　Myelodysplasia

NO → Physiologic genu varum ③ (bowlegs)
Physiologic genu valgum ④ (knock-knees)

Nelson chapters 681, 697
Personal Strategies chapter 46

NEUROLOGY

Chapter 50 Headaches

Headaches are common and usually benign. Reassurance that their child does not have a serious underlying cause for the headache is often the reason parents seek medical attention.

(1) A thorough history should define the quality and pattern of the complaint as well as inciting factors, recent trauma, response to medications, and associated visual or sensory disturbances.

Older children are often able to describe their headache; nonverbal children may become irritable, rub their eyes and head, vomit, or seek a darkened environment.

Increased intracranial pressure (ICP) causes headaches due to traction on the dura and intracranial blood vessels. Many but not all structural (i.e., organic) causes of headaches do cause increased ICP. Historical "red flags" suggestive of increased ICP include pain that is present in the morning or awakens the patient from sleep; increased pain with cough, straining, or position change; altered sensorium or personality; or a patient's description of "the worst headache of my life." Worrisome physical findings include abnormal neurologic findings, meningeal signs, papilledema, and altered sensorium.

A family history of migraines can be particularly helpful. Up to 80% of patients with migraine headaches will have a positive family history. Inquire about aneurysms as well. A headache diary may be helpful in classifying chronic or recurrent headaches.

In addition to a thorough neurologic examination, the physical examination should include a blood pressure evaluation, a thorough ENT examination including dentition, and an assessment of visual acuity.

(2) Patients with a recurrent headache disorder often present with a first acute severe headache. Migraines are most common in this scenario. Migraines are classically characterized by a positive family history for migraines, associated nausea, vomiting or abdominal pain, relief with rest, photophobia, and an aura or a transient neurologic disturbance. Neurologic deficits may occur with complicated migraines. Imaging may not be indicated if the family history and clinical presentation suggest migraine. Neuroimaging should be strongly considered when there is no family history of migraine.

(3) Complicated migraines are accompanied by neurologic deficits that occur during and after the headache. Basilar artery migraines are characterized by an intense occipital headache and frequently include ataxia, nausea, vomiting, and visual changes. Ophthalmoplegic migraine headaches are accompanied by cranial nerve (usually third) palsies. Hemiplegic migraines include unilateral motor and sensory symptoms. In migraine equivalent syndromes (e.g., acute confusional state, cyclic vomiting, benign paroxysmal vertigo), headache is not usually the predominant complaint. Neuroimaging to rule out CNS pathology may be indicated in the presence of an unusual constellation of neurologic signs or symptoms.

(4) Magnetic resonance imaging facilitates detection of vascular malformations, posterior fossa lesions, and certain smaller lesions that may not be identified by CT. Computed tomography is often the initial study because it is more commonly available, plus imaging time is shorter.

(5) Brain abscesses should be considered, especially in children with right-to-left cardiac shunts, chronic middle ear or sinus infections, and history of recent chronic persistent headaches.

(6) Hydrocephalus causes generalized pain that may be acute or gradual in onset and mild or severe in quality, depending on how rapidly the hydrocephalus is progressing. Headaches usually occur in the morning and lessen after arising.

(7) Third ventricle cysts may function as a ball-valve mechanism causing intermittent severe headaches due to transient increases in ICP. Other cysts (e.g., arachnoid, epidermoid, and dermoid) may cause progressive headaches similar to those from tumors.

(8) Headache often accompanies fever of any cause. Neurologic abnormalities, altered mental status, or meningeal signs (e.g., nuchal rigidity, Kernig and Brudzinski signs) warrant an evaluation to rule out meningitis.

(9) Chronic headaches may occur as part of a postconcussive or post-traumatic syndrome beginning shortly after a head injury and persisting up to several years. About 70% of patients will be asymptomatic after 1 year, but 15% remain symptomatic after 3 years. A neck injury (whiplash) may cause similar chronic symptoms. Cervical spine films with or without neuroimaging should be done acutely. Subsequent neuroimaging may be indicated to rule out a chronic subdural hematoma, which is rare.

(10) Muscle tension or muscle contraction headaches may be triggered by stress, fatigue, or hunger. They may be occasional or chronic. Chronic headaches are more likely in older children and adolescents. The pain is typically described as a constant squeezing pain located in a band around the head that escalates over the course of the day. Neurologic examination is always normal, and rarely nausea and photophobia may occur. Psychosocial factors can often be identified.

(11) The classic migraine is a unilateral throbbing headache that is preceded by an aura (blurred vision, scotomas, flashing lights, zigzag lines, hemianopia). Nausea, vomiting, pallor, and sensitivity to light, movement, and noise are common. Rarely, transient sensory disturbances (e.g., numbness, tingling, hemiparesis, aphasia) may occur. Migraines can be triggered by strenuous exertion or athletic activity.

(12) Common migraines are more frequent in school-aged children than are classic migraines. They are not preceded by an aura, although patients may feel ill or fatigued before the onset. The

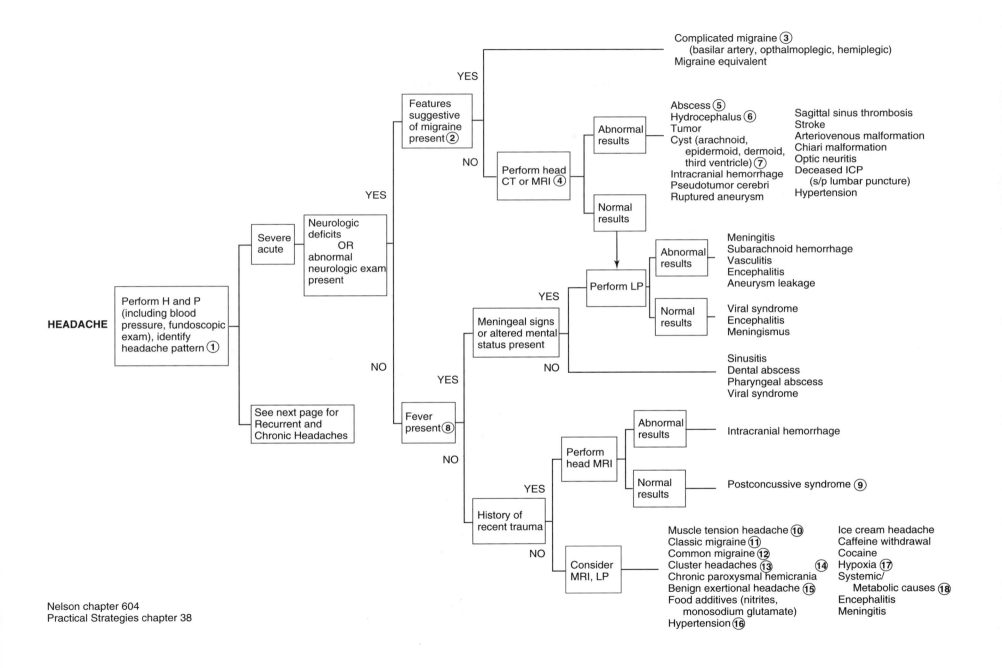

HEADACHE

Perform H and P (including blood pressure, fundoscopic exam), identify headache pattern ①

Severe acute

Neurologic deficits OR abnormal neurologic exam present

See next page for Recurrent and Chronic Headaches

YES

Features suggestive of migraine present ②

YES — Complicated migraine ③ (basilar artery, opthalmoplegic, hemiplegic) Migraine equivalent

NO

Perform head CT or MRI ④

Abnormal results
- Abscess ⑤
- Hydrocephalus ⑥
- Tumor
- Cyst (arachnoid, epidermoid, dermoid, third ventricle) ⑦
- Intracranial hemorrhage
- Pseudotumor cerebri
- Ruptured aneurysm
- Sagittal sinus thrombosis
- Stroke
- Arteriovenous malformation
- Chiari malformation
- Optic neuritis
- Deceased ICP (s/p lumbar puncture)
- Hypertension

Normal results

Perform LP

Abnormal results
- Meningitis
- Subarachnoid hemorrhage
- Vasculitis
- Encephalitis
- Aneurysm leakage

Normal results
- Viral syndrome
- Encephalitis
- Meningismus

NO

Fever present ⑧

YES

Meningeal signs or altered mental status present

YES — Perform LP

NO
- Sinusitis
- Dental abscess
- Pharyngeal abscess
- Viral syndrome

NO

History of recent trauma

YES

Perform head MRI

Abnormal results — Intracranial hemorrhage

Normal results — Postconcussive syndrome ⑨

NO

Consider MRI, LP
- Muscle tension headache ⑩
- Classic migraine ⑪
- Common migraine ⑫
- Cluster headaches ⑬
- Chronic paroxysmal hemicrania ⑭
- Benign exertional headache ⑮
- Food additives (nitrites, monosodium glutamate)
- Hypertension ⑯
- Ice cream headache
- Caffeine withdrawal
- Cocaine
- Hypoxia ⑰
- Systemic/ Metabolic causes ⑱
- Encephalitis
- Meningitis

Nelson chapter 604
Practical Strategies chapter 38

pain may develop acutely or gradually and is usually throbbing and poorly localized. Nausea, vomiting, pallor, and sensitivity to light are common and patients generally seek out a quiet place to sleep.

13 Cluster headaches are rare in children. Pain onset is rapid, and the pain is usually localized to the eyes and temporal region and is accompanied by lacrimation, rhinorrhea, sweating, and nasal congestion. The pain lasts 30 to 90 minutes and repeats several times each day. Attacks are clustered over weeks to months. The affected patient tends to walk around in an agitated state.

14 Chronic paroxysmal hemicrania is a disorder characterized by frequent brief unilateral headaches accompanied by ipsilateral conjunctival injection and tearing. Headaches last about 10 minutes and may recur up to 10 to 20 times daily. Onset is typically in adulthood, although older children and adolescents can be affected. Neuroimaging should be performed to rule out vascular malformations.

15 Benign exertional headaches can be triggered by exercise or exertion in people who do not suffer from migraines.

16 Both acute and chronic hypertension may cause headaches, although most children with chronic hypertension are asymptomatic. Acute headaches due to hypertension may rarely be the presenting symptom of glomerulonephritis.

17 Hypoxia due to chronic lung disease, obstructive sleep apnea, or high altitudes may cause headaches due to dilation of cerebral arteries.

18 Evaluation for underlying systemic or metabolic disorders (e.g., endocrine, hematologic, renal) should be based on clinical presentation.

19 Cough headaches are caused by a transient rise in ICP due to activities that increase intrathoracic pressure (e.g., exertion, coughing, bending). Symptoms are brief and resolve in seconds. They are often benign, but neuroimaging is done to rule out rare life-threatening causes (e.g., tumors, Chiari malformations, colloid cyst of the third ventricle).

20 Pseudotumor cerebri or benign intracranial hypertension occurs as a constant or intermittent headache. Papilledema is usually present, and there may be a history of an enlarged blind spot and constricted visual fields. Diplopia due to paralysis of the abducens nerve is also common. The disorder is more common in older children and adolescents, females, and obese individuals. Neuroimaging is indicated before lumbar puncture to rule out intracranial processes. Except for papilledema and an increased CSF opening pressure, the findings in the physical examination, neuroimaging studies, and CSF studies are usually normal.

21 Eyestrain due to a latent disturbance in convergence may cause a headache of muscular origin owing to trying to maintain a conjugate gaze. Eyestrain due to refractive errors is a popular theory but actually an infrequent cause of headache in children. Rare ocular causes of headache include increased intraocular pressure, tumor, and inflammation.

22 Headache may occur after a seizure or rarely as a manifestation of a seizure.

23 Occipital neuralgia is occipital pain due to irritation of the greater occipital nerve (i.e., a continuation of C2). The posterior scalp is tender with decreased sensation and the sensation of "pins and needles."

24 Temporomandibular joint syndrome most commonly causes unilateral pain. The pain may be constant or associated with opening the mouth and is accompanied by a clicking sound.

25 Analgesic rebound causes headaches in patients taking analgesics daily or on most days. The headache occurs due to a vicious cycle of pain and analgesic use followed by more pain and more analgesic use as the effect wears off.

26 Low-level carbon monoxide poisoning should be suspected in children with chronic headaches.

BIBLIOGRAPHY

Fenichel GM: Clinical Pediatric Neurology, 3rd ed. Philadelphia: WB Saunders, 1997.
Forsyth R, Farrell K: Headache in childhood. Pediatr Rev 20:39–45, 1999.

HEADACHE (continued)

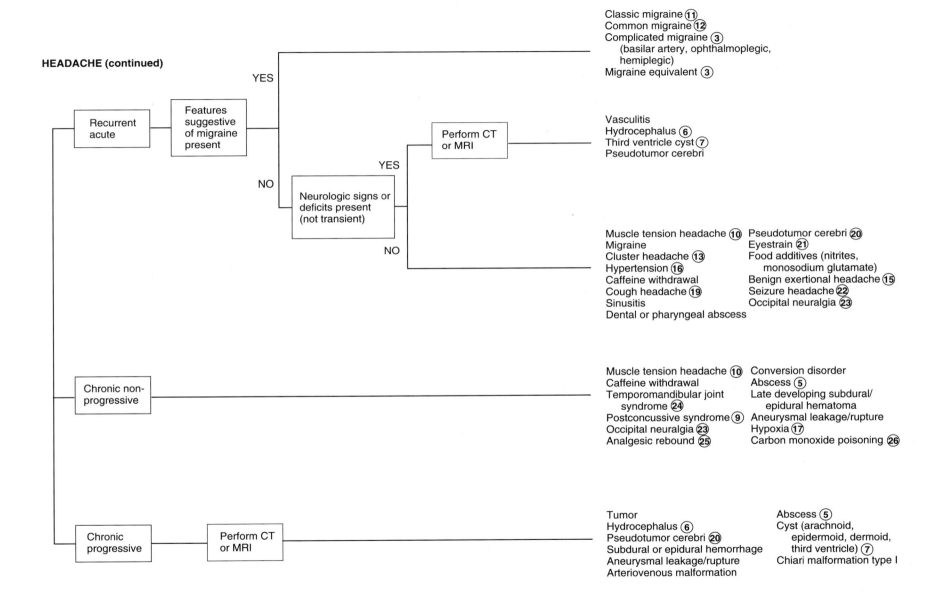

Recurrent acute

Features suggestive of migraine present

YES →
Classic migraine (11)
Common migraine (12)
Complicated migraine (3)
(basilar artery, ophthalmoplegic, hemiplegic)
Migraine equivalent (3)

NO →
Neurologic signs or deficits present (not transient)

YES →
Perform CT or MRI →
Vasculitis
Hydrocephalus (6)
Third ventricle cyst (7)
Pseudotumor cerebri

NO →
Muscle tension headache (10)
Migraine
Cluster headache (13)
Hypertension (16)
Caffeine withdrawal
Cough headache (19)
Sinusitis
Dental or pharyngeal abscess

Pseudotumor cerebri (20)
Eyestrain (21)
Food additives (nitrites, monosodium glutamate)
Benign exertional headache (15)
Seizure headache (22)
Occipital neuralgia (23)

Chronic non-progressive →
Muscle tension headache (10)
Caffeine withdrawal
Temporomandibular joint syndrome (24)
Postconcussive syndrome (9)
Occipital neuralgia (23)
Analgesic rebound (25)

Conversion disorder
Abscess (5)
Late developing subdural/epidural hematoma
Aneurysmal leakage/rupture
Hypoxia (17)
Carbon monoxide poisoning (26)

Chronic progressive →
Perform CT or MRI →
Tumor
Hydrocephalus (6)
Pseudotumor cerebri (20)
Subdural or epidural hemorrhage
Aneurysmal leakage/rupture
Arteriovenous malformation

Abscess (5)
Cyst (arachnoid, epidermoid, dermoid, third ventricle) (7)
Chiari malformation type I

Chapter 51 **Seizures and Other Paroxysmal Disorders**

A seizure is a paroxysmal disturbance in brain function that manifests as an alteration in motor activity, level of consciousness, or autonomic function. Seizures are classified according to whether they are generalized or partial (only a portion of the cerebral cortex is involved in partial seizures), and whether consciousness is preserved or impaired. Epilepsy defines a disorder of recurrent seizures unprovoked by trauma, fever, or other insults. Epilepsy may be idiopathic or a symptom of a recognizable underlying disorder. Status epilepticus is the occurrence of prolonged or recurrent seizures for 30 minutes or longer. A number of nonepileptic paroxysmal disorders occur in childhood and must be distinguished from epileptic seizures.

(1) A description of the event is the most valuable part of the evaluation because physical findings are rare and diagnostic studies may not be conclusive. Inquire about the occurrence of an aura, a postictal state, a loss of sphincter control, and any inciting events (trauma, fever, crying). Obtain the medical history, including a birth and developmental history. Inquire about medication use. In children with a known seizure disorder, specifically ask about medication compliance. Neurocutaneous lesions (café-au-lait spots, ash leaf macules) should be noted on the physical examination.

(2) A febrile seizure is a seizure in a child between 6 months and 5 years of age in association with a fever and in the absence of a CNS infection. Additional criteria for simple febrile seizures include a child with a previously normal neurologic status and no recurrence of the seizure during the febrile illness. There may be a positive family history of febrile seizures. Complex febrile seizures are defined as focal or prolonged (longer than 15 minutes) or occurring in a flurry of repetitive episodes during the febrile illness.

(3) A focal seizure, an abnormal neurologic examination, or a very prolonged seizure should prompt a thorough evaluation for a CNS infection. For children experiencing a focal seizure, an electroencephalogram may specifically aid in the diagnosis of herpes simplex virus encephalitis. A CT should be obtained for all children with a focal seizure.

(4) Lumbar puncture should be strongly considered in young children because meningeal signs in this age group are not reliable indicators of meningitis. Lumbar puncture should also be carefully considered in children who have recently received an antibiotic that might mask signs and symptoms of meningitis.

(5) Current guidelines recommend a simplified approach to the child with a first febrile seizure. Although a first febrile seizure may be the first manifestation of a seizure disorder, the majority of simple febrile seizures are benign events and an extensive workup is reserved for children with other risk factors.

In children experiencing a simple febrile seizure without suspicion of meningitis, evaluation should be limited to identifying the underlying source of the fever. Routine laboratory evaluation, neuroimaging, and performance of an EEG are not indicated.

(6) Evaluation of the infant younger than 2 months of age with seizures requires consideration of causes mostly unique to the neonatal age group, such as metabolic, toxic, structural, ischemic, traumatic, infectious.

(7) Head banging (i.e., jactatio capitis nocturna) is a common behavior of rhythmic to-and-fro movements of the head and body. Children have no memory of this behavior, which typically occurs as they are going to sleep.

(8) Benign nocturnal myoclonus describes sudden jerking movements of the limbs during sleep. These movements are normal in people of all ages and occur primarily in the early stages of sleep. Evaluation is not necessary.

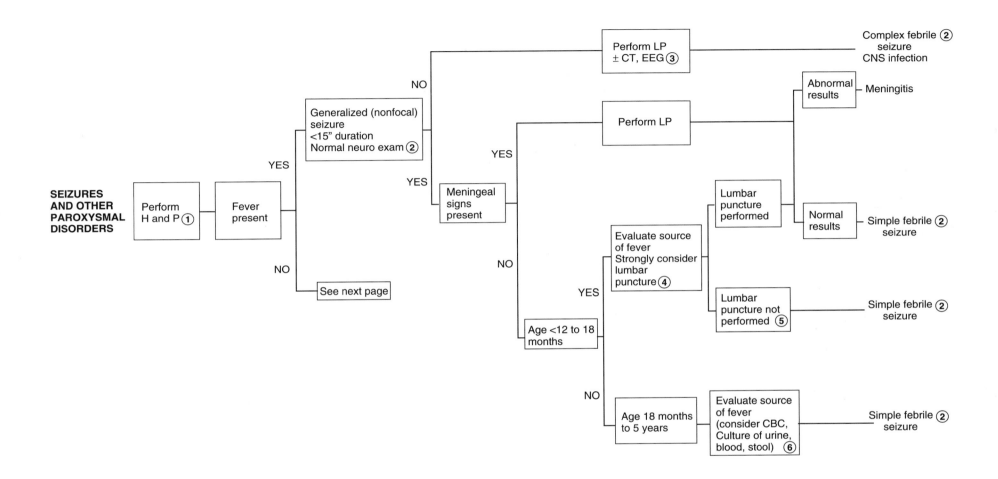

SEIZURES AND OTHER PAROXYSMAL DISORDERS

Perform H and P ①

Fever present

YES → Generalized (nonfocal) seizure <15" duration Normal neuro exam ②

NO → See next page

NO → Perform LP ± CT, EEG ③ → Complex febrile ② seizure CNS infection

YES → Meningeal signs present

YES → Perform LP → Abnormal results — Meningitis

→ Normal results — Simple febrile ② seizure

NO → Age <12 to 18 months

YES → Evaluate source of fever Strongly consider lumbar puncture ④

Lumbar puncture performed

Lumbar puncture not performed ⑤ — Simple febrile ② seizure

NO → Age 18 months to 5 years → Evaluate source of fever (consider CBC, Culture of urine, blood, stool) ⑥ — Simple febrile ② seizure

Nelson chapters 602, 603
Practical Strategies chapter 40

Seizures and Other Paroxysmal Disorders *(continued)*

(9) Benign partial epilepsies of childhood are a classification of idiopathic focal seizure disorders in children with normal findings on neurologic examinations and neuroimaging studies. A family history is often positive for epilepsy. An EEG is necessary for diagnosis and shows characteristic findings. The most common variant is benign rolandic epilepsy. This disorder typically appears as a brief hemifacial seizure (generalization occurs rarely) that awakens the child from sleep. Drooling is common, and consciousness is preserved. The EEG shows centrotemporal spikes. Neuroimaging may not be necessary in cases clearly meeting the criteria for this variant.

(10) Breath-holding spells should be distinguished from seizures before proceeding with the evaluation for seizures. In breath-holding spells, breathing stops in expiration. Cyanotic breath-holding spells (i.e., cyanotic infant syncope) usually occur during crying usually due to frustration or anger. Apnea, cyanosis, and posturing with or without a brief loss of consciousness typically occur. Pallid breath-holding spells with pallor and loss of tone are often precipitated by a painful event. Brief tonic-clonic movements may occur with either type of episode. Breath-holding spells typically occur between 6 and 18 months of age, although they may be seen up to age 6 years. Children recover quickly from breath-holding spells with no neurologic sequelae. No diagnostic evaluation is indicated.

(11) Partial seizures occur due to excessive neuronal activation of a portion of the brain. Manifestations may include somatosensory or autonomic symptoms, focal motor signs, or automatisms (i.e., semi-purposeful movements). EEGs reveal focal epileptiform discharges, and neuroimaging is usually indicated to rule out anatomic lesions.

(12) Infants affected with startle disease may experience apnea, an exaggerated startle response, and a generalized stiffening on awakening. A few children may continue to experience an exaggerated startle response with stiffening and falling throughout life.

(13) Shuddering or shivering attacks are brief episodes of sudden flexion of the head and neck accompanied by fine tremulous contractions of the musculature. A family history of essential tremor is common.

(14) Episodes of fluctuating hemiparesis occur in alternating hemiplegia of childhood. Other involuntary movements, nystagmus, or autonomic disturbances may accompany the episodes. Diagnosis is clinical.

(15) Benign paroxysmal vertigo most commonly occurs in toddlers. Children experience brief episodes of sudden vertigo, ataxia, and pallor. Children frequently fall to the floor, refusing to stand or walk, even though no loss of consciousness occurs. Nystagmus is usually evident. Neurologic evaluation is typically normal, except for abnormal vestibular function noted on ice water caloric testing.

(16) Paroxysmal head-nodding, torticollis, and nystagmus characterize spasmus nutans. Neuroimaging is recommended to rule out tumors.

(17) Repetitive purposeless movements are often exhibited by autistic or handicapped children, especially in environments with a low level of stimulation. They may be difficult to distinguish clinically from seizure activity. Masturbation in young children is also sometimes mistaken as seizures by parents.

(18) Any individual experiencing a nonfebrile nonfocal seizure should have an MRI and EEG done if they are younger than 2 years old or older than 18 years. For children between 2 and 18 years, a nonurgent EEG should be obtained. Clinical judgment is then used to determine the need for an MRI. If the EEG shows a focal spike pattern, an MRI should be performed. Anyone experiencing a focal seizure should always undergo an MRI and EEG. Laboratory evaluation is not indicated for an isolated nonfocal seizure unless the presentation suggests the seizure is symptomatic of an underlying disorder (e.g., trauma, dehydration).

(19) Evaluation of a suspected acute symptomatic seizure is determined by the clinical presentation. Neuroimaging (preferably MRI) is indicated in any child with partial (focal) seizures. It should also be considered in cases of head trauma followed by a seizure, and when a child is found unconscious and it is not clear whether the trauma or seizure caused the loss of consciousness.

(20) Multiple types of seizures and seizure disorders (i.e., epilepsies) are classified by their clinical and EEG characteristics. Many are associated with underlying syndromes or risk factors such as hypoxic-ischemic encephalopathy or congenital malformations. Interictal EEGs are normal in 40% of patients with epilepsy. The diagnostic yield is improved when activation procedures, including hyperventilation, photic simulation, and sleep, are included.

(21) Generalized seizures involve both cerebral hemispheres, resulting in bilateral symptoms and EEG changes. Consciousness is impaired in most types of generalized seizures. Some myoclonic and atonic seizures are exceptions.

(22) Myoclonic movements due to muscle spasms may be benign or extremely ominous. Infantile spasms are the most serious variant. Infants begin experiencing rapid "jackknifing" contractions of the neck, trunk, and limbs followed by a brief sustained tonic contraction. Onset is most common between 4 and 7 months of age, and the spasms often occur in clusters. Hypsarrhythmia is the characteristic finding on EEG. An EEG is necessary to distinguish infantile spasms from benign myoclonus of infancy, which is a benign condition, and myoclonic epilepsy that may occur as a benign primary epilepsy or a severe disorder with progressive neurologic deterioration.

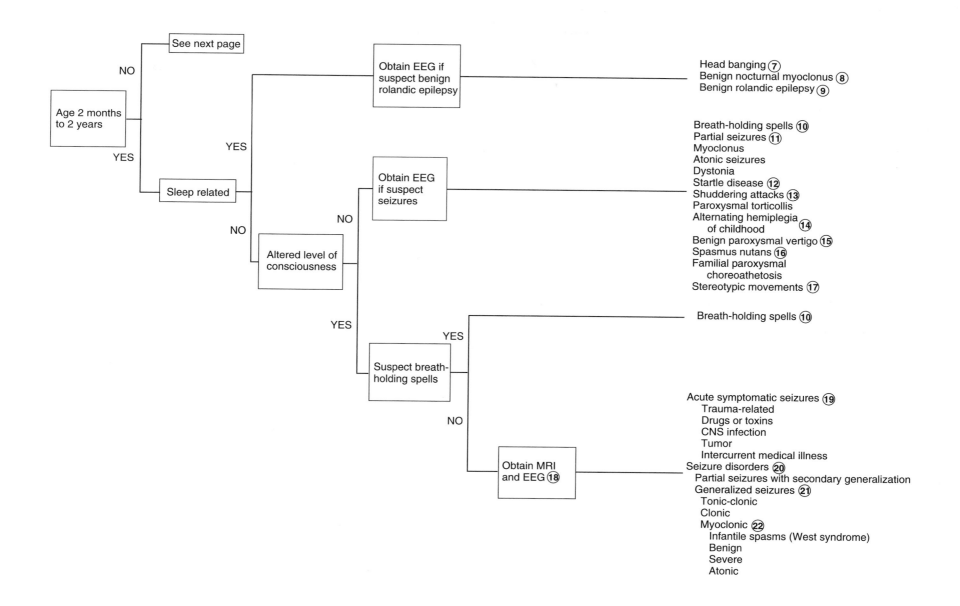

(23) Narcolepsy is characterized by recurrent short sleep attacks. It is usually accompanied by cataplexy (i.e., a sudden collapse due to loss of muscle tone) and induced by laughter, excitement, or startle.

(24) Night terrors are an incomplete sudden arousal from non–rapid eye movement sleep, occurring about 2 hours after sleep onset, accompanied by inconsolable screaming and crying. They occur most often in preschoolers and early school-aged children. Children appear awake but have no memory of the event.

(25) Rarely, prolonged episodes of hyperventilation may result in loss of consciousness and some seizure activity.

(26) Absence epilepsy is a generalized seizure disorder occurring as staring spells sometimes with automatisms in children between 3 and 12 years of age. Hyperventilation will often reproduce the event. Diagnosis is by characteristic 3-Hz spike-and-wave complexes on the EEG.

BIBLIOGRAPHY

AAP Practice Parameter: The neurodiagnostic evaluation of the child with a first simple febrile seizure. Pediatrics 97:769, 1996.
Fenichel GM: Clinical Pediatric Neurology, 3rd ed. Philadelphia: WB Saunders, 1997.
Golden GS: Nonepileptic paroxysmal events in childhood. Pediatr Clin North Am 39:715–725, 1992.

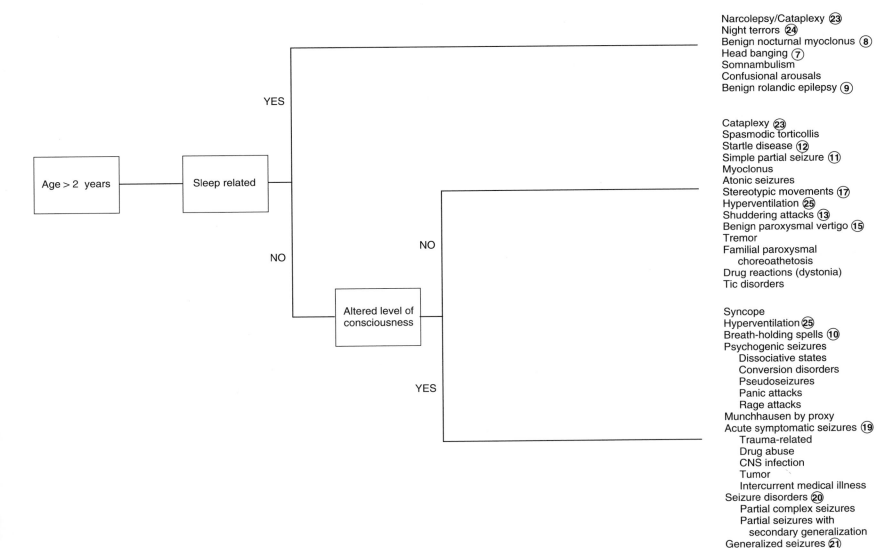

Narcolepsy/Cataplexy ㉓
Night terrors ㉔
Benign nocturnal myoclonus ⑧
Head banging ⑦
Somnambulism
Confusional arousals
Benign rolandic epilepsy ⑨

Cataplexy ㉓
Spasmodic torticollis
Startle disease ⑫
Simple partial seizure ⑪
Myoclonus
Atonic seizures
Stereotypic movements ⑰
Hyperventilation ㉕
Shuddering attacks ⑬
Benign paroxysmal vertigo ⑮
Tremor
Familial paroxysmal
　　choreoathetosis
Drug reactions (dystonia)
Tic disorders

Syncope
Hyperventilation ㉕
Breath-holding spells ⑩
Psychogenic seizures
　　Dissociative states
　　Conversion disorders
　　Pseudoseizures
　　Panic attacks
　　Rage attacks
Munchhausen by proxy
Acute symptomatic seizures ⑲
　　Trauma-related
　　Drug abuse
　　CNS infection
　　Tumor
　　Intercurrent medical illness
Seizure disorders ⑳
　　Partial complex seizures
　　Partial seizures with
　　　secondary generalization
Generalized seizures ㉑
　　Absence ㉖
　　Tonic-clonic
　　Clonic
　　Myoclonic
　　Atonic

Age > 2 years

Sleep related

Altered level of
consciousness

YES

NO

NO

YES

Chapter 52 Involuntary Movements

Involuntary movements can be the primary or secondary manifestation of numerous neurologic disorders. Classification can be difficult. Careful observation by an experienced practitioner is usually necessary to classify the movement and diagnose the disorder. Diagnosis is often further complicated because many disorders occur with a movement that is prominent initially, but, as the disorder evolves, is overshadowed by a different symptom.

(1) Distinguishing movement disorders from seizures is often the first diagnostic challenge because many movement disorders are also paroxysmal. Characteristics suggestive of seizures include (1) symptoms that persist or worsen during sleep, (2) brief, nonstereotypical movements, (3) altered level of consciousness, and (4) accompanying epileptiform activity on EEG. An EEG should be performed whenever a seizure disorder is suspected. If seizures are deemed unlikely, identifying or classifying the type of abnormal movement is the next step in narrowing the differential diagnosis. Videotaping is a helpful diagnostic aid.

(2) Hypokinesia or parkinsonism (bradykinesia, rigidity, tremor, abnormal posture) is rare in childhood. It may occur in children recovering from encephalitis or head trauma or as a component of rare genetic disorders.

(3) Choreiform movements are rapid random jerking movements of any part of the body. The movements are characterized by an inability to maintain a sustained muscle contraction (hand grip, tongue protrusion) because of interruption by choreiform movements. Diagnosis is often delayed because children try to disguise the movements. A history of fidgetiness or hyperactivity is common. Choreoathetosis describes a slow writhing movement accompanying chorea. Ballismus (also a form of chorea) describes high amplitude flinging of the extremities.

(4) Mild choreiform movements typically manifest as only fine movements of the extended arms and hands. These movements are not functionally significant and resolve spontaneously.

(5) Tardive dyskinesia refers to drug-induced choreiform movements. Facial movements (e.g., tongue protrusion, lip smacking, puckering, grimacing) are the usual manifestations. The onset is late (months to years) in the course of drug therapy and is not considered a dose-related reaction. The diagnosis is clinical and should be suspected in children taking neuroleptic drugs (e.g., phenothiazines, haloperidol, metoclopramide). Other drugs that have been implicated are anticonvulsants, antiemetics, oral contraceptives, theophylline, and stimulants.

(6) Sydenham chorea is a rare neurologic component of rheumatic fever. It occurs several months after the acute β-hemolytic streptococcal infection and may be accompanied by encephalopathy and hypotonia. Serum titers of anti-DNAase B and antihyaluronidase (AH) may be more reliable than antistreptolysin O titers for documenting recent infection. Cardiac evaluation (EKG, echocardiogram) should be done to rule out rheumatic carditis, which occurs in one third of cases.

(7) Severe choreoathetosis is seen in 1% to 10% of children after bypass surgery for congenital heart disease. Diagnosis is clinical.

(8) Benign familial (hereditary) chorea is an autosomal dominant disorder appearing early in childhood with continuous and not episodic or paroxysmal chorea and possibly intention tremor, dysarthria, hypotonia, or athetosis. Development may be delayed, but intelligence is normal. Diagnosis is clinical. The family history may be overlooked if incomplete expression of the disorder occurs in parents.

(9) Familial paroxysmal choreoathetosis is similar to benign familial chorea and characterized by nonepileptic paroxysmal attacks of choreoathetosis, dystonia, or ballismus.

(10) Wilson disease (hepatolenticular degeneration) is an autosomal recessive disorder characterized by liver failure and neurologic symptoms. About 40% of patients present with neurologic symptoms. The most common neurologic manifestation is dystonia. Dysarthria, chorea, rigidity, postural abnormalities, tremors, and drooling may also develop. Diagnosis is by elevated serum ceruloplasmin level and liver biopsy showing increased copper content. The Kayser-Fleischer ring, a yellow-brown ring around the cornea, is pathognomonic.

(11) Huntington disease is an autosomal dominant disorder. Presentation in childhood is rare. Rigidity and dystonia are the most common pediatric manifestations, although chorea, mental deterioration, behavioral problems, and seizures may also occur.

(12) Dystonia is a slow writhing or twisting movement resulting in abnormal posture of the limbs or trunk or grimacing of the face. It may be focal, segmental, or generalized. When the arm and leg on one side of the body are affected, the condition is called hemidystonia. Dystonia is caused by simultaneous contracture of agonist and antagonist muscles. Hypertrophy of affected muscles becomes evident over time. Electromyography is necessary for diagnosis in most cases.

(13) Transient paroxysmal dystonia of infancy is a nonfamilial disorder characterized by abnormal posturing and limb dystonia. Episodes present in the first several months of life, increase in frequency, then gradually diminish and disappear within several years. Children remain neurologically and developmentally normal.

(14) Torsion dystonia (previously called idiopathic dystonia musculorum deformans) in children typically begins with unilateral foot or leg involvement presenting as toe-walking and progresses to generalized involvement. An autosomal recessive variant of the disorder is significantly more common in Ashkenazi Jews.

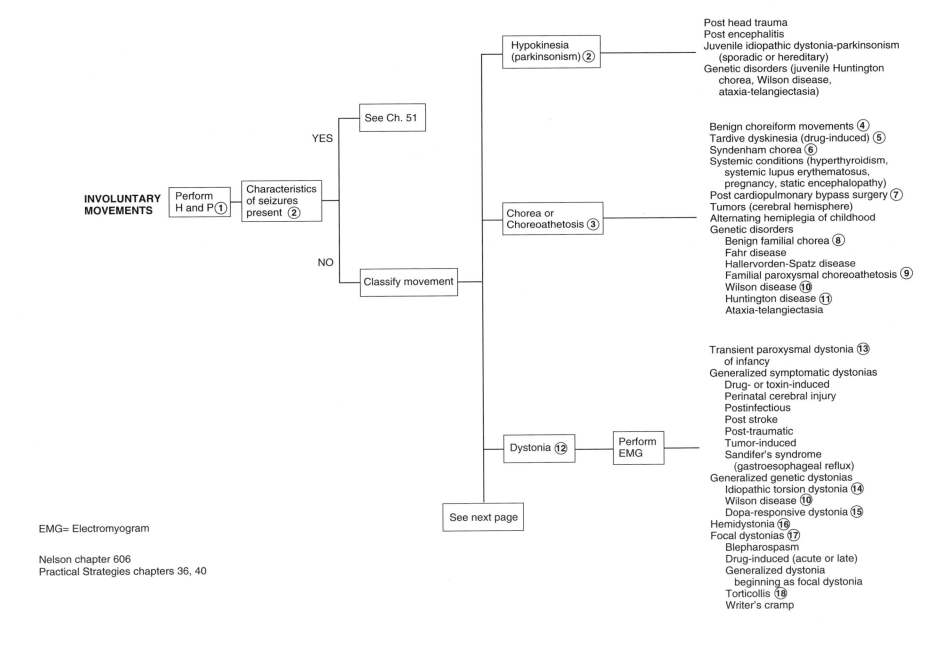

INVOLUNTARY MOVEMENTS — Perform H and P ① — Characteristics of seizures present ②

YES — See Ch. 51

NO — Classify movement

Hypokinesia (parkinsonism) ②
Post head trauma
Post encephalitis
Juvenile idiopathic dystonia-parkinsonism
    (sporadic or hereditary)
Genetic disorders (juvenile Huntington
    chorea, Wilson disease,
    ataxia-telangiectasia)

Chorea or Choreoathetosis ③
Benign choreiform movements ④
Tardive dyskinesia (drug-induced) ⑤
Syndenham chorea ⑥
Systemic conditions (hyperthyroidism,
    systemic lupus erythematosus,
    pregnancy, static encephalopathy)
Post cardiopulmonary bypass surgery ⑦
Tumors (cerebral hemisphere)
Alternating hemiplegia of childhood
Genetic disorders
    Benign familial chorea ⑧
    Fahr disease
    Hallervorden-Spatz disease
    Familial paroxysmal choreoathetosis ⑨
    Wilson disease ⑩
    Huntington disease ⑪
    Ataxia-telangiectasia

Dystonia ⑫ — Perform EMG
Transient paroxysmal dystonia ⑬
    of infancy
Generalized symptomatic dystonias
    Drug- or toxin-induced
    Perinatal cerebral injury
    Postinfectious
    Post stroke
    Post-traumatic
    Tumor-induced
    Sandifer's syndrome
        (gastroesophageal reflux)
Generalized genetic dystonias
    Idiopathic torsion dystonia ⑭
    Wilson disease ⑩
    Dopa-responsive dystonia ⑮
Hemidystonia ⑯
Focal dystonias ⑰
    Blepharospasm
    Drug-induced (acute or late)
    Generalized dystonia
        beginning as focal dystonia
    Torticollis ⑱
    Writer's cramp

See next page

EMG= Electromyogram

Nelson chapter 606
Practical Strategies chapters 36, 40

Involuntary Movements *(continued)*

(15) Dopa-responsive dystonia (Segawa disease) is an autosomal dominant disorder presenting between ages 4 and 8 years with a gait disturbance caused by leg dystonia eventually followed by abnormal posturing of upper extremities, cogwheel rigidity, masklike facies, and bradykinesia. Diagnosis may be through clinical or by chromosomal analysis.

(16) Evaluation with an MRI is indicated for hemidystonia to rule out intracranial lesions.

(17) Focal dystonia involving eye closing in children is usually drug induced. It needs to be distinguished from tics.

(18) When torticollis is associated with dystonia in the face or limbs, an MRI is indicated to rule out intracranial and cervical spine disorders.

(19) Myoclonus describes brief involuntary jerking muscle movements that may occur spontaneously or in response to a stimulus. Myoclonus may be rhythmic or nonrhythmic and focal or generalized and must be distinguished from tics and tremor. It diminishes but does not necessarily disappear during sleep. It may be benign (physiologic), associated with CNS injury, or a symptom of a more severe, progressive neurologic disorder.

(20) Nocturnal or sleep myoclonus is a benign form of myoclonus occurring with sleep or just before awakening or during times of increased stress.

(21) Benign myoclonus of infancy is characterized by clusters of jerks of the head, neck, and arms. It is distinguished from the more ominous infantile myoclonic spasms by normal development and normal EEG.

(22) Essential myoclonus is a chronic condition of jerking (e.g., focal, segmental, generalized) that may be sporadic or familial. Facial, trunk, and proximal muscles are typically affected, and no other neurologic problems are associated. Diagnosis is clinical. EEGs and imaging studies are normal.

(23) Prominent myoclonic movements on awakening characterize juvenile myoclonic epilepsy of Janz. Characteristic EEG findings are spike-and-wave complexes at 3.5 to 6 Hz.

(24) Myoclonus-opsoclonus syndrome (i.e., myoclonic encephalopathy of infancy) is a condition characterized by opsoclonus (i.e., flurries of conjugate eye movements) and severe myoclonic jerking of the trunk and head. It may occur as an idiopathic disorder, due to encephalitis, or as a manifestation of occult neural crest tumors, most commonly due to neuroblastoma.

(25) Tremor is an involuntary, rhythmic continuous oscillatory (i.e., to-and-fro) movement. A low level physiologic tremor is normal in all people. It may be exacerbated by stress, anxiety, and certain medications.

(26) Jitteriness is common in normal full-term infants, and it may last for a few weeks. Organic causes must be considered and include hypoxic-ischemic encephalopathy, drug withdrawal, hypoglycemia, hypomagnesemia, hypocalcemia, and intracranial hemorrhage. Normal jitteriness can be stopped by gently touching and flexing the moving limb. Staring and eye deviation do not occur with normal jitteriness.

(27) Essential (familial) tremor is an inherited condition that affects only the limb being used.

(28) Tics (i.e., habit spasms) are brief, complex, stereotyped movements or vocal utterances. They are distinguished from chorea by the stereotypical appearance, plus they (unlike chorea) can be voluntarily suppressed for brief periods. Transient tics, typically eye-blinking or facial movements, may last several weeks or up to 1 year and are often associated with a positive family history.

(29) Tourette syndrome is a life-long condition of verbal and motor tics that begins between 2 and 15 years of age. Attention deficit disorder and obsessive compulsive behaviors occur in many cases. Symptoms are typically exacerbated by stress. Diagnosis is clinical.

(30) Mirror movements are involuntary movements of one side of the body that mirror intentional movements of the opposite side of the body. They are normal starting in infancy and may persist up to 10 years of age.

BIBLIOGRAPHY

Butler IF: Movement disorders of children. Pediatr Clin North Am 39:727–742, 1992.

Fenichel GM: Clinical Pediatric Neurology, 3rd ed. Philadelphia: WB Saunders Company, 1997.

INVOLUNTARY MOVEMENTS
(continued)

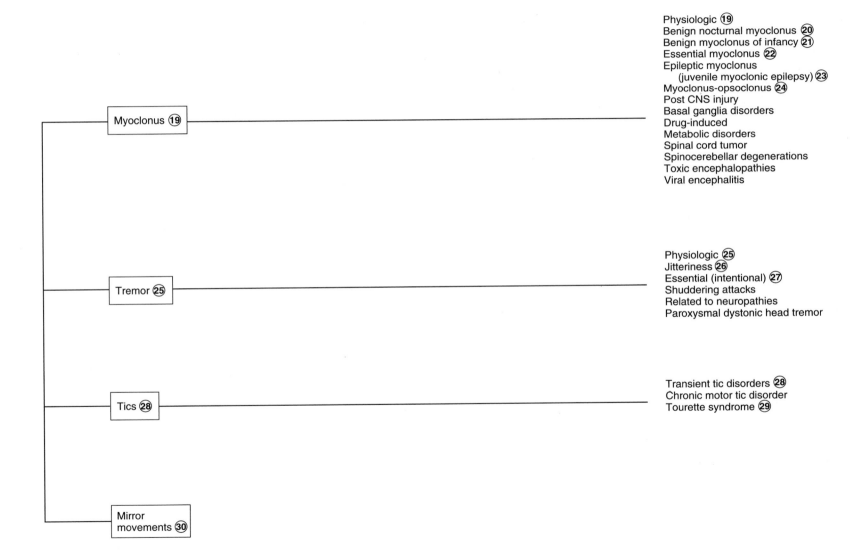

Myoclonus ⑲
- Physiologic ⑲
- Benign nocturnal myoclonus ⑳
- Benign myoclonus of infancy ㉑
- Essential myoclonus ㉒
- Epileptic myoclonus
  (juvenile myoclonic epilepsy) ㉓
- Myoclonus-opsoclonus ㉔
- Post CNS injury
- Basal ganglia disorders
- Drug-induced
- Metabolic disorders
- Spinal cord tumor
- Spinocerebellar degenerations
- Toxic encephalopathies
- Viral encephalitis

Tremor ㉕
- Physiologic ㉕
- Jitteriness ㉖
- Essential (intentional) ㉗
- Shuddering attacks
- Related to neuropathies
- Paroxysmal dystonic head tremor

Tics ㉘
- Transient tic disorders ㉘
- Chronic motor tic disorder
- Tourette syndrome ㉙

Mirror movements ㉚

Chapter 53 **Hypotonia and Weakness**

Weakness is generally a complaint of the older child. Young infants are more likely to present with hypotonia than weakness. Although the two frequently occur together, they are not synonymous. Any component of the nervous system may be responsible. Brain disorders are more common in hypotonic infants, whereas neuromuscular disorders are more likely in older children.

1 Perinatal events are important in the evaluation of hypotonia. Intrauterine movements and birth weight may be helpful in assessing neonates. A feeding and developmental history is more relevant for infants and toddlers. A history of traumatic or precipitous birth may be a risk factor for intracranial hemorrhage. Occasionally, characteristic facies or physical stigmata will suggest the diagnosis (e.g., Down syndrome, Prader-Willi syndrome).

The degree and distribution of the hypotonia and weakness are significant to the diagnosis. Hypotonic infants manifest significant joint hyperextensibility (scarf sign) and abnormal postural reflexes (traction response, axillary suspension, ventral suspension). They usually have markedly diminished spontaneous movements. Exaggerated or persistent primitive reflexes (e.g., Moro, asymmetric tonic neck reflex) and brisk tendon reflexes suggest cerebral hypotonia. For the older child presenting with weakness, inquire about fatigability, falling, school (i.e., cognitive) performance, and possibility of ingestions. A family history may also be helpful.

In toddlers and older children, strength can be assessed by observation of various tasks (e.g., standing on one foot, running, climbing stairs, rising to stand from a sitting or lying position [Gowers sign]). Strength can also be measured more objectively when the child is old enough to cooperate.

2 When considering a floppy infant, signs or symptoms suggestive of a cerebral disorder include seizures, impaired level of consciousness, poor feeding, jitteriness, dysmorphic features, organ malformations, fisting of hands, brisk deep tendon reflexes, clonus, and autonomic dysfunction.

3 Cerebral palsy is a static encephalopathy, a nonprogressive clinical disorder characterized by varying degrees of mental and motor impairment. Rarely, hypotonia is prominent or persistent. In most cases hypotonia will progress to spasticity and dyskinetic movements. Although perinatal hypoxia or asphyxia is a commonly identified cause of cerebral palsy, most cases are likely due to undetected prenatal events.

4 Creatine phosphokinase (CPK) is released by damaged or degenerating muscle fibers. Electromyography (EMG) measures the electric potentials during various states of muscle contractions and may demonstrate certain types of muscle diseases. Muscle biopsy can distinguish between neurogenic and myopathic processes, and histochemical studies will identify specific metabolic myopathies.

More specialized molecular and biochemical testing may be necessary when metabolic disorders or progressive encephalopathies are suggested. The evaluation for a metabolic disorder should include blood for a CBC, electrolytes, pH, glucose, ammonia, lactate, carnitine, and amino acids and urine for ketones, reducing substances, organic acids, amino acids, and carnitine.

5 Spinal muscular atrophies cause progressive weakness in infants, sometimes starting in the prenatal period. Juvenile variants of this disorder occur beyond infancy. Diagnosis is by EMG, DNA probes, and muscle biopsy.

6 Myasthenia gravis occurs owing to the presence of anti-acetylcholine receptor antibodies, which produce a blockade at the neuromuscular junction. It may appear as a transient neonatal condition due to placentally acquired antibodies. A permanent form of the disease may also begin in infancy, but is less common, or childhood. Ptosis and extraocular muscle weakness are the most common symptoms. Rapid fatigue of muscles with worsening symptoms as the day progresses is characteristic. Diagnosis is confirmed by the presence of anti-acetylcholine antibodies and symptomatic improvement with the edrophonium (i.e., Tensilon) test.

7 Hypotonia and weakness are almost universal findings in infants with Down syndrome. The strength improves, but the hypotonia persists as they grow older. Infants with Prader-Willi syndrome present with marked hypotonia in infancy. Characteristic phenotypic features (e.g., brachycephaly, almond-shaped palpebrae, short stature, small hands and feet) and the pathologic food-seeking behaviors become evident later in childhood. Weakness improves in these children, although the hypotonia persists.

8 In congenital myotonic dystrophy, severe hypotonia, weakness, swallowing and sucking difficulties, and congenital joint contractures are evident at birth. In childhood-onset myotonic dystrophy, myotonia (i.e., a disturbance of muscle relaxation) may be the first symptom. It may precede the distal weakness by several years. Facial weakness is also characteristic. Genetic testing is available for definitive diagnosis when the EMG is inconclusive.

9 Systemic disorders may cause hypotonia due to a disturbance of cerebral function. The onset may be acute or insidious. Depending on the clinical picture, laboratory studies to assess serum electrolytes, renal function, and thyroid function and to rule out infection should be considered. A lumbar puncture and CSF evaluation may be necessary to rule out certain suspected infectious causes. If symptoms have been chronic or other neurologic abnormalities exist, a metabolic investigation should also be done. Cytogenetic (chromosomal) studies may be helpful if a genetic disorder is suspected.

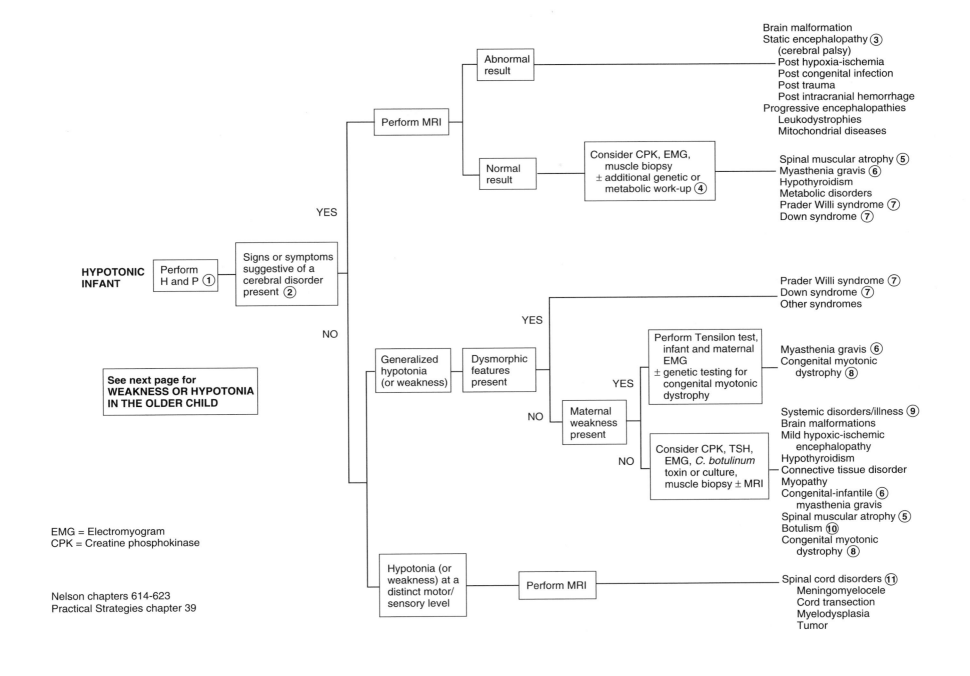

HYPOTONIC INFANT

Perform H and P (1) → Signs or symptoms suggestive of a cerebral disorder present (2)

YES → Perform MRI

- Abnormal result →
  - Brain malformation
  - Static encephalopathy (3) (cerebral palsy)
  - Post hypoxia-ischemia
  - Post congenital infection
  - Post trauma
  - Post intracranial hemorrhage
  - Progressive encephalopathies
  - Leukodystrophies
  - Mitochondrial diseases

- Normal result → Consider CPK, EMG, muscle biopsy ± additional genetic or metabolic work-up (4) →
  - Spinal muscular atrophy (5)
  - Myasthenia gravis (6)
  - Hypothyroidism
  - Metabolic disorders
  - Prader Willi syndrome (7)
  - Down syndrome (7)

NO → Generalized hypotonia (or weakness) → Dysmorphic features present

- **YES** →
  - Prader Willi syndrome (7)
  - Down syndrome (7)
  - Other syndromes

- **NO** → Maternal weakness present
  - **YES** → Perform Tensilon test, infant and maternal EMG ± genetic testing for congenital myotonic dystrophy →
    - Myasthenia gravis (6)
    - Congenital myotonic dystrophy (8)
  - **NO** → Consider CPK, TSH, EMG, *C. botulinum* toxin or culture, muscle biopsy ± MRI →
    - Systemic disorders/illness (9)
    - Brain malformations
    - Mild hypoxic-ischemic encephalopathy
    - Hypothyroidism
    - Connective tissue disorder
    - Myopathy
    - Congenital-infantile (6) myasthenia gravis
    - Spinal muscular atrophy (5)
    - Botulism (10)
    - Congenital myotonic dystrophy (8)

Hypotonia (or weakness) at a distinct motor/sensory level → Perform MRI →
- Spinal cord disorders (11)
  - Meningomyelocele
  - Cord transection
  - Myelodysplasia
  - Tumor

See next page for WEAKNESS OR HYPOTONIA IN THE OLDER CHILD

EMG = Electromyogram
CPK = Creatine phosphokinase

Nelson chapters 614-623
Practical Strategies chapter 39

10 Infantile botulism most commonly occurs in infants between 2 and 6 months of age. Source of the spores carrying the toxin of *Clostridium botulinum* may be honey, corn syrup, soil, or dust. Infants present with a descending paralysis. Cranial nerve symptoms are typically noted first. A recent history including poor feeding, constipation, weak cry and smile, hypotonia, ptosis, and mydriasis is common. Diagnosis is confirmed by recovery of the organism or toxin from stool, blood, or food sources. Older children can present with food-borne botulism due to ingestion of preformed toxin in poorly canned foods.

11 Spinal cord disorders often occur as hyperreflexia, clonus, positive Babinski sign, and defined sensory loss in the extremities. Hypotonia may be the prominent acute sign in infants. The diagnosis should be considered in infants with hypotonia after a difficult delivery. In older children disorders include traumatic transection, spinal cord tumor, transverse myelitis, and epidural spinal abscesses. Hypotonia is subsequently replaced by hypertonia.

12 Metabolic disorders usually appear in the neonatal period, although partial or incomplete errors may not appear until later. A complaint of hypotonia combined with a history of recurrent bouts of lethargy, vomiting, acidosis, and other neurologic findings should prompt appropriate metabolic screening laboratory studies.

13 Duchenne muscular dystrophy, an X-linked recessive disorder, is the most common type of muscular dystrophy. Diagnosis is usually in late infancy or early childhood when the child presents with a hyperlordotic posture and Gowers sign by age 3 years, followed by a Trendelenburg gait, muscle atrophy, and pseudohypertrophy of the calves. Diagnosis is based on the history, examination, and elevated CPK and is confirmed by muscle biopsy.

14 Guillain-Barré syndrome is an acute demyelinating polyneuropathy characterized by an ascending motor weakness and areflexia. Respiratory compromise may occur if respiratory muscles are involved. The syndrome frequently follows an upper respiratory tract infection or *Campylobacter* diarrhea. Evaluation reveals abnormal nerve conduction velocity. CSF protein may be elevated in the absence of pleocytosis.

15 The most common causes of progressive distal weakness are neuropathies, most of which are familial. Dysesthesias (e.g., painful tingling and burning sensations) often accompany the weakness. Autonomic symptoms (e.g., orthostatic hypotension, gastrointestinal dysmotility, abnormal sweating) may be present, and deep tendon reflexes are usually markedly diminished relative to the degree of weakness. Diagnosis of these disorders is by nerve conduction velocity studies and EMG. A lumbar puncture and an evaluation of the CSF may be necessary to rule out certain suspected infectious causes. For example, nonpolio enteroviruses may cause poliomyelitis-like disease.

16 Several species of North American ticks carry a toxin that can cause a paralysis clinically similar to Guillain-Barré syndrome. Tendon reflexes are usually diminished. Sensation is preserved, but burning or tingling may occur.

17 Scapulohumeral or scapuloperoneal syndromes have characteristics of both nerve and muscle disease. Patients present with proximal arm and distal leg weakness.

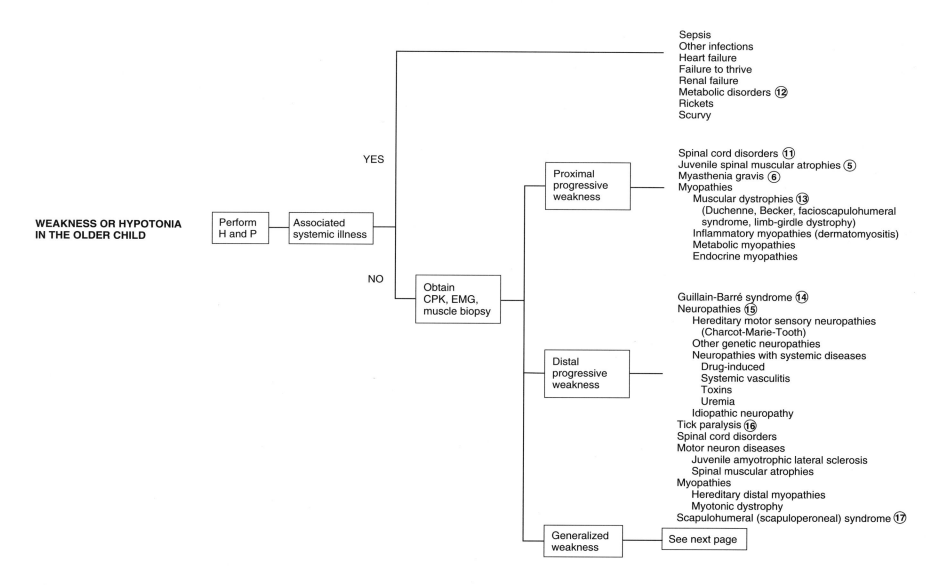

WEAKNESS OR HYPOTONIA IN THE OLDER CHILD

Perform H and P → Associated systemic illness

YES

Sepsis
Other infections
Heart failure
Failure to thrive
Renal failure
Metabolic disorders ⑫
Rickets
Scurvy

NO

Obtain CPK, EMG, muscle biopsy

Proximal progressive weakness

Spinal cord disorders ⑪
Juvenile spinal muscular atrophies ⑤
Myasthenia gravis ⑥
Myopathies
　Muscular dystrophies ⑬
　　(Duchenne, Becker, facioscapulohumeral
　　syndrome, limb-girdle dystrophy)
　Inflammatory myopathies (dermatomyositis)
　Metabolic myopathies
　Endocrine myopathies

Distal progressive weakness

Guillain-Barré syndrome ⑭
Neuropathies ⑮
　Hereditary motor sensory neuropathies
　　(Charcot-Marie-Tooth)
　Other genetic neuropathies
　Neuropathies with systemic diseases
　　Drug-induced
　　Systemic vasculitis
　　Toxins
　　Uremia
　Idiopathic neuropathy
Tick paralysis ⑯
Spinal cord disorders
Motor neuron diseases
　Juvenile amyotrophic lateral sclerosis
　Spinal muscular atrophies
Myopathies
　Hereditary distal myopathies
　Myotonic dystrophy
Scapulohumeral (scapuloperoneal) syndrome ⑰

Generalized weakness → See next page

EMG = Electromyogram
CPK = Creatine phosphokinase

(18) Transverse myelitis appears acutely with hypotonia and weakness. There is an identifiable motor-sensory level, impaired bowel and bladder function, hyperreflexia, and abnormal Babinski sign. Spinal MRI shows abnormal signal intensity of the involved level, and CSF examination shows a mild pleocytosis and elevated protein level.

(19) In periodic paralysis, patients experience episodes of severe weakness, often followed by partial or complete paralysis. Episodes are usually related to hypokalemia or hyperkalemia and may be primary (i.e., genetically transmitted) or secondary (i.e., most commonly due to potassium losses via the urinary tract—hyperaldosteronism, renal tubular defects) or gastrointestinal tract (e.g., severe chronic diarrhea, prolonged vomiting or use of gastrointestinal drains, fistulas).

(20) Joint hyperextensibility and hypotonia out of proportion to the degree of weakness suggest a connective tissue disorder (e.g., Ehlers-Danlos). Diagnosis of many of these disorders is clinical, although molecular genetic testing is available for an increasing number of these disorders.

BIBLIOGRAPHY

Fenichel GM: Clinical Pediatric Neurology, 3rd ed. Philadelphia: WB Saunders Company, 1997.

**WEAKNESS OR HYPOTONIA
IN THE OLDER CHILD
(continued)**

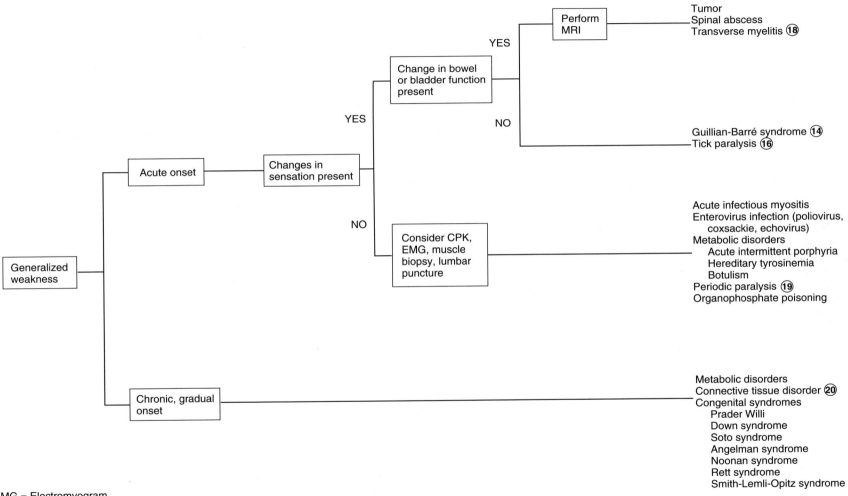

EMG = Electromyogram
CPK = Creatine phosphokinase

Chapter 54 Ataxia

Ataxia is a disturbance of the fine control of movement and posture that is normally coordinated by the cerebellum.

(1) It is important to determine not only the nature of the complaint but also whether it is acute or intermittent versus chronic or progressive. Inquire about associated symptoms (e.g., systemic illness, nystagmus, vertigo). Be aware that a slowly developing ataxia may be noticed acutely. Consider that any acute ataxia could be the initial presentation of an episodic or a recurrent disorder.

The physical examination should include a careful neurological assessment, particularly of cerebellar function and muscle strength. Muscle weakness may be misinterpreted as cerebellar dysfunction. A positive Romberg sign implies an abnormality of the posterior column pathways or vestibular function but not a cerebellar function.

(2) Ataxia occurs in approximately 50% of patients who experience basilar artery migraines. Visual loss, vertigo, tinnitus, alternating hemiparesis, and paresthesias may also occur. An EEG will help to rule out seizure activity and may reveal occipital intermittent rhythmic delta activity during and shortly after an attack.

(3) In benign paroxysmal vertigo, true ataxia does not occur but the vertigo is so severe that the child collapses on the floor. Infants and preschool children are most often affected. Episodes are brief, consciousness is not impaired, and headache is absent. Diagnosis is clinical.

(4) Hartnup disease is an autosomal recessive disorder of tryptophan metabolism. Most children with the disorder remain asymptomatic. Cutaneous photosensitivity is the major clinical manifestation when symptoms do occur; emotional instability, episodic ataxia, and occasionally diarrhea may also occur.

(5) Hereditary ataxias are often diagnosed using the family history and clinical features. The abnormal gene and gene products remain unidentified for many, although specialized testing is becoming available for an increasing number of these disorders. Referral to a neurologist is recommended.

(6) Ataxia due to brain tumors may be chronic or acute due to bleeding or rapid development of hydrocephalus.

(7) Ataxia or an unsteady gait may be prominent after a head injury. Neurologic examination is otherwise normal. Symptoms of postconcussion syndrome may last 1 to 6 months. Diagnosis is clinical. Imaging at the time of the injury is recommended to rule out intracranial hemorrhage. Toxicology screening should always be considered.

(8) Drug ingestion is one of the most common causes of acute ataxia. Ataxia may be a more prominent syndrome than altered mental status in certain ingestions (e.g., anticonvulsants, lead, alcohol). Overuse of antihistamines may exacerbate unsteadiness or ataxia that occurs due to otitis media. Alcohol and drug abuse must be considered in adolescents. Urine toxicology screens detect a limited number of substances. Specific screens for suspected agents should be performed.

(9) Ataxia-telangiectasia affects primarily the nervous and immune systems. It should be suspected in young children with ataxia, chronic sinopulmonary infections, and disturbance of voluntary gaze. Telangiectases are usually a late development. Diagnosis is by detection of immunologic deficits.

(10) Friedreich ataxia is an autosomal recessive disorder characterized by ataxia, dysarthric speech, nystagmus, and skeletal abnormalities. Onset is between 2 and 16 years. Diagnosis is mostly clinical. Electrophysiologic studies are often abnormal. A cardiac evaluation should be performed.

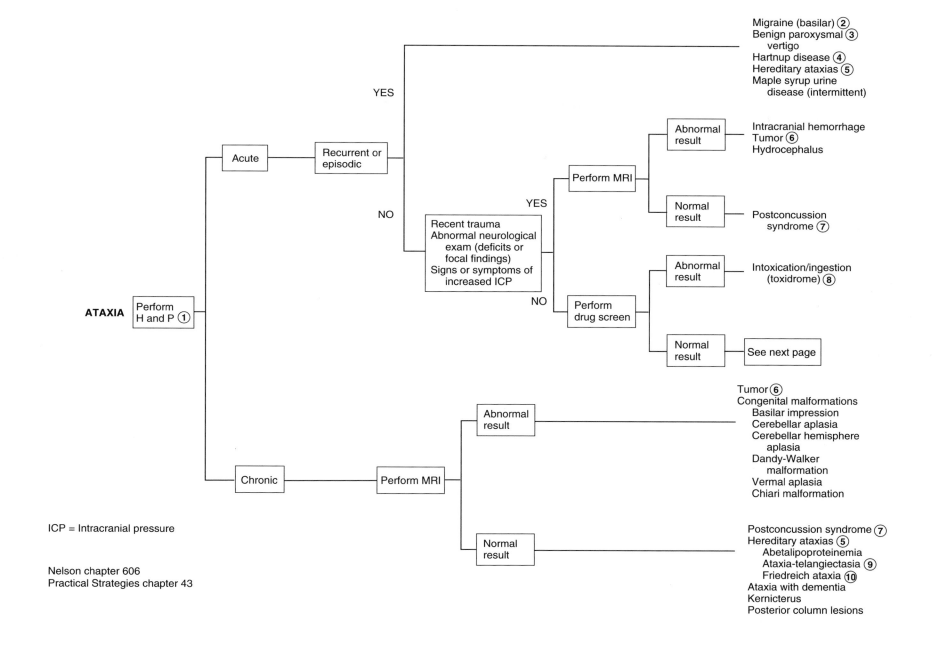

ATAXIA — Perform H and P ①

Acute

Recurrent or episodic

YES →
Migraine (basilar) ②
Benign paroxysmal ③
vertigo
Hartnup disease ④
Hereditary ataxias ⑤
Maple syrup urine
disease (intermittent)

NO →
Recent trauma
Abnormal neurological exam (deficits or focal findings)
Signs or symptoms of increased ICP

YES → Perform MRI
- Abnormal result → Intracranial hemorrhage
Tumor ⑥
Hydrocephalus
- Normal result → Postconcussion syndrome ⑦

NO → Perform drug screen
- Abnormal result → Intoxication/ingestion (toxidrome) ⑧
- Normal result → See next page

Chronic → Perform MRI
- Abnormal result →
Tumor ⑥
Congenital malformations
Basilar impression
Cerebellar aplasia
Cerebellar hemisphere aplasia
Dandy-Walker malformation
Vermal aplasia
Chiari malformation
- Normal result →
Postconcussion syndrome ⑦
Hereditary ataxias ⑤
Abetalipoproteinemia
Ataxia-telangiectasia ⑨
Friedreich ataxia ⑩
Ataxia with dementia
Kernicterus
Posterior column lesions

ICP = Intracranial pressure

Nelson chapter 606
Practical Strategies chapter 43

Ataxia *(continued)*

11 Severe vertigo, vomiting, and association with middle ear infections or nonspecific viral infections characterize acute labyrinthitis. Unilateral hearing loss and nystagmus may also be present.

12 Acute cerebellar ataxia (i.e., acute postinfectious cerebellitis) is a common cause of acute ataxia in children. Preceding illness is identified in approximately 80% of cases. Varicella is a common agent. The ataxia develops 2 to 3 weeks after the illness. The onset is acute and maximal at onset. Vomiting may occur early, and nystagmus or dysarthria may be present, but the sensorium is always clear. The diagnosis is one of exclusion. A drug screen should always be performed and an imaging study considered.

The exception to immediate imaging may be the child who develops ataxia shortly after a vari-cella infection. In acute cerebellar ataxia, improvement should begin within a few days. Full recovery may take weeks to months. Imaging should definitely be performed in those children if rapid improvement of the ataxia does not occur. If any changes in mental status, fever, or other neurologic symptoms (e.g., seizures, areflexia, weakness) are present, further evaluation should be performed. CSF results if obtained are often normal or show a slight pleocytosis at the onset. An elevation of protein level occurs later.

13 Ataxia and cranial nerve dysfunction characterize brain stem encephalitis. Evaluation of the CSF shows pleocytosis, normal glucose levels, and normal or slightly elevated protein levels.

14 The Miller-Fisher syndrome is considered a variant of Guillain-Barré syndrome. Ataxia, ophthalmoplegia, and areflexia occur after a viral illness. CSF examination shows an initial cellular response followed by an elevation of protein.

15 Myoclonic-encephalopathy-neuroblastoma syndrome is characterized by opsoclonus, myoclonic ataxia, and encephalopathy. (See Ch. 9.) It may occur as an isolated entity, but occult neuroblastoma must be ruled out.

16 Acute episodic ataxia ("pseudoataxia") may rarely be the only clinical manifestation of seizure activity. EEG is diagnostic.

BIBLIOGRAPHY

Fenichel GM: Clinical Pediatric Neurology, 3rd ed. Philadelphia, WB Saunders Company, 1997.

Friday JH: Ataxia. In Fleisher G, Ludwig S (eds): Textbook of Pediatric Emergency Medicine, 4th ed, p 153. Baltimore, Williams & Wilkins, 2000.

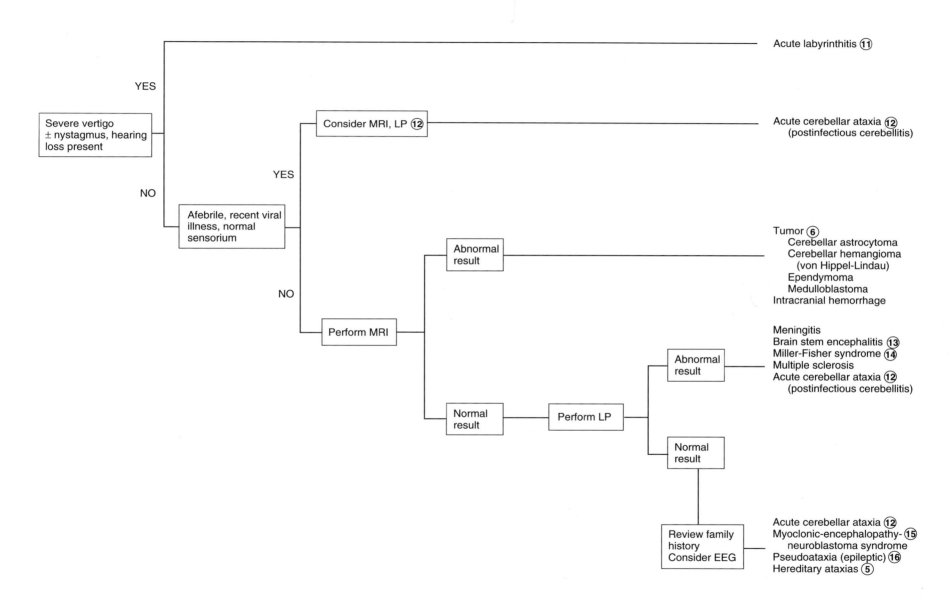

Acute labyrinthitis ⑪

Severe vertigo ± nystagmus, hearing loss present

YES

NO

Afebrile, recent viral illness, normal sensorium

YES

Consider MRI, LP ⑫

Acute cerebellar ataxia ⑫
(postinfectious cerebellitis)

NO

Perform MRI

Abnormal result

Tumor ⑥
    Cerebellar astrocytoma
    Cerebellar hemangioma
      (von Hippel-Lindau)
    Ependymoma
    Medulloblastoma
Intracranial hemorrhage

Normal result

Perform LP

Abnormal result

Meningitis
Brain stem encephalitis ⑬
Miller-Fisher syndrome ⑭
Multiple sclerosis
Acute cerebellar ataxia ⑫
    (postinfectious cerebellitis)

Normal result

Review family history
Consider EEG

Acute cerebellar ataxia ⑫
Myoclonic-encephalopathy- ⑮
    neuroblastoma syndrome
Pseudoataxia (epileptic) ⑯
Hereditary ataxias ⑤

An alteration in consciousness (i.e., awareness of self and environment) may range from delirium (e.g., irritability, confusion, agitation) to coma. A delirious state is often characterized by alternating periods of lucidity and frequently progresses to lethargy or coma.

(1) A child presenting with any alteration in consciousness must be emergently stabilized before a search is started for the cause. The patient must then be evaluated to rule out a potentially life-threatening intracranial process that requires urgent treatment. The Glasgow Coma Scale (GCS) is the most widely used tool for assessing and monitoring changes in mental status. The GCS is a better way to describe altered levels of consciousness when compared with less specific terms such as stuporous, obtunded, or lethargic.

The history should include a recent review of systems and a history of trauma, medications, and possible toxic ingestions.

Certain components of the physical examination may suggest an underlying systemic disorder. For example, certain skin lesions may suggest neurocutaneous disorders, Addison disease, or infectious conditions. Hepatomegaly can suggest hepatic failure (e.g., Reye syndrome) or heart failure. Fractured extremities raise the possibility of a fat embolism. Toxidromes (e.g., apnea and pinpoint pupils for opiates) help identify a possible ingestion.

A patient's breathing pattern may aid in the diagnosis of altered mental status. Hyperventilation occurs with toxic-metabolic encephalopathies, increased intracranial pressure, and metabolic acidosis. Hypoventilation occurs with many drug ingestions. Other breathing patterns (e.g., Cheyne-Stokes, apneustic breathing) may indicate specific sites of CNS dysfunction. The odor of the breath may be helpful. Many disorders and certain ingestions are accompanied by a characteristic odor.

(2) A history of a traumatic head injury should prompt an evaluation for a progressive intracranial process. Other worrisome signs and symptoms include a bulging fontanel, retinal hemorrhages, focal neurologic findings, and signs of brain stem dysfunction (e.g., abnormal respiratory pattern and abnormal corneal, oculocephalic, or oculovestibular reflexes). Signs of increased intracranial pressure include a unilateral fixed or dilated pupil, ptosis, Cushing triad (hypertension, bradycardia, apnea), cranial nerve VI palsy, papilledema, and history of vomiting, headache, or ataxia.

(3) Shaken baby syndrome usually occurs in children younger than 12 months. Children often have no external signs of trauma, although retinal hemorrhages and bulging fontanel may be evident on examination. Neuroimaging reveals subdural hematomas. A complete evaluation for other injuries is indicated when abuse is suspected.

(4) A lumbar puncture is *contraindicated* in children if they have any of the following : (1) cardiorespiratory compromise, (2) focal neurologic findings, (3) signs of increased intracranial pressure other than a bulging fontanel, and (4) skin or soft tissue infection overlying the site of the lumbar puncture.

(5) An intravenous dose of naloxone is recommended to potentially treat this rapidly reversible cause of altered mental status.

(6) Depending on the suspected cause, laboratory tests to be considered are a CBC, blood culture, sodium, and blood urea nitrogen determinations, and arterial blood gas analysis. Additional laboratory studies to consider are liver function tests; blood ammonia level; calcium, magnesium, and phosphorus levels; and serum osmolality. An osmolal gap and anion gap should be calculated. (See Ch. 82.) When the physical examination and laboratory studies do not help reveal a diagnosis, a head CT should be obtained. An EEG may be helpful if encephalitis, encephalopathy, or a seizure disorder is suspected.

(7) Poisonings are common in children. A sudden onset of altered mental status, seizures, and vomiting, especially with a preceding period of confusion or delirium, should raise suspicion for a possible ingestion. Toxicology screens may be helpful, although they may be of limited value because they are not standardized. If certain agents are suspected, tests for them should be specifically requested. An EKG may reveal conduction abnormalities, common with certain ingestions, that may aid in the diagnosis. Many toxins cause a characteristic toxidrome of symptoms that may aid in their identification. Level of consciousness, pupillary examination, and vital signs are the most helpful components in identifying a toxidrome.

(8) Inborn errors of metabolism usually occur in the neonate with vomiting, lethargy, or seizures, although partial or incomplete errors may not occur until later childhood or adolescence. A patient or family history of recurrent episodes of lethargy, vomiting, personality changes, or frequent hospitalizations should raise suspicion for a metabolic disorder and prompt an appropriate laboratory evaluation. (See also Ch. 22.)

In older infants and children, altered mental status may be due to electrolyte abnormalities (e.g., hypernatremia, hyponatremia, hypocalcemia).

(9) A sudden onset of encephalopathy, shock, seizures, coagulopathy, bleeding, and hepatic and renal impairment occurs in hemorrhagic shock-encephalopathy.

(10) Reye syndrome is characterized by an acute onset of vomiting, combativeness, and mental status changes ranging from delirium to coma. Hepatic enzyme levels and serum ammonia levels are elevated. Hypoglycemia and metabolic acidosis may occur. The syndrome typically occurs after a viral infection (varicella, influenza B, influenza A) and has been strongly associated with aspirin use.

BIBLIOGRAPHY

Fenichel GM: Clinical Pediatric Neurology, 3rd ed. Philadelphia: WB Saunders Company, 1997.

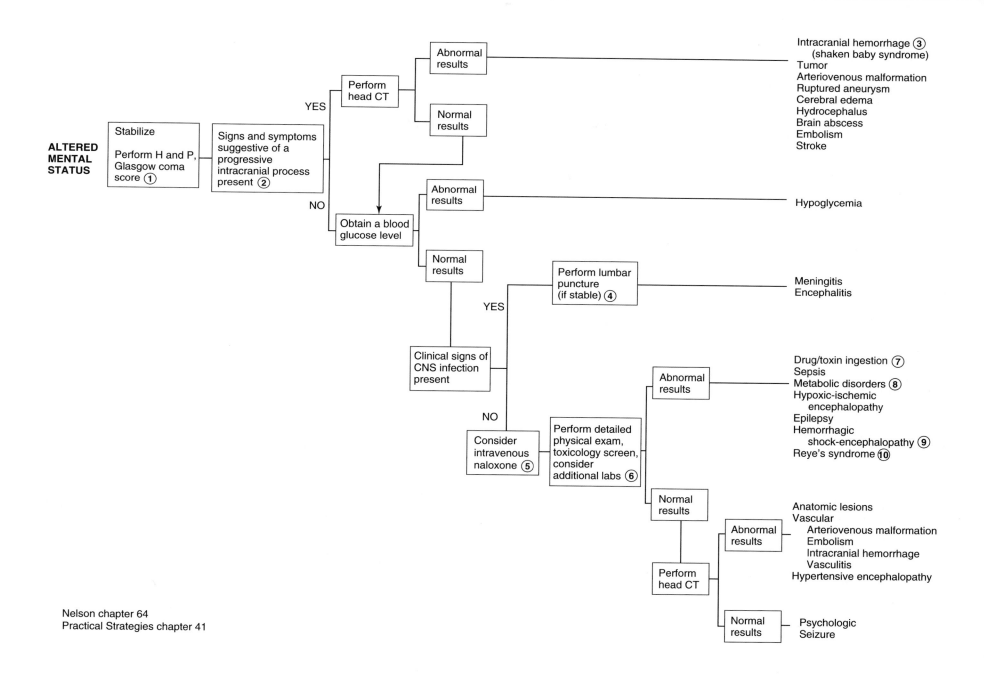

ALTERED MENTAL STATUS

Stabilize

Perform H and P, Glasgow coma score ①

Signs and symptoms suggestive of a progressive intracranial process present ②

YES → Perform head CT

- Abnormal results → Intracranial hemorrhage ③ (shaken baby syndrome)
  Tumor
  Arteriovenous malformation
  Ruptured aneurysm
  Cerebral edema
  Hydrocephalus
  Brain abscess
  Embolism
  Stroke
- Normal results →

NO → Obtain a blood glucose level

- Abnormal results → Hypoglycemia
- Normal results →

Clinical signs of CNS infection present

YES → Perform lumbar puncture (if stable) ④ → Meningitis
Encephalitis

NO → Consider intravenous naloxone ⑤ → Perform detailed physical exam, toxicology screen, consider additional labs ⑥

- Abnormal results → Drug/toxin ingestion ⑦
  Sepsis
  Metabolic disorders ⑧
  Hypoxic-ischemic encephalopathy
  Epilepsy
  Hemorrhagic shock-encephalopathy ⑨
  Reye's syndrome ⑩
- Normal results → Perform head CT
  - Abnormal results → Anatomic lesions
    Vascular
      Arteriovenous malformation
      Embolism
      Intracranial hemorrhage
      Vasculitis
    Hypertensive encephalopathy
  - Normal results → Psychologic
    Seizure

Nelson chapter 64
Practical Strategies chapter 41

Chapter 56 **Hearing Loss**

A growing proportion of children in the United States are being screened for hearing at birth. Children with acquired or late-onset hearing loss may present with a more subtle problem, such as poor school performance. Sometimes children with effusion or eustachian tube dysfunction present with a complaint of hearing loss. The role of the primary care practitioner is to identify the hearing loss and follow through on appropriate referrals for comprehensive evaluation and treatment. Identifying hearing loss as early as possible is critical to minimizing the adverse effects on speech and language and school performance.

(1) Approximately 15% of newborns weighing less than 1500 g or born before 32 weeks' gestation have hearing loss. Known risk factors for hearing loss include congenital infections, ototoxic drugs, meningitis, asphyxia, and persistent fetal circulation. Prenatal exposure to alcohol, trimethadione, and mercury and maternal deficiency of iodine are also associated with hearing loss. For older children, inquire about noise exposure, trauma, and toxic ingestions or exposures.

A family history positive for kidney abnormalities, different colored eyes, white forelock of hair, night blindness, cardiac arrhythmias, or sudden cardiac death, as well as deafness, should raise suspicion for hereditary causes of hearing loss.

On the physical examination, microphthalmia or retinitis may suggest a congenital infection (e.g., cytomegalovirus infection, rubella).

A history of absent or delayed language milestones is significant in the evaluation of hearing loss. Some general "red flags" suggesting language delays include (1) not startling to loud sounds by 3 months, (2) not vocalizing by 6 months, (3) not localizing speech or other sounds by 9 months, (4) not babbling multiple sounds or syllables by 12 months, (5) not saying "mama" or "dada" specifically by 13 months, and (6) less than 50% of speech understandable by 24 months.

(2) Mild conductive hearing loss is common with otitis media and normally improves with the resolution of the effusion. Small tympanic membrane perforations have little effect on hearing, but large perforations may.

(3) Tympanometry provides information about tympanic membrane compliance and middle ear pressure. Before age 6 months, the excessive compliance of the ear canal limits the usefulness of the test.

Newborn screening programs rely on otoacoustic emissions testing and brain stem auditory evoked response (BAER) to test infant hearing. The BAER test provides more information regarding frequencies of hearing affected. Once a child can cooperate, pure tone audiometry with bone and air conduction results is recommended. Referral for behavioral observation audiometry or a BAER test may be indicated for the child too young to complete pure tone audiometry.

(4) A temporary shift in hearing threshold after exposure to potentially injurious sounds can precede permanent noise-induced hearing loss (NIHL). NIHL has been attributed to high levels of continuous noise (e.g., music, recreational vehicles, power tools) and high intensity sounds of short duration (e.g., gunfire, firecrackers).

(5) Many centers provide a multidisciplinary approach to hearing loss, including evaluation and treatment by the audiologist, otolaryngologist, and speech pathologist. Genetics consultation may be helpful when a syndrome is suspected.

(6) Approximately 80% of cases are inherited as autosomal recessive traits. Two thirds of cases are not part of any syndrome. Hearing impairment associated with some genetic disorders may not manifest until later in childhood.

(7) Effects of ototoxic drugs may not appear until up to 6 months after exposure to the drug. Aminoglycosides and diuretics are the most common offenders. Lead toxicity is also a cause of hearing loss.

(8) Both conductive and sensorineural hearing loss have been reported in children who experience head trauma. Resolution over 6 months is the norm.

(9) Hearing loss due to congenital syphilis may not appear until after age 2 years. Some children with congenital cytomegalovirus (CMV) suddenly lose residual hearing at age 4 to 5 years. Hearing loss due to asymptomatic CMV may occur at any time up to 5 years of age.

(10) The tympanogram in otitis media with effusion is typically rounded or flat.

(11) Guidelines for management of the young child (age 1 to 3 years) with otitis media with effusion are available.

BIBLIOGRAPHY

Roizen NJ: Etiology of hearing loss in children: Nongenetic causes. Pediatr Clin North Am 46:49–64, 1999.

Stool SE, Berg AO, et al: Managing Otitis Media with Effusion in Young Children. Quick Reference Guide for Clinicians. AHCPR publication 94-0622. US Department of Health and Human Services, July 1994. (Summary published in Pediatrics 94:766–773, 1994.)

Tomaski SM, Grundfast KM: A stepwise approach to the diagnosis and treatment of hereditary hearing loss. Pediatr Clin North Am 46:35–48, 1999.

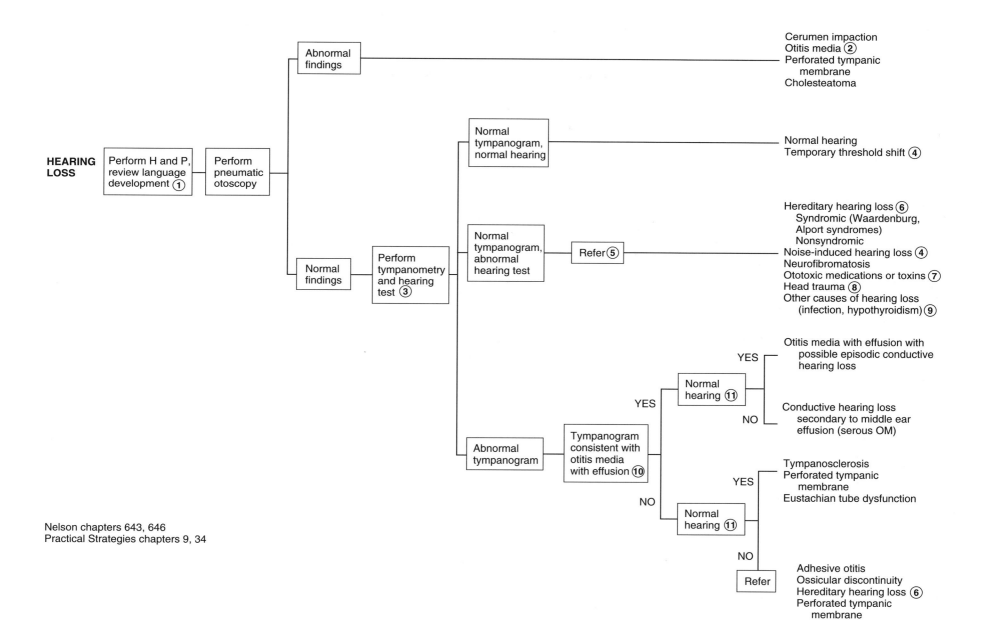

HEARING LOSS

Perform H and P, review language development ① → Perform pneumatic otoscopy

Abnormal findings → Cerumen impaction
Otitis media ②
Perforated tympanic membrane
Cholesteatoma

Normal findings → Perform tympanometry and hearing test ③

Normal tympanogram, normal hearing → Normal hearing
Temporary threshold shift ④

Normal tympanogram, abnormal hearing test → Refer ⑤ → Hereditary hearing loss ⑥
  Syndromic (Waardenburg, Alport syndromes)
  Nonsyndromic
Noise-induced hearing loss ④
Neurofibromatosis
Ototoxic medications or toxins ⑦
Head trauma ⑧
Other causes of hearing loss (infection, hypothyroidism) ⑨

Abnormal tympanogram → Tympanogram consistent with otitis media with effusion ⑩

YES → Normal hearing ⑪
  YES → Otitis media with effusion with possible episodic conductive hearing loss
  NO → Conductive hearing loss secondary to middle ear effusion (serous OM)

NO → Normal hearing ⑪
  YES → Tympanosclerosis
    Perforated tympanic membrane
    Eustachian tube dysfunction
  NO → Refer → Adhesive otitis
    Ossicular discontinuity
    Hereditary hearing loss ⑥
    Perforated tympanic membrane

Nelson chapters 643, 646
Practical Strategies chapters 9, 34

DERMATOLOGY

Chapter 57 Alopecia

Alopecia is the absence or loss of hair. Hypotrichosis (i.e., very sparse or thin hair) occurs along with alopecia in many conditions.

(1) The history and physical examination often reveal the diagnosis. A family history of hereditary disorders may include hair abnormalities. Inquire about recent stressors (e.g., surgery, illness). Most diagnoses can be confirmed by microscopic examination of a hair pull (i.e., a tuft of hair gently removed to include the roots), potassium hydroxide (KOH) examination, culture, or biopsy.

(2) Sebaceous nevi of Jadassohn are small well-demarcated yellowish orange plaques. They remain relatively flat through infancy and childhood. Hormonal stimulation during adolescence causes an increase in size with a potential for malignant changes. The nevi should be removed before or during adolescence.

(3) Alopecia along the frontal and occipital sutures is characteristic of the Hallermann-Streiff syndrome (i.e., oculomandibulocephaly).

(4) Congenital triangular alopecia overlying the frontotemporal suture may not be noticed until age 2 to 3 years. The base of the triangular area (3 to 5 cm) abuts on the anterior hairline.

(5) Ectodermal dysplasia is characterized by a primary defect of teeth, skin, and appendageal structures (e.g., hair, nails, eccrine and sebaceous glands). Hidrotic and hypohidrotic or anhidrotic ectodermal dysplasias are examples.

(6) Congenital structural defects of the hair shaft appear as alopecia or hypotrichosis with short, fragile hair that does not appear to grow.

(7) Loose anagen hair of childhood is a condition of actively growing but loosely anchored hairs. It is most often seen in young (2 to 5 years old), blond females. They present with diffuse or patchy alopecia, apparent lack of hair growth, and hairs that are easily pulled from the head.

(8) Tinea capitis can occur with patchy or diffuse scaling, localized or "black dot" alopecia, or kerion. Alopecia may be the chief complaint, especially if the patient is regularly using moisturizing hair or scalp preparations. *Trichophyton tonsurans* is the dermatophyte currently responsible for the majority of tinea capitis infections. T. tonsurans does not fluoresce under black light. A culture is often needed for diagnosis and is probably the method of choice for the primary care practitioner. Diagnosis may be made by examination of a KOH preparation of scale or involved hair, but this method is not very sensitive. Kerions are boggy, pustular plaques that develop as a hypersensitivity reaction to the dermatophyte. The reaction is inflammatory, and cultures of the purulent matter are usually negative for bacteria.

(9) Infections that can result in scarring and alopecia include cellulitis, impetigo, folliculitis, and varicella. Bockhart impetigo is a superficial folliculitis that commonly affects the scalp, face, buttocks, and extremities.

(10) Alopecia areata is a disorder characterized by well-circumscribed round or oval patches of hair loss on the scalp and other sites. The affected surface usually appears normal. When the condition is diffuse over the scalp it is called alopecia universalis; when it is diffuse over the body including eyebrows and eyelashes, it is alopecia totalis.

(11) Hair styling resulting in prolonged or extensive traction can cause nonscarring alopecia along the margins of tightly braided or styled hair. Pustules and folliculitis are often present.

(12) Avulsion may be a manifestation of child abuse.

(13) Occipital hair loss occurring in a young infant is a form of traction alopecia. Some hair loss occurs normally early in the newborn period. Rubbing the head on a sheet or mattress simply exaggerates this normal phase of hair loss. Young infants may demonstrate a "halo scalp ring alopecia" around the edge of a caput succedaneum or cephalohematoma.

(14) Telogen effluvium is a sudden diffuse loss of hair that is commonly associated with a history of a recent stressor (e.g., illness, surgery). The stressor causes an interruption of the normal cycle of hair growth that becomes most evident 2 to 4 months later when growth resumes and pushes out the resting hairs. Other inciting stressors are medications, febrile illnesses, crash diets, anesthesia, parturition, endocrine disorders, and severe stress.

(15) Toxic alopecia (i.e., anagen effluvium) is acute severe hair loss due to radiation or chemotherapy.

(16) Androgenetic (male pattern) baldness can occur any time after adolescence. The condition can occasionally affect females.

BIBLIOGRAPHY

Hurwitz S: Clinical Pediatric Dermatology, 2nd ed. Philadelphia: WB Saunders Company, 1993.

Levy ML: Disorders of the hair and scalp. Pediatr Clin North Am 38:905–919, 1991.

Weston WL, Lane AT: Color Textbook of Pediatric Dermatology, 2nd ed. St. Louis: Mosby-Year Book, 1996.

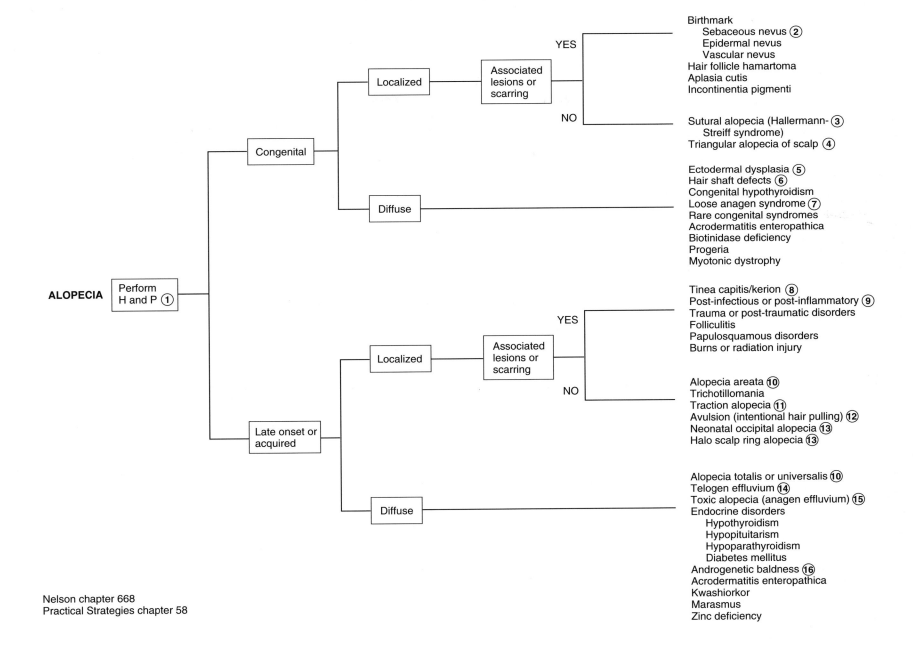

ALOPECIA — Perform H and P ①

- **Congenital**
  - **Localized** — Associated lesions or scarring
    - **YES**
      - Birthmark
        - Sebaceous nevus ②
        - Epidermal nevus
        - Vascular nevus
      - Hair follicle hamartoma
      - Aplasia cutis
      - Incontinentia pigmenti
    - **NO**
      - Sutural alopecia (Hallermann-Streiff syndrome) ③
      - Triangular alopecia of scalp ④
  - **Diffuse**
    - Ectodermal dysplasia ⑤
    - Hair shaft defects ⑥
    - Congenital hypothyroidism
    - Loose anagen syndrome ⑦
    - Rare congenital syndromes
    - Acrodermatitis enteropathica
    - Biotinidase deficiency
    - Progeria
    - Myotonic dystrophy

- **Late onset or acquired**
  - **Localized** — Associated lesions or scarring
    - **YES**
      - Tinea capitis/kerion ⑧
      - Post-infectious or post-inflammatory ⑨
      - Trauma or post-traumatic disorders
      - Folliculitis
      - Papulosquamous disorders
      - Burns or radiation injury
    - **NO**
      - Alopecia areata ⑩
      - Trichotillomania
      - Traction alopecia ⑪
      - Avulsion (intentional hair pulling) ⑫
      - Neonatal occipital alopecia ⑬
      - Halo scalp ring alopecia ⑬
  - **Diffuse**
    - Alopecia totalis or universalis ⑩
    - Telogen effluvium ⑭
    - Toxic alopecia (anagen effluvium) ⑮
    - Endocrine disorders
      - Hypothyroidism
      - Hypopituitarism
      - Hypoparathyroidism
      - Diabetes mellitus
    - Androgenetic baldness ⑯
    - Acrodermatitis enteropathica
    - Kwashiorkor
    - Marasmus
    - Zinc deficiency

Nelson chapter 668
Practical Strategies chapter 58

Chapter 58 Vesicles and Bullae

Vesicles are small fluid-filled lesions; bullae are large vesicles (>1 cm). Fluid may be clear or hemorrhagic. Vesiculobullous lesions (blisters) may be infectious or noninfectious. Noninfectious lesions may be induced by trauma or spontaneous. Many of the vesiculobullous disorders are rare in children but need to be considered in the diagnosis of chronic blistering disorders. Many are clinically indistinguishable from others; skin biopsy, immunofluorescence, and electron microscopy are often necessary to make the definitive diagnosis.

The usefulness of the algorithm is limited (without photographs) to categorizing potential diagnoses based on some broad clinical criteria. Reference to a dermatology textbook or reference will often be necessary to confirm suspected diagnoses.

(1) A Tzanck smear, culture, or polymerase chain reaction for herpes simplex virus should be obtained to confirm the diagnosis.

(2) Epidermolysis bullosa constitutes a group of inherited blistering disorders. One acquired variant is also recognized. Most variants become evident in the neonatal period with blisters developing in areas of trauma or pressure. One variant (i.e., Weber-Cockayne) may not appear until adolescence or adulthood, with blisters developing on the hands and feet after significant trauma or friction.

(3) Incontinentia pigmenti is a hereditary disorder with multisystem involvement that mainly affects females. Cutaneous manifestations develop in the first 2 weeks of life with crops of vesicles or bullae developing on the trunk or extremities. Evolution to verrucous lesions followed by characteristic pigmentation changes subsequently occurs. The hair, eyes, central nervous system, and teeth are also affected.

(4) Epidermolytic hyperkeratosis is a form of ichthyosis characterized by large bullae occurring shortly after birth. Hyperkeratosis and scaling develop in the first few months of life.

(5) Congenital erosive and vesicular dermatosis is a rare nonhereditary disorder appearing at birth with extensive erosive and bullous lesions.

(6) Staphylococcal scalded skin syndrome is an exfoliative dermatitis characterized by diffuse tender erythema, flaccid bullae, sheets of desquamating skin, and positive Nikolsky sign. The face, neck, groin, and axillae are most commonly affected.

(7) Sucking blisters may be located on the dorsal surfaces of the forearm, hands, or fingers.

(8) Bullous impetigo most commonly affects infants and young children. The diaper area is the most commonly affected site in neonates.

(9) Vesicles are a common manifestation of scabies in infants and young children, especially on the palms and soles. Severe pruritus is characteristic.

(10) Erythema multiforme is a vesiculobullous eruption that is probably a hypersensitivity reaction triggered by a variety of drugs, infections, and toxic substances. Characteristic target lesions have a dusky center, pale inner ring, and erythematous outer rim. Stevens-Johnson syndrome is a more serious variant of erythema multiforme involving at least two mucous membranes, as well as the skin.

(11) Linear IgA disease (i.e., chronic bullous disease of children) usually occurs in the preschool years. A widespread eruption of large bullae with a variable degree of pruritus occurs; commonly affected sites include the perioral and periocular regions, scalp, lower abdomen, buttocks, and anogenital region. Sometimes the bullae develop in an annular or rosette-like configuration surrounding a central crust ("cluster of jewels").

(12) Dermatitis herpetiformis is most likely to occur in the 2- to 7-year-old age group. In this disorder, recurrent outbreaks of papules and vesicles occur in a symmetric distribution on the extensor surfaces. The outbreaks are extremely pruritic and tender. Hemorrhagic bullae on the palms and soles occasionally occur.

(13) Pemphigus refers to severe, chronic blistering disorders that usually appear in adulthood. Oral lesions and localized bullae may precede more extensive involvement for weeks or months.

(14) Hand-foot-mouth syndrome is a viral (Coxsackie) illness characterized by a prodrome of fever, anorexia, and sore throat followed by an enanthem of small ulcerating oral vesicles. The characteristic exanthem of oval vesicles, primarily on the hands and feet, follows the enanthem. Vesicles can also be seen with other enteroviral infections.

(15) Toxic epidermal necrolysis is a severe exfoliative dermatitis characterized by extensive erythema, bullae, and exfoliation of large sheets of skin. The disorder occurs in infants and children younger than 5 years old, although it is uncommon in the neonatal period.

BIBLIOGRAPHY

Hurwitz S: Clinical Pediatric Dermatology, 2nd ed. Philadelphia: WB Saunders Company, 1993.
Weston WL, Lane AT: Color Textbook of Pediatric Dermatology, 2nd ed. St. Louis: Mosby–Year Book, 1996.

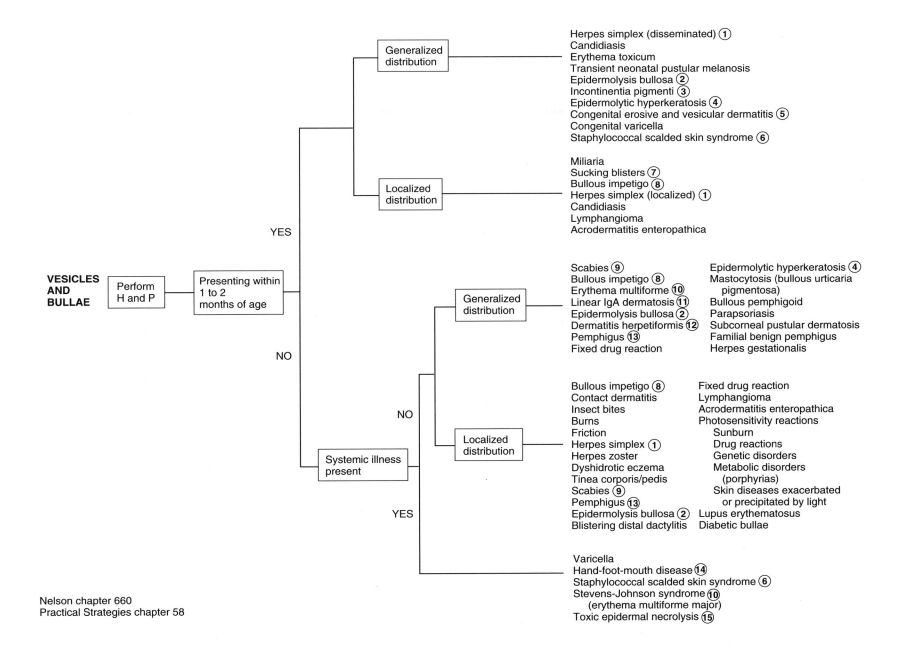

VESICLES AND BULLAE — Perform H and P — Presenting within 1 to 2 months of age

YES

Generalized distribution
- Herpes simplex (disseminated) ①
- Candidiasis
- Erythema toxicum
- Transient neonatal pustular melanosis
- Epidermolysis bullosa ②
- Incontinentia pigmenti ③
- Epidermolytic hyperkeratosis ④
- Congenital erosive and vesicular dermatitis ⑤
- Congenital varicella
- Staphylococcal scalded skin syndrome ⑥

Localized distribution
- Miliaria
- Sucking blisters ⑦
- Bullous impetigo ⑧
- Herpes simplex (localized) ①
- Candidiasis
- Lymphangioma
- Acrodermatitis enteropathica

NO — Systemic illness present

NO

Generalized distribution
- Scabies ⑨
- Bullous impetigo ⑧
- Erythema multiforme ⑩
- Linear IgA dermatosis ⑪
- Epidermolysis bullosa ②
- Dermatitis herpetiformis ⑫
- Pemphigus ⑬
- Fixed drug reaction
- Epidermolytic hyperkeratosis ④
- Mastocytosis (bullous urticaria pigmentosa)
- Bullous pemphigoid
- Parapsoriasis
- Subcorneal pustular dermatosis
- Familial benign pemphigus
- Herpes gestationalis

Localized distribution
- Bullous impetigo ⑧
- Contact dermatitis
- Insect bites
- Burns
- Friction
- Herpes simplex ①
- Herpes zoster
- Dyshidrotic eczema
- Tinea corporis/pedis
- Scabies ⑨
- Pemphigus ⑬
- Epidermolysis bullosa ②
- Blistering distal dactylitis
- Fixed drug reaction
- Lymphangioma
- Acrodermatitis enteropathica
- Photosensitivity reactions
  - Sunburn
  - Drug reactions
  - Genetic disorders
  - Metabolic disorders (porphyrias)
  - Skin diseases exacerbated or precipitated by light
  - Lupus erythematosus
  - Diabetic bullae

YES
- Varicella
- Hand-foot-mouth disease ⑭
- Staphylococcal scalded skin syndrome ⑥
- Stevens-Johnson syndrome ⑩ (erythema multiforme major)
- Toxic epidermal necrolysis ⑮

Nelson chapter 660
Practical Strategies chapter 58

Chapter 59 *Fever and Rash*

There are many disease processes that feature fever and rash occurring together. It is important to narrow the differential diagnosis with a comprehensive and careful history and physical examination. The causes include infections, vasculitides, and hypersensitivity disorders. Laboratory tests should be ordered according to the presumptive diagnosis based on the results of the history and physical examination. Many rashes are pathognomonic for certain diseases (e.g., varicella), and testing is usually not indicated.

(1) History should include the following features of the rash: presence of pruritus or pain, appearance in relationship to the fever, evolution and progression, and distribution. A history of ill contacts, recent travel, exposures (to pets, wildlife, insects), medications and intravenous drug use, transfusions, and sexual activity should be obtained. A history suggestive of an underlying immune deficiency should be sought. (See Ch. 78.)

Examination should include a general assessment of the patient to determine the severity of the illness, including vital signs and height of fever.

Tachycardia and tachypnea in a patient with fever and rash may indicate sepsis, particularly if there is altered mental status. The development of hypotension may indicate septic shock.

(2) The appearance of the rash (e.g., papular, vesicular, petechial) and the presence of associated enanthems (i.e., eruptions on mucosal surfaces) often suggest the diagnosis. The distribution of the rash should be noted: whether generalized or localized, symmetric or asymmetric, or centripetal or centrifugal.

(3) Petechial rashes and particularly purpuric rashes in a febrile child should always alert the physician to potentially life-threatening infections, especially in a child younger than 2 years. These children require an immediate and careful evaluation. Sepsis due to *Neisseria meningitidis*, as well as other organisms, is of particular concern. Purpura may be associated with disseminated intravascular coagulation (DIC), severe thrombocytopenia, or vasculitides.

(4) In a patient with a petechial or purpuric rash, a CBC should be obtained. Other tests (e.g., coagulation studies, blood culture, and cerebrospinal fluid evaluation) may be considered, depending on clinical presentation. Thrombocytopenia may be associated with many infections including viral ones. (See Ch. 63.) If coagulation studies are abnormal, DIC should be suspected. Even with a normal platelet count and coagulation studies, a WBC count $> 15,000/mm^3$, absolute band count > 500 cells/mm^3, and CSF white cell count > 7 cells/mm^3 suggest an increased risk for bacterial or rickettsial infection.

(5) Enteroviruses are a common cause of petechial rashes. The patients usually do not appear ill and may not require extensive testing. However, they must be observed closely. The presence of purpura demands a complete investigation, including blood and CSF cultures, coagulation studies, and empirical treatment of bacterial causes.

(6) In children with Henoch-Schönlein purpura, the rash usually begins as urticarial lesions, later becoming raised and purpuric, but it may be petechial.

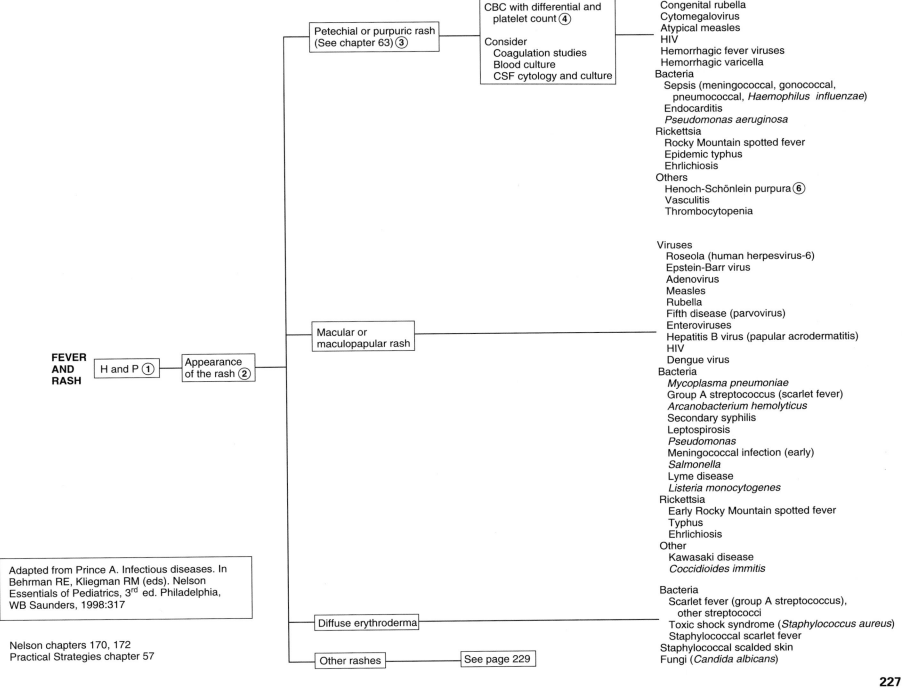

FEVER AND RASH

H and P (1) → Appearance of the rash (2)

Petechial or purpuric rash (See chapter 63) (3) →

CBC with differential and platelet count (4)

Consider
    Coagulation studies
    Blood culture
    CSF cytology and culture

→ Enterovirus (5)
Congenital rubella
Cytomegalovirus
Atypical measles
HIV
Hemorrhagic fever viruses
Hemorrhagic varicella
Bacteria
    Sepsis (meningococcal, gonococcal,
        pneumococcal, *Haemophilus influenzae*)
    Endocarditis
    Pseudomonas aeruginosa
Rickettsia
    Rocky Mountain spotted fever
    Epidemic typhus
    Ehrlichiosis
Others
    Henoch-Schönlein purpura (6)
    Vasculitis
    Thrombocytopenia

Macular or maculopapular rash →

Viruses
    Roseola (human herpesvirus-6)
    Epstein-Barr virus
    Adenovirus
    Measles
    Rubella
    Fifth disease (parvovirus)
    Enteroviruses
    Hepatitis B virus (papular acrodermatitis)
    HIV
    Dengue virus
Bacteria
    Mycoplasma pneumoniae
    Group A streptococcus (scarlet fever)
    Arcanobacterium hemolyticus
    Secondary syphilis
    Leptospirosis
    Pseudomonas
    Meningococcal infection (early)
    Salmonella
    Lyme disease
    Listeria monocytogenes
Rickettsia
    Early Rocky Mountain spotted fever
    Typhus
    Ehrlichiosis
Other
    Kawasaki disease
    Coccidioides immitis

Diffuse erythroderma →

Bacteria
    Scarlet fever (group A streptococcus),
        other streptococci
    Toxic shock syndrome (*Staphylococcus aureus*)
    Staphylococcal scarlet fever
Staphylococcal scalded skin
Fungi (*Candida albicans*)

Other rashes → See page 229

Adapted from Prince A. Infectious diseases. In Behrman RE, Kliegman RM (eds). Nelson Essentials of Pediatrics, 3rd ed. Philadelphia, WB Saunders, 1998:317

Nelson chapters 170, 172
Practical Strategies chapter 57

227

(7) *Pseudomonas aeruginosa* causes the classic skin lesions of ecthyma gangrenosum. The lesions begin as pink macules, progressing to hemorrhagic nodules and ulcers. The ulcers classically have ecchymotic, gangrenous centers with eschar formation and are surrounded by a red areola.

(8) The typical rash of erythema chronicum migrans is pathognomonic for Lyme disease. It begins as a red macule or papule and expands in an annular pattern to an average diameter of 15 cm. Patients frequently test as seronegative at this time.

(9) Erysipelas is characterized by a well-demarcated, bright red, painful lesion. The skin appears infiltrated, and the borders are raised and firm.

(10) Koplik spots are pathognomonic for measles. They are a white or bluish-white enanthem found on the buccal mucosa near the lower molars.

(11) The Jones criteria must be fulfilled to make a diagnosis of rheumatic fever. Major criteria include erythema marginatum, polyarthritis, carditis, chorea, and subcutaneous nodules; minor criteria include fever, arthralgia, previous rheumatic fever, leukocytosis, elevated erythrocyte sedimentation rate/C-reactive protein, and prolonged PR interval. One major plus two minor criteria or two major criteria with evidence of recent group A streptococcal disease strongly suggests the diagnosis.

BIBLIOGRAPHY

Sood SK: Lyme disease. Pediatr Infect Dis J 18:936–944, 1999.

FEVER AND RASH (continued)

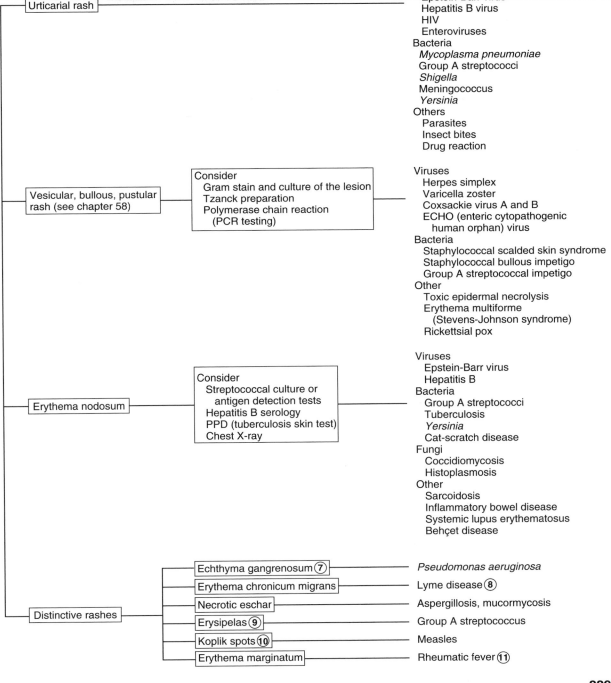

Urticarial rash ── Epstein-Barr virus
Hepatitis B virus
HIV
Enteroviruses
Bacteria
  Mycoplasma pneumoniae
  Group A streptococci
  Shigella
  Meningococcus
  Yersinia
Others
  Parasites
  Insect bites
  Drug reaction

Vesicular, bullous, pustular rash (see chapter 58) ── Consider
  Gram stain and culture of the lesion
  Tzanck preparation
  Polymerase chain reaction
    (PCR testing)

Viruses
  Herpes simplex
  Varicella zoster
  Coxsackie virus A and B
  ECHO (enteric cytopathogenic
    human orphan) virus
Bacteria
  Staphylococcal scalded skin syndrome
  Staphylococcal bullous impetigo
  Group A streptococcal impetigo
Other
  Toxic epidermal necrolysis
  Erythema multiforme
    (Stevens-Johnson syndrome)
  Rickettsial pox

Erythema nodosum ── Consider
  Streptococcal culture or
    antigen detection tests
  Hepatitis B serology
  PPD (tuberculosis skin test)
  Chest X-ray

Viruses
  Epstein-Barr virus
  Hepatitis B
Bacteria
  Group A streptococci
  Tuberculosis
  Yersinia
  Cat-scratch disease
Fungi
  Coccidiomycosis
  Histoplasmosis
Other
  Sarcoidosis
  Inflammatory bowel disease
  Systemic lupus erythematosus
  Behçet disease

Distinctive rashes ──
  Echthyma gangrenosum (7) ── *Pseudomonas aeruginosa*
  Erythema chronicum migrans ── Lyme disease (8)
  Necrotic eschar ── Aspergillosis, mucormycosis
  Erysipelas (9) ── Group A streptococcus
  Koplik spots (10) ── Measles
  Erythema marginatum ── Rheumatic fever (11)

Adapted from Prince A. Infectious diseases. In Behrman RE, Kliegman RM (eds). Nelson Essentials of Pediatrics, 3rd ed. Philadelphia, WB Saunders, 1998:317

Nelson chapters 170, 172
Practical Strategies chapter 57

229

HEMATOLOGY

Lymphadenopathy is the presence of one or more enlarged lymph nodes measuring > 1 cm in diameter (inguinal nodes > 1.5 cm, epitrochlear lymph nodes > 0.5 cm). It may be due to (1) *reactive lymphadenopathy,* a common and normal function of lymph nodes characterized by hyperplasia in response to antigenic stimuli; (2) *lymphadenitis,* an inflammatory response to bacteria or their products, accompanied by erythema, warmth, and tenderness; (3) *malignancy* by primary origin in the node or secondary to metastases; and (4) rare lipid *storage disorders.*

① A good history is essential. The age of the child may indicate the cause. Adenopathy in neonates may be due to infections *in utero* (cytomegalovirus, syphilis, toxoplasmosis, human immunodeficiency virus [HIV]). In toddlers, adenopathy is due to either focal infections that drain to the affected node or systemic viral infections. Malignancy is more likely to be a cause of lymphadenopathy in older children. Immunodeficiency may predispose children to opportunistic infections or malignancies. Certain medications (e.g., procainamide, sulfasalazine, phenytoin, or tetracycline) may cause a lupus-like illness and adenopathy. Family history may suggest infections such as HIV, syphilis, tuberculosis, group A β-hemolytic streptococci, or mononucleosis. Birth and travel history may indicate exposure to endemic infections (e.g., tuberculosis, histoplasmosis), as well as consumption of infected foods (e.g., *Brucella, Mycobacterium* from unpasteurized milk products). Diagnostic clues may be revealed by social history (socioeconomic status or ethnicity), family diet (consumption of raw meats), and presence of family pets (cat-scratch disease, toxoplasmosis from kitty litter). Adolescents must be asked about sexual activity, risk factors for HIV, and exposure to sexually transmitted diseases (i.e., syphilis). Lymphogranuloma venereum may cause inguinal lymphadenopathy. An acute onset may suggest infection, whereas an insidious onset accompanied by systemic symptoms (e.g., anorexia,

weight loss, fevers, night sweats) suggests a disease such as tuberculosis or *Hodgkin disease.*

On physical examination, all areas that may be involved must be palpated, including cervical, preauricular/postauricular, axillary, epitrochlear, inguinal, and supraclavicular. Location of the node may be helpful in diagnosis, whether lymphadenopathy is localized or generalized. Localized lymphadenopathy often indicates involvement in the area of lymphatic drainage. Supraclavicular lymphadenopathy is usually a red flag for mediastinal tumors or infections or for metastatic abdominal tumors. Palpation of the nodes is helpful, with erythema, warmth, and tenderness indicating adenitis. Tender, nonerythematous, soft nodes may indicate a viral or a systemic infection. Firm or hard, rubbery, nontender nodes may indicate infiltrating tumors. Hard, matted, fixed, nontender nodes indicate tumor or fibrosis after acute infection.

② Reactive adenopathy is usually a transient response to infections of the upper respiratory tract or skin. Pharyngeal infections commonly cause cervical lymphadenopathy. Common viral agents include adenovirus, parainfluenza, influenza, rhinovirus, and enterovirus. Cytomegalovirus (CMV) and Epstein-Barr virus (EBV) may cause a localized or generalized lymphadenopathy. Bacterial causes include group A β-hemolytic streptococci or oral anaerobes such as *Fusobacterium.* Scalp infections such as tinea capitis may cause occipital lymphadenopathy.

③ If there is pharyngitis associated with cervical adenitis, a throat culture or rapid streptococcal antigen detection test may be done to help diagnose group A β-hemolytic streptococci. Viral causes include EBV, herpes simplex, and enteroviruses.

④ An acute-onset, unilateral adenitis is usually bacterial in origin and may form an abscess. Bacterial infections of skin and soft tissue (e.g., abscess, cellulitis, erysipelas, and fasciitis) are primarily caused by group A β-hemolytic streptococci or *Staphylococcus aureus.* Foot injuries through

old sneakers or shoes may cause inguinal adenitis because of infection with *Pseudomonas aeruginosa.*

⑤ Subacute or chronic adenitis may be due to mycobacterial infections. Tuberculosis is increasing in incidence in children and is usually associated with hilar adenopathy, with the lungs as the primary source of the infection. A positive tuberculin skin test and a chest X-ray may confirm tuberculosis. Induration of > 15 mm is considered positive in a child older than age 4 years with no risk factors. In children with known contacts with tuberculosis, or who are clinically suspected to have tuberculosis, on immunosuppressive therapy, or who have immunosuppressive conditions, including HIV infection, induration > 5 mm is considered positive. Children at increased risk of disseminated disease or increased environmental exposure to tuberculosis are considered positive at > 10 mm induration. Cervical adenitis is usually due to atypical mycobacteria, primarily *Mycobacterium avium-intracellulare, M. kansasii, M. scrofulaceum,* and *M. marinum.* Diagnosis is determined using acid-fast staining and culture of the excised node or by fine-needle aspiration. An indeterminate tuberculin skin test with 5 to 9 mm of induration suggests infection with atypical mycobacteria. With modern methods of milk pasteurization, *M. bovis,* a previously common cause of cervical adenitis, is rarely seen.

⑥ Cat-scratch disease, caused by a gram-negative bacillus, *Bartonella henselae,* occurs after exposure to a scratch or bite of a cat, with development of a papule at the site of trauma, followed in 7 to 14 days by regional lymphadenitis, usually axillary. Other symptoms include low-grade fever and malaise. The lymph nodes usually regress spontaneously within several weeks. Some 10% may have a purulent drainage that is culture negative. Serologic tests, such as indirect fluorescent antibody (IFA) and enzyme-linked immunosorbent assay (ELISA) IgM tests, are the preferred

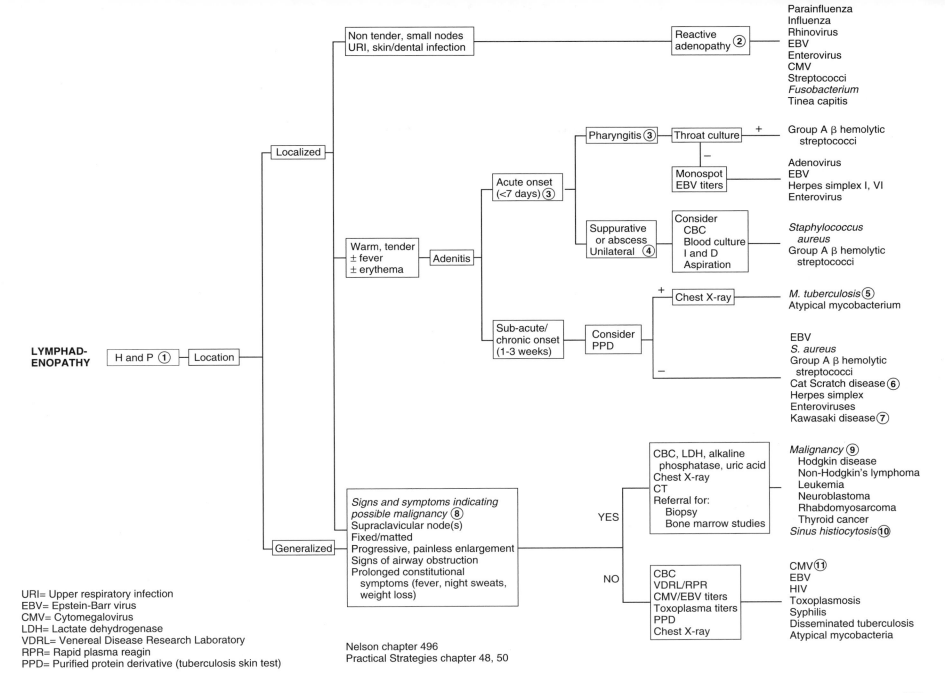

LYMPHAD-ENOPATHY — H and P ① — Location

Localized

Non tender, small nodes
URI, skin/dental infection — Reactive adenopathy ②
- Parainfluenza
- Influenza
- Rhinovirus
- EBV
- Enterovirus
- CMV
- Streptococci
- *Fusobacterium*
- Tinea capitis

Warm, tender
± fever
± erythema — Adenitis

Acute onset (<7 days) ③

Pharyngitis ③ — Throat culture
- (+) Group A β hemolytic streptococci
- (−) Monospot EBV titers
  - Adenovirus
  - EBV
  - Herpes simplex I, VI
  - Enterovirus

Suppurative or abscess Unilateral ④ — Consider CBC, Blood culture, I and D, Aspiration
- *Staphylococcus aureus*
- Group A β hemolytic streptococci

Sub-acute/chronic onset (1-3 weeks) — Consider PPD — Chest X-ray
- (+) *M. tuberculosis* ⑤, Atypical mycobacterium
- (−)
  - EBV
  - *S. aureus*
  - Group A β hemolytic streptococci
  - Cat Scratch disease ⑥
  - Herpes simplex
  - Enteroviruses
  - Kawasaki disease ⑦

Generalized

Signs and symptoms indicating possible malignancy ⑧
- Supraclavicular node(s)
- Fixed/matted
- Progressive, painless enlargement
- Signs of airway obstruction
- Prolonged constitutional symptoms (fever, night sweats, weight loss)

YES — CBC, LDH, alkaline phosphatase, uric acid; Chest X-ray; CT; Referral for: Biopsy, Bone marrow studies
- *Malignancy* ⑨
  - Hodgkin disease
  - Non-Hodgkin's lymphoma
  - Leukemia
  - Neuroblastoma
  - Rhabdomyosarcoma
  - Thyroid cancer
- *Sinus histiocytosis* ⑩

NO — CBC; VDRL/RPR; CMV/EBV titers; Toxoplasma titers; PPD; Chest X-ray
- CMV ⑪
- EBV
- HIV
- Toxoplasmosis
- Syphilis
- Disseminated tuberculosis
- Atypical mycobacteria

URI= Upper respiratory infection
EBV= Epstein-Barr virus
CMV= Cytomegalovirus
LDH= Lactate dehydrogenase
VDRL= Venereal Disease Research Laboratory
RPR= Rapid plasma reagin
PPD= Purified protein derivative (tuberculosis skin test)

Nelson chapter 496
Practical Strategies chapter 48, 50

methods of verifying the diagnosis. Polymerase chain reaction (PCR) testing is the most sensitive. Diagnosis is confirmed by biopsy of the node showing granulomas, central necrosis, and organisms seen on Warthin-Starry silver stain.

(7) Kawasaki disease is determined clinically in children by noting 5 consecutive days of high fever accompanied by at least four of the following five conditions: cervical lymphadenopathy, oral mucosal erythema, conjunctivitis without exudates, rash, and extremity changes, such as edema and desquamation in the absence of known causes of these signs. The lymph node is typically single and large but is not consistently present.

(8) If any of the "red flags" are present, malignancy is suspected and the necessary evaluation should be done. This may include examination of the CBC for anemia, thrombocytopenia, leukopenia, or leukocytosis and for blast cells. Because of a tumor burden, there may be an elevation of lactate dehydrogenase, alkaline phosphatase, and uric acid levels. A chest X-ray may show mediastinal lymphadenopathy, which is suggestive of lymphoma. A CT scan may also be considered. Close clinical follow-up should be done to watch for progression of symptoms. If cancer is suspected, a referral should be made to the appropriate specialist for biopsy or for bone marrow studies.

(9) *Hodgkin disease* usually occurs as painless cervical or supraclavicular lymphadenopathy in older children and adolescents. Approximately 30% have systemic symptoms (e.g., fatigue, weight loss, fevers, night sweats). Pruritus, hemolytic anemia, and chest pain after alcohol ingestion are clues. Diagnosis is confirmed by lymph node biopsy and/or bone marrow aspiration. Non-Hodgkin lymphoma usually occurs as supraclavicular, cervical, or axillary adenopathy. In children in the United States, B-cell lymphomas originate in the abdomen with inguinal or iliac lymphadenopathy.

About half of children with acute lymphoblastic leukemia present with adenopathy at the time of diagnosis. Systemic signs and symptoms (e.g., fever, malaise, weight loss, pallor, bone pain, petechiae, hepatosplenomegaly) may be present. The CBC may show anemia, thrombocytopenia, leukocytosis or leukopenia, and circulating blast cells. Acute myelogenous leukemia is less common in children but appears similarly. Several other malignancies, including disseminated neuroblastoma, rhabdomyosarcoma, and thyroid cancer, may occur as localized or generalized lymphadenopathy.

(10) Sinus histiocytosis is a rare disorder with massive cervical lymphadenopathy, fever, elevated erythrocyte sedimentation rate, leukocytosis, and hypergammaglobulinemia. It may be diagnosed using biopsy and tends to resolve spontaneously.

(11) Generalized lymphadenopathy may be due to viral infections. HIV-infected children may have systemic symptoms, failure to thrive, and evidence of opportunistic infections. EBV and CMV may both cause generalized lymphadenopathy. Syphilis caused by the spirochete *Treponema pallidum* results in both localized and generalized lymphadenopathy. In primary syphilis there is usually localized inguinal adenopathy; in secondary syphilis there is usually generalized lymph node involvement. Epitrochlear involvement is suggestive. Diagnostic tests include rapid plasma reagin (RPR), Venereal Disease Research Laboratory (VDRL), and fluorescent treponemal antibody absorption (FTA-ABS). (See Ch. 41.) *Toxoplasma gondii* is a parasite of cats and can be acquired by humans from contact with cat feces or by eating raw meat. Although the infection may be transmitted to the fetus, lymphadenopathy is uncommon in the newborn and is more common in older children and young adults. Disseminated tuberculosis may present as generalized lymphadenopathy, pulmonary infiltrates, and systemic symptoms. Atypical mycobacteria may cause generalized lymphadenopathy in HIV-infected children.

BIBLIOGRAPHY

Margileth AM: Sorting out the causes of lymphadenopathy. Contemp Pediatr 12:23–40, 1995.

Margileth AM: Lymphadenopathy: When to diagnose and treat. Contemp Pediatr 12:71–89, 1995.

Peter G (ed): 1997 Red Book: Report of the Committee on Infectious Diseases, 24th ed. American Academy of Pediatrics, Elk Grove, IL. 1997.

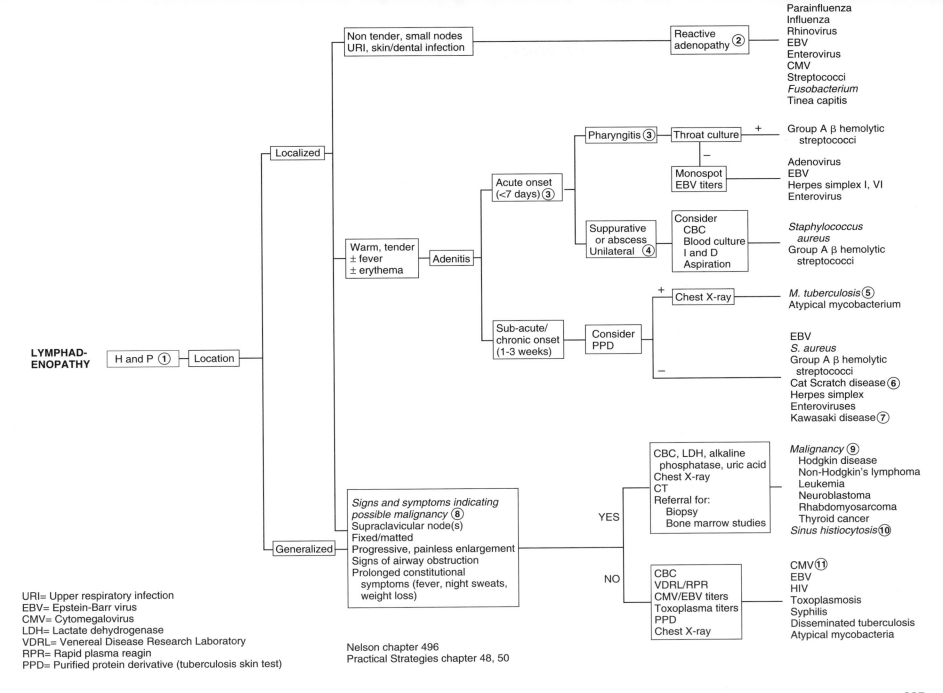

LYMPHAD-ENOPATHY — H and P ① — Location

Localized

Non tender, small nodes URI, skin/dental infection → Reactive adenopathy ②
- Parainfluenza
- Influenza
- Rhinovirus
- EBV
- Enterovirus
- CMV
- Streptococci
- *Fusobacterium*
- Tinea capitis

Warm, tender ± fever ± erythema — Adenitis

Acute onset (<7 days) ③

Pharyngitis ③ → Throat culture
- \+ Group A β hemolytic streptococci
- − Monospot EBV titers
  - Adenovirus
  - EBV
  - Herpes simplex I, VI
  - Enterovirus

Suppurative or abscess Unilateral ④ → Consider CBC / Blood culture / I and D / Aspiration
- *Staphylococcus aureus*
- Group A β hemolytic streptococci

Sub-acute/ chronic onset (1-3 weeks) → Consider PPD → Chest X-ray
- \+ *M. tuberculosis* ⑤ / Atypical mycobacterium
- − EBV / *S. aureus* / Group A β hemolytic streptococci / Cat Scratch disease ⑥ / Herpes simplex / Enteroviruses / Kawasaki disease ⑦

Generalized

Signs and symptoms indicating possible malignancy ⑧
Supraclavicular node(s)
Fixed/matted
Progressive, painless enlargement
Signs of airway obstruction
Prolonged constitutional symptoms (fever, night sweats, weight loss)

YES → CBC, LDH, alkaline phosphatase, uric acid / Chest X-ray / CT / Referral for: Biopsy / Bone marrow studies
- *Malignancy* ⑨
  - Hodgkin disease
  - Non-Hodgkin's lymphoma
  - Leukemia
  - Neuroblastoma
  - Rhabdomyosarcoma
  - Thyroid cancer
- *Sinus histiocytosis* ⑩

NO → CBC / VDRL/RPR / CMV/EBV titers / Toxoplasma titers / PPD / Chest X-ray
- CMV ⑪
- EBV
- HIV
- Toxoplasmosis
- Syphilis
- Disseminated tuberculosis
- Atypical mycobacteria

URI= Upper respiratory infection
EBV= Epstein-Barr virus
CMV= Cytomegalovirus
LDH= Lactate dehydrogenase
VDRL= Venereal Disease Research Laboratory
RPR= Rapid plasma reagin
PPD= Purified protein derivative (tuberculosis skin test)

Nelson chapter 496
Practical Strategies chapter 48, 50

Anemia is defined as a decrease in hemoglobin concentration of more than 2 standard deviations below the mean. Normal values of hemoglobin and hematocrit vary with age. A term infant has a normal hemoglobin level of 15 to 21 g/dl, followed by a physiologic nadir of 9.5 to 10 g/dl around 2 months of age. This is exaggerated in premature infants.

(1) History should include iron sources in the diet. Infants with excessive intake (>24 oz/day) of cow's milk or low-iron formula are at risk. Allergy to cow's milk may also cause occult gastrointestinal blood losses. Goat's milk is associated with folate deficiency, and vitamin B_{12} deficiency occurs in those on macrobiotic diets. Increased iron requirements occur as a result of increased menstrual blood losses, pregnancy, and in prematurity. Impaired absorption of iron may be associated with malabsorptive syndromes such as inflammatory bowel disease or celiac disease. Pica may suggest lead poisoning. A neonatal history of hyperbilirubinemia may indicate a congenital hemolytic anemia, especially if there is a family history of anemia, splenectomy, or cholecystectomy. Medications may lead to hemolysis, as in glucose-6-phosphate dehydrogenase (G6PD) deficiency. Infections and chronic disease are also associated with anemia. Travel history may reveal infections such as malaria.

Physical examination may indicate an acute onset. Chronic anemia may affect growth. Chronic hemolytic anemias cause expansion of bone marrow with prominent cheek bones, frontal bossing, and dental malocclusion. Splenomegaly may be present. Lymphadenopathy and hepatosplenomegaly occur with infiltrative disease of the bone marrow. Examination may also reveal signs of chronic inflammation or systemic disease. A careful skin examination may reveal bruising or purpura.

(2) An increased reticulocyte count implies that there is hemolysis or blood loss. The reticulocyte count is expressed as a percent of the total number of RBCs. In patients with moderate/severe anemia, this may appear elevated. It is therefore expressed as the corrected reticulocyte count (reticulocyte count × hemoglobin/normal hemoglobin for age). The mean corpuscular volume (MCV) is used to categorize anemias into microcytic, normocytic, and macrocytic. Examination of the peripheral blood smear is important in diagnosis of anemias. Hypersegmentation of polymorphonuclear cells and macrocytosis indicates megaloblastic disease. Classic findings specific to diseases include spherocytes in spherocytic anemia and immune-mediated hemolytic anemia, sickle cells in sickle cell anemia, and Howell-Jolly bodies in asplenic patients. Blister or bite cells are seen in G6PD deficiency. Target cells can be found in iron deficiency, hemoglobinopathies, and thalassemia. In malaria there are intraerythrocytic parasites. Bone marrow examination provides a definitive diagnosis in sideroblastic anemia, aplastic anemias, and malignancies.

(3) Iron deficiency is the most common cause of anemia in children. If it is suggested by history and CBC (↓ hemoglobin, ↑ red blood cell distribution width, ↓ MCV), a therapeutic trial of iron may be considered (3–6 mg/kg/day of elemental iron). An increase in hemoglobin of 1 g/dl within 2 to 4 weeks confirms the diagnosis. Laboratory confirmation of iron-deficiency anemia by low serum iron, high total iron-binding capacity (TIBC), and low ferritin is necessary in children who are at low risk for iron deficiency.

(4) β-Thalassemia trait is most common in children of Mediterranean or African descent. The red blood cell distribution width is normal, and hemoglobin A_2 is increased. Children with β-thalassemia major (Cooley anemia) present during infancy with severe anemia, increase in reticulocyte counts, and features of bone marrow expansion. Children with β-thalassemia trait are asymptomatic. α-Thalassemia may occur as an asymptomatic carrier state; as a trait with mild anemia and microcytosis; as hemoglobin H disease with a moderate hemolytic anemia, microcytosis, reticulocytosis, and splenomegaly; or as Barts disease, which is generally incompatible with life. Hemoglobin H and Barts disease usually occur in Asians. α-Thalassemia is usually a diagnosis of exclusion because DNA sequencing is rarely done outside a laboratory setting. In thalassemia trait and sideroblastic anemia, TIBC is normal and iron and ferritin are normal or increased.

(5) Lead poisoning (i.e., plumbism) is often associated with iron deficiency, which enhances the absorption of lead.

(6) Anemia of chronic disease may be microcytic or normocytic, with increased erythrocyte sedimentation rate and decreased serum iron and TIBC. The ferritin may be increased due to an inflammatory state.

(7) Iron-deficiency anemia may be normocytic in the early stages. Acute infections may cause a transient mild anemia. Transient red blood cell hypoplasia may occur in patients with hemolytic anemias after infection with parvovirus B19. Transient erythroblastopenia of childhood is a temporary arrest of red blood cell production and occurs predominantly in children aged 6 months to 3 years. Chronic renal disease may cause anemia due to a deficiency of erythropoietin.

(8) Leukemia and metastatic malignancy may cause bone marrow infiltration and normocytic anemia with thrombocytopenia and either leukocytosis or leukopenia. Acquired aplastic anemia may be postinfectious (hepatitis, EBV), drug related (chloramphenicol, anticonvulsants), toxin related (benzene), or idiopathic. It is characterized by anemia, neutropenia, and thrombocytopenia. There is hypoplasia of the bone marrow.

(9) Megaloblastic anemia (large RBCs with abnormal WBCs and platelets) due to vitamin B_{12} or folate deficiency is rare in children. Breast-fed infants of strictly vegetarian mothers may have vitamin B_{12} deficiency. Malabsorption of vitamin B_{12} may be due to an intrinsic factor deficiency

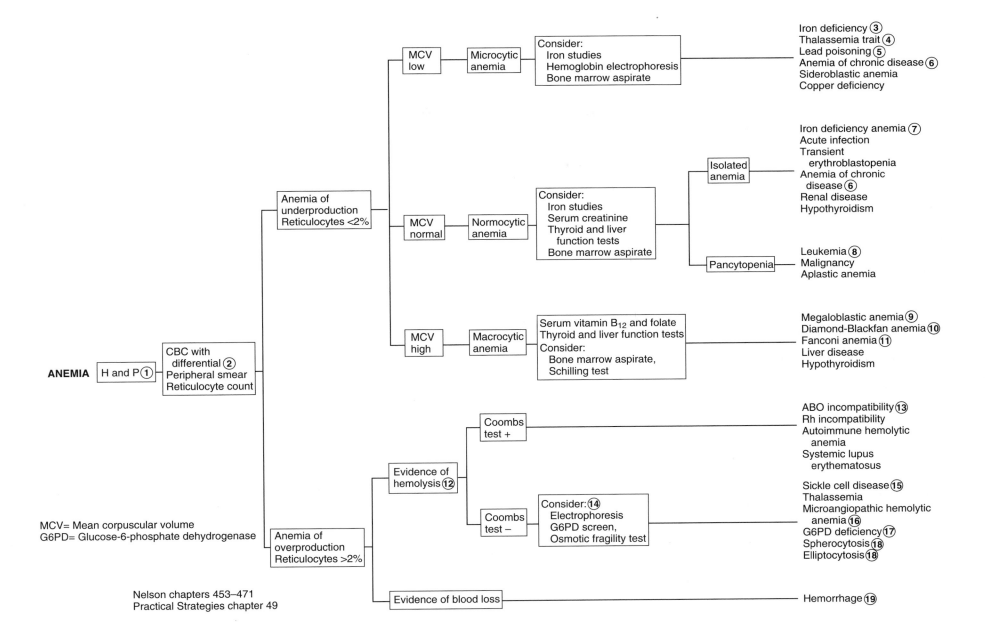

ANEMIA — H and P ①

CBC with differential ② / Peripheral smear / Reticulocyte count

Anemia of underproduction Reticulocytes <2%

- MCV low → Microcytic anemia → Consider: Iron studies, Hemoglobin electrophoresis, Bone marrow aspirate →
  - Iron deficiency ③
  - Thalassemia trait ④
  - Lead poisoning ⑤
  - Anemia of chronic disease ⑥
  - Sideroblastic anemia
  - Copper deficiency

- MCV normal → Normocytic anemia → Consider: Iron studies, Serum creatinine, Thyroid and liver function tests, Bone marrow aspirate →
  - Isolated anemia →
    - Iron deficiency anemia ⑦
    - Acute infection
    - Transient erythroblastopenia
    - Anemia of chronic disease ⑥
    - Renal disease
    - Hypothyroidism
  - Pancytopenia →
    - Leukemia ⑧
    - Malignancy
    - Aplastic anemia

- MCV high → Macrocytic anemia → Serum vitamin B₁₂ and folate / Thyroid and liver function tests / Consider: Bone marrow aspirate, Schilling test →
  - Megaloblastic anemia ⑨
  - Diamond-Blackfan anemia ⑩
  - Fanconi anemia ⑪
  - Liver disease
  - Hypothyroidism

Anemia of overproduction Reticulocytes >2%

- Evidence of hemolysis ⑫
  - Coombs test + →
    - ABO incompatibility ⑬
    - Rh incompatibility
    - Autoimmune hemolytic anemia
    - Systemic lupus erythematosus
  - Coombs test − → Consider: ⑭ Electrophoresis, G6PD screen, Osmotic fragility test →
    - Sickle cell disease ⑮
    - Thalassemia
    - Microangiopathic hemolytic anemia ⑯
    - G6PD deficiency ⑰
    - Spherocytosis ⑱
    - Elliptocytosis ⑱

- Evidence of blood loss → Hemorrhage ⑲

MCV= Mean corpuscular volume
G6PD= Glucose-6-phosphate dehydrogenase

Nelson chapters 453–471
Practical Strategies chapter 49

(e.g., congenital pernicious anemia) or to resection of the terminal ileum, or it may occur with involvement of the terminal ileum with inflammatory bowel disease. Congenital pernicious anemia due to deficiency of intrinsic factor is rare and may be diagnosed using the Schilling test. Resection or inflammatory disease of the small bowel may cause folate deficiency. Infants fed goat's milk may be folate deficient. Increased folate requirements may occur in chronic hemolytic anemia (i.e., sickle cell).

(10) Congenital hypoplastic anemia (Diamond-Blackfan anemia) occurs in the first year of life as severe anemia and reticulocytopenia. The RBCs have elevated MCVs and increased fetal hemoglobin.

(11) Fanconi anemia may occur with pancytopenia and physical stigmata such as thumb and radial anomalies. RBCs have fetal characteristics (e.g., increased MCV and fetal hemoglobin).

(12) Hemolytic disorders are characterized by shortened RBC survival and reticulocytosis. There may be icterus, splenomegaly, gallstones, and significant family or neonatal history. Laboratory findings include abnormal cell morphology; increased red blood cell distribution width, indirect bilirubin, urine urobilinogen, and lactate dehydrogenase; decreased serum haptoglobin; and hemoglobinuria.

(13) A positive Coombs test indicates an immune-mediated anemia. Isoimmune hemolytic anemia is the most common cause of neonatal anemia. Rh incompatibility is rare because of administration of Rh immune globulin to Rh-negative mothers. When it occurs it causes severe hemolysis and can occur as intrauterine hydrops fetalis or severe jaundice. The direct Coombs test is strongly positive. ABO incompatibility occurs when the mother is blood group O and the fetus group A or B and is usually less severe. Acquired autoimmune hemolytic anemia may occur with an underlying immunologic dysfunction (e.g., HIV, lymphoma) or after an acute infection, usually viral. It may be drug related (e.g., penicillins, cephalosporins) or idiopathic. The direct Coombs test result is positive, and spherocytes are seen on peripheral smear. Cold agglutinin disease occurs most commonly after infections from *Mycoplasma pneumoniae* or viruses. It is characterized by increased cold agglutinin antibodies, which cause hemolysis after exposure to cold. Paroxysmal cold hemoglobinuria and, rarely, infectious mononucleosis also cause anemia with cold exposure.

(14) In children with a negative Coombs test, other tests should be considered based on history, physical findings, and the CBC and smear. These may include hemoglobin electrophoresis, glucose-6-phosphate dehydrogenase screening, and osmotic fragility tests.

(15) Sickle cell hemoglobinopathies are most common in children of Central African descent and less common in children of Mediterranean or Arabic descent. Sickle cell disease may occur combined with hemoglobin C or β-thalassemia, causing a less severe disorder. Diagnosis is by hemoglobin electrophoresis.

(16) Microangiopathic hemolytic anemia may be associated with disseminated intravascular coagulation or hemolytic-uremic syndrome. It can also present as thrombocytopenia in Kasabach-Merritt syndrome (i.e., a consumptive coagulopathy seen with large hemangiomas) and thrombotic thrombocytopenic purpura.

(17) G6PD deficiency is an RBC enzyme defect. It is an X-linked disorder and occurs most often in patients of African or Mediterranean descent. Characteristic findings include "bite cells" and inclusion bodies called Heinz bodies. There is increased susceptibility of RBCs to oxidant injury due to infections, medications (sulfonamides, antimalarials, nitrofurantoin, nalidixic acid, chloramphenicol, methylene blue, vitamin K analogs), toxins (mothballs, large doses of vitamin C, benzene), and foods (fava beans).

(18) Membrane defects include hereditary spherocytosis and elliptocytosis. Presenting features are anemia, jaundice, and splenomegaly. Diagnosis is confirmed by an osmotic fragility test.

(19) A significant acute or subacute blood loss leads to anemia. The RBC morphology and size remain normal. It may require 3 to 5 days to produce an elevated reticulocyte count. Transfusion may be required to replace large blood losses when there are clinical manifestations such as fatigue, lightheadedness, tachycardia, dyspnea, or heart failure.

BIBLIOGRAPHY

Berliner N, Duffy TP, Abelson HT: Approach to the adult and child with anemia. In Hoffman R, Benz EJ, Shattil SJ (eds): Hematology, 2nd ed. New York:Churchill Livingstone, 1995.

Sackey K: Hemolytic anemia: I and II. Pediatr Rev 20:152–159, 204–208, 1999.

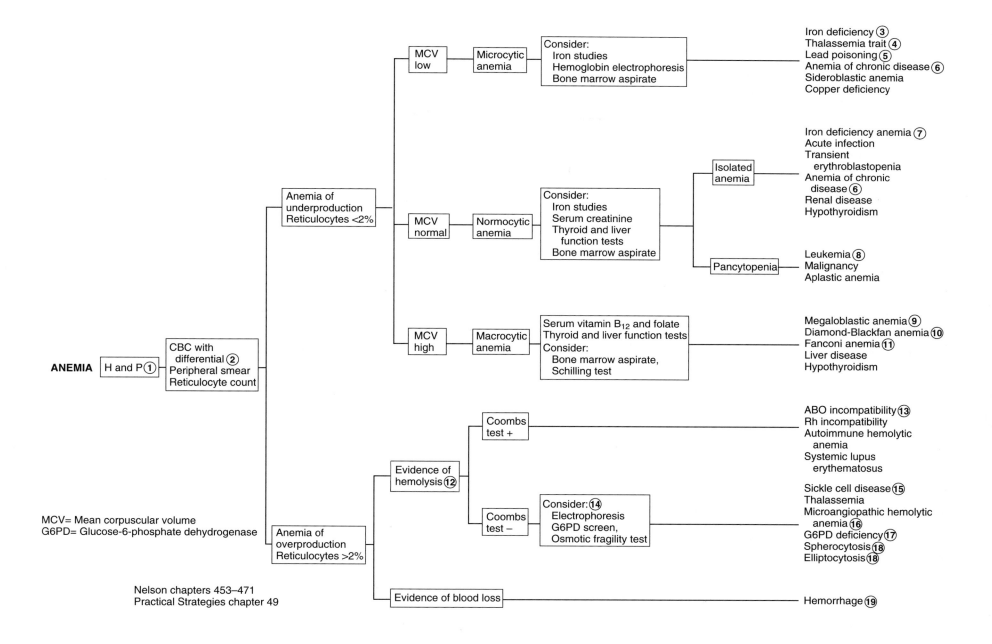

ANEMIA → H and P ①

CBC with differential ②
Peripheral smear
Reticulocyte count

Anemia of underproduction
Reticulocytes <2%

MCV low → Microcytic anemia → Consider:
Iron studies
Hemoglobin electrophoresis
Bone marrow aspirate
→ Iron deficiency ③
Thalassemia trait ④
Lead poisoning ⑤
Anemia of chronic disease ⑥
Sideroblastic anemia
Copper deficiency

MCV normal → Normocytic anemia → Consider:
Iron studies
Serum creatinine
Thyroid and liver function tests
Bone marrow aspirate

→ Isolated anemia → Iron deficiency anemia ⑦
Acute infection
Transient erythroblastopenia
Anemia of chronic disease ⑥
Renal disease
Hypothyroidism

→ Pancytopenia → Leukemia ⑧
Malignancy
Aplastic anemia

MCV high → Macrocytic anemia → Serum vitamin B₁₂ and folate
Thyroid and liver function tests
Consider:
Bone marrow aspirate,
Schilling test
→ Megaloblastic anemia ⑨
Diamond-Blackfan anemia ⑩
Fanconi anemia ⑪
Liver disease
Hypothyroidism

Anemia of overproduction
Reticulocytes >2%

→ Evidence of hemolysis ⑫

Coombs test + → ABO incompatibility ⑬
Rh incompatibility
Autoimmune hemolytic anemia
Systemic lupus erythematosus

Coombs test – → Consider: ⑭
Electrophoresis
G6PD screen,
Osmotic fragility test
→ Sickle cell disease ⑮
Thalassemia
Microangiopathic hemolytic anemia ⑯
G6PD deficiency ⑰
Spherocytosis ⑱
Elliptocytosis ⑱

→ Evidence of blood loss → Hemorrhage ⑲

MCV= Mean corpuscular volume
G6PD= Glucose-6-phosphate dehydrogenase

Nelson chapters 453–471
Practical Strategies chapter 49

Bleeding disorders are caused by a disturbance in the normal hemostasis. Components of the hemostatic mechanism include platelets, anticoagulant proteins, procoagulant proteins, and components of the vessel walls.

1 History should include age and acuity at onset of bleeding; the triggers; whether bleeding was immediate or delayed; and whether it was prolonged. Severity of bleeding must be determined, such as nosebleeds requiring cautery or packing or surgeries requiring transfusions. Perinatal history should include details regarding bruising or petechiae, bleeding with circumcision, cephalhematoma, CNS or gastrointestinal bleeding, unexplained anemia or jaundice, or bleeding after cord separation. A history of vitamin K administration and maternal drugs should be obtained. In adolescent girls a history of dysfunctional uterine bleeding would be important. A detailed family history should be obtained, including maternal obstetric history of bleeding. Medications such as aspirin, other nonsteroidal antiinflammatory drugs (NSAIDs), anticoagulants, antibiotics, and anticonvulsants may be associated with bleeding.

The bleeding site may indicate the etiology. Acute mucocutaneous bleeding may indicate idiopathic thrombocytopenic purpura. Generalized bleeding may be associated with disseminated intravascular coagulation (DIC), vitamin K deficiency, liver disease, or uremia.

Various findings on physical examination may be helpful in determining the etiology. Heart murmurs may indicate endocarditis; arthropathy is suggestive of hemophilia; joint laxity is seen with Ehlers-Danlos syndrome; and thumb or radial anomalies are seen with Fanconi anemia or TAR (thrombocytopenia–absent radius) syndrome. Hepatosplenomegaly may indicate liver disease, and lymphadenopathy, a malignancy. Skin findings include hematomas, petechiae, ecchymoses, telangiectasia, purpura, poor wound healing, lax skin, and varicose veins.

2 The critical evaluation for a bleeding disorder should begin with a few specific laboratory tests. A CBC including a platelet count may reveal thrombocytopenia or anemias. Prothrombin time (PT) and partial thromboplastin time (PTT) are dependent on all coagulation factors except factor XIII. A clotting factor deficiency or the presence of an inhibitor can prolong PT and PTT. Testing for an inhibitor is done by mixing one part of patient plasma with one part pooled plasma; if the PT or PTT corrects, there is a factor deficiency; if it does not correct, an inhibitor is present. Inhibitors include anticoagulants (e.g., heparin), autoantibodies against clotting factors, and lupus type anticoagulants. Fibrinogen function is measured by thrombin time or fibrinogen activity. Bleeding time indirectly measures platelet number and function and platelet–vessel wall interaction. A measure of von Willebrand factor (vWf) function should also be considered since other screening laboratory results may be normal in von Willebrand disease. If the patient is on medications that might interfere with hemostasis, tests should be done or repeated off the medications before proceeding with any further investigations.

3 If bleeding time is prolonged, a test for vWf function should be done to exclude von Willebrand disease. If the test result is normal, platelet aggregation studies should be done. Primary defects include Glanzmann thrombasthenia (deficiency of a fibrinogen receptor) with normal platelet counts and Bernard-Soulier syndrome (deficiency of the von Willebrand receptor) with mild thrombocytopenia. Platelet function defects may also be due to medications (e.g., aspirin, NSAIDs, alcohol, high doses of penicillin, valproate, and others).

4 The most common cause of lifelong symptoms of mucocutaneous bleeding is von Willebrand disease due to deficiency of vWf, which is prevalent in approximately 1% of children. Inheritance is typically autosomal dominant. The vWf is a protein required for platelet plug formation; it is also a carrier for factor VIII. In severe deficiency of vWf there is also deficient factor VIII. PTT and bleeding time are often, but not always, abnormal, and so screening for vWf should always be considered when evaluating bleeding disorders. The PTT corrects with 1:1 mixing with pooled plasma. In addition, stress, medications, trauma, and difficult venipuncture may increase vWf levels. Levels of vWf are dependent on blood type and may be influenced by age. Interpretation of tests requires a qualified laboratory and often the assistance of a hematologist.

5 Deficiency of factor VIII is hemophilia A, and that of factor IX is hemophilia B or Christmas disease. These are transmitted as X-linked traits; therefore, family history of bleeding in males in the mother's family should be obtained. Hemophilia A or B usually occur as bleeding into muscles or joints and easy bruising. Because factor VIII does not cross the placenta, bleeding may occur during the neonatal period. Factor XI deficiency, or hemophilia C, has autosomal recessive transmission. Factor XII or Hageman factor deficiency causes prolonged PTT but is usually asymptomatic.

6 Inhibitors may be directed against a specific coagulation factor or a reaction site in the coagulation pathway. Inhibitors against specific factors usually affect factors VIII, IX, or XI, causing prolonged PTT with normal PT. Lupus anticoagulant is directed against a reaction site and causes prolonged PT and PTT; it is more likely to cause thrombosis than bleeding.

7 Vitamin K deficiency is common in neonates, malnourished children, those receiving broad-spectrum antibiotics, and children with cholestatic liver disease. Vitamin K deficiency may present as generalized bleeding into skin, gastrointestinal tract, and central nervous system. Dicumarol and rat poison (superwarfarin) also act by affecting vitamin K and, therefore, vitamin K–dependent factors II, VII, IX, and X.

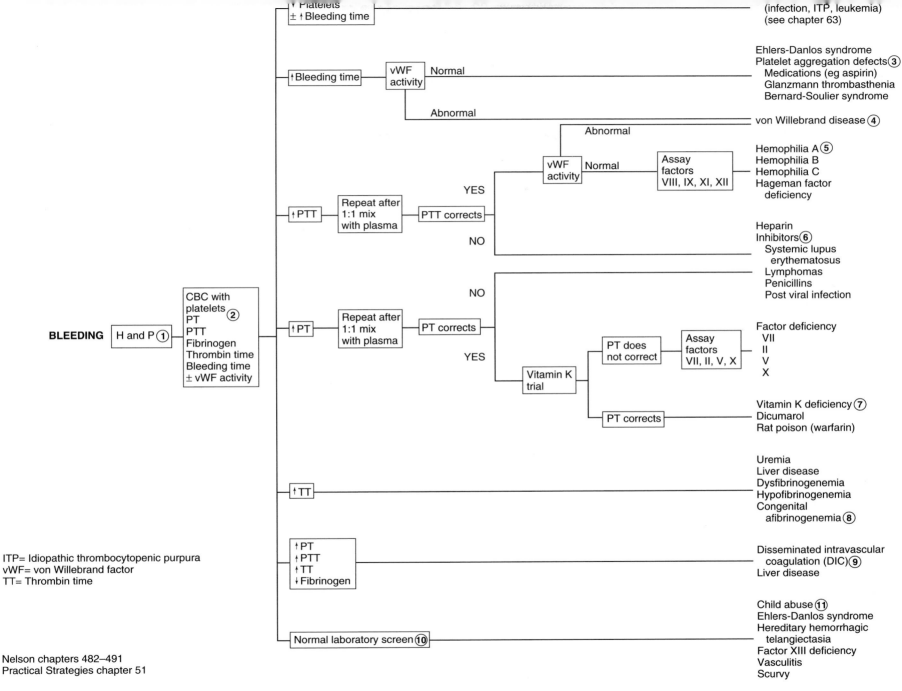

↓ Platelets
± ↑ Bleeding time — (infection, ITP, leukemia)
(see chapter 63)

↑Bleeding time → vWF activity — Normal — Ehlers-Danlos syndrome
Platelet aggregation defects ③
  Medications (eg aspirin)
  Glanzmann thrombasthenia
  Bernard-Soulier syndrome

Abnormal — von Willebrand disease ④

Abnormal → vWF activity — Normal → Assay factors VIII, IX, XI, XII — Hemophilia A ⑤
Hemophilia B
Hemophilia C
Hageman factor
  deficiency

↑PTT → Repeat after 1:1 mix with plasma → PTT corrects — YES

NO — Heparin
Inhibitors ⑥
  Systemic lupus
    erythematosus
  Lymphomas
  Penicillins
  Post viral infection

BLEEDING H and P ① → CBC with platelets ②
PT
PTT
Fibrinogen
Thrombin time
Bleeding time
± vWF activity

↑PT → Repeat after 1:1 mix with plasma → PT corrects — NO

YES → Vitamin K trial → PT does not correct → Assay factors VII, II, V, X — Factor deficiency
VII
II
V
X

PT corrects — Vitamin K deficiency ⑦
Dicumarol
Rat poison (warfarin)

↑TT — Uremia
Liver disease
Dysfibrinogenemia
Hypofibrinogenemia
Congenital
  afibrinogenemia ⑧

↑PT
↑PTT
↑TT
↓Fibrinogen — Disseminated intravascular coagulation (DIC) ⑨
Liver disease

Normal laboratory screen ⑩ — Child abuse ⑪
Ehlers-Danlos syndrome
Hereditary hemorrhagic
  telangiectasia
Factor XIII deficiency
Vasculitis
Scurvy

ITP= Idiopathic thrombocytopenic purpura
vWF= von Willebrand factor
TT= Thrombin time

Nelson chapters 482–491
Practical Strategies chapter 51

241

8 Congenital afibrinogenemia is a rare disorder. Although the blood is incoagulable, hemorrhage is rarely spontaneous and usually occurs with trauma or surgery.

9 DIC is a generalized consumption of clotting factors, anticoagulant proteins, and platelets. It is usually triggered by a severe illness, hypoxia, acidosis, tissue necrosis, and endothelial damage and may be accompanied by shock. It may appear as a hemorrhagic or thrombotic disorder or both. Liver failure affects all coagulation factors except factor VIII. In both DIC and liver failure there is prolonged PT, PTT, and thrombin time and decreased fibrinogen. Fibrin degradation products are elevated in DIC and are normal or elevated in liver failure. Platelets are decreased in DIC but may be normal or decreased with liver failure.

10 von Willebrand disease and, less commonly, platelet aggregation defects may be present despite normal studies. A screen for vWf activity and, if truly suggestive of a bleeding disorder, platelet aggregation studies should be considered.

11 Significant bruising or bleeding with normal laboratory studies should prompt consideration of child abuse. It may also be seen with diseases affecting vessel walls such as Ehlers-Danlos syndrome and hereditary hemorrhagic telangiectasia. Factor XIII deficiency often occurs in infancy as bleeding after separation of the umbilical stump and later as intracranial, gastrointestinal, and intraarticular bleeding. Results of routine coagulation studies are normal.

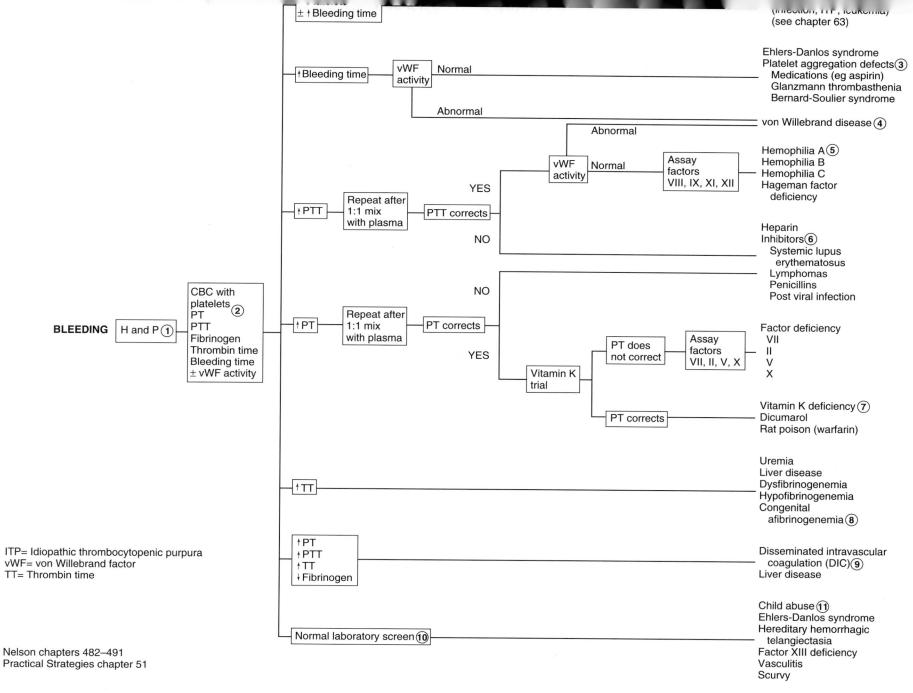

BLEEDING H and P ①

CBC with platelets ②
PT
PTT
Fibrinogen
Thrombin time
Bleeding time
± vWF activity

± ↑ Bleeding time → (Infection, ITP, leukemia) (see chapter 63)

↑ Bleeding time → vWF activity
- Normal → Ehlers-Danlos syndrome
  Platelet aggregation defects ③
  Medications (eg aspirin)
  Glanzmann thrombasthenia
  Bernard-Soulier syndrome
- Abnormal → von Willebrand disease ④

↑ PTT → Repeat after 1:1 mix with plasma → PTT corrects
- YES → vWF activity
  - Abnormal
  - Normal → Assay factors VIII, IX, XI, XII → Hemophilia A ⑤
    Hemophilia B
    Hemophilia C
    Hageman factor deficiency
- NO → Heparin
  Inhibitors ⑥
  Systemic lupus erythematosus
  Lymphomas
  Penicillins
  Post viral infection

↑ PT → Repeat after 1:1 mix with plasma → PT corrects
- NO
- YES → Vitamin K trial
  - PT does not correct → Assay factors VII, II, V, X → Factor deficiency
    VII
    II
    V
    X
  - PT corrects → Vitamin K deficiency ⑦
    Dicumarol
    Rat poison (warfarin)

↑ TT → Uremia
Liver disease
Dysfibrinogenemia
Hypofibrinogenemia
Congenital afibrinogenemia ⑧

↑ PT
↑ PTT
↑ TT
↓ Fibrinogen → Disseminated intravascular coagulation (DIC) ⑨
Liver disease

Normal laboratory screen ⑩ → Child abuse ⑪
Ehlers-Danlos syndrome
Hereditary hemorrhagic telangiectasia
Factor XIII deficiency
Vasculitis
Scurvy

ITP= Idiopathic thrombocytopenic purpura
vWF= von Willebrand factor
TT= Thrombin time

Nelson chapters 482–491
Practical Strategies chapter 51

243

Petechiae are pinpoint, flat, red lesions caused by capillary bleeding into the skin. Purpura are red, purple, or brown lesions of the skin or mucosa that are raised and may be palpable. Petechiae are often caused by thrombocytopenia, but they may also be caused by platelet function defects or blood vessel defects. The presence of purpura often implies disseminated intravascular coagulation (DIC). Thrombocytopenia is a decrease in platelet count by 2 standard deviations below the mean ($<150,000/mm^3$). Platelet counts $> 50,000/mm^3$ are rarely associated with clinical bleeding in the absence of trauma. When the platelet count is as low as 20,000 to 30,000/mm^3 there may be spontaneous bleeding.

(1) History should include that of trauma. Localized petechiae may occur with trauma and predominantly on the face with prolonged crying or emesis and may not require further evaluation. History of menorrhagia, bleeding during surgery, and exposure to toxins, drugs, or radiation should be obtained, as well as noting the presence of infections or systemic illness. Bloody diarrhea may be indicative of hemolytic-uremic syndrome (HUS). Congenital anomalies may be associated with platelet defects, as well as some familial conditions. Lymphadenopathy or hepatosplenomegaly may indicate infiltrative processes. Examination for joint laxity (Ehlers-Danlos syndrome) and thumb and radial anomalies (Fanconi anemia or TAR [thrombocytopenia–absent radius] syndrome) should be done. In addition to petechiae and purpura, skin findings may include hematomas, ecchymoses, telangiectases, poor wound healing, and lax skin.

(2) A CBC and review of peripheral smear is important. Clumping or aggregation of platelets due to interaction with anticoagulants in collection tubes or due to platelet cold agglutinins should be identified. Thrombocytopenia may be hypoproductive, characterized by small platelets, or destructive with large platelets. Hypoproductive conditions often involve the marrow and are associated with anemia and neutropenia. Peripheral smear may also show fragmented red blood cells consistent with microangiopathy (DIC, HUS). Leukocytosis suggests sepsis, blasts suggest leukemia, and leukocyte inclusions, congenital thrombocytopenias.

(3) A common cause of thrombocytopenia in a well-appearing child is idiopathic thrombocytopenic purpura (ITP). The platelet count is usually $< 20,000/mm^3$, and the presence of megakaryocytes indicates a rapid turnover of platelets. History may reveal a preceding viral illness. Mucosal bleeding such as epistaxis and from the gastrointestinal tract may be present. Marrow examination should be considered in children with atypical presentation or with hepatosplenomegaly or lymphadenopathy. (See Ch. 60.) In adolescents, particularly in girls, an antinuclear antibody (ANA) test may be considered to rule out systemic lupus erythematosus (SLE). HIV infection may also occur initially as thrombocytopenia, and the appropriate laboratory studies should be obtained if this is suggested. Drugs that may cause thrombocytopenia include quinidine, carbamazepine, phenytoin, sulfonamides, trimethoprim-sulfamethoxazole, and chloramphenicol.

(4) Thrombocytopenia with small platelets (i.e., hypoproductive) may be associated with congenital syndromes. TAR syndrome is associated with severe thrombocytopenia, aplasia of the radii and thumbs, and renal and cardiac anomalies. It is a familial condition and may appear in the neonatal period. Similar features may be present in Fanconi pancytopenia, which usually presents in the third or fourth year of life. Wiskott-Aldrich syndrome, an X-linked recessive trait, includes eczema, thrombocytopenia, hemorrhage, and immunologic defects, resulting in frequent infections.

Immunoglobulin levels are often helpful in making the diagnosis. Kasabach-Merritt syndrome occurs in children with large cavernous hemangiomas of the trunk, extremities, or abdominal organs where platelets are trapped in the vascular bed. Peripheral smear shows thrombocytopenia and red blood cell fragments; bone marrow examination shows the normal number of megakaryocytes.

(5) Fever and a petechial/purpuric rash should always alert the physician to the possibility of serious bacterial infection, in particular, infection with *Neisseria meningitidis*. Serious infections with other bacteria and rickettsial diseases can also produce this type of rash. Thrombocytopenia may or may not be present. A number of viral infections also occur as petechial rashes. Most common of these is enterovirus infection, but rubella virus, measles virus, varicella virus, Ebstein-Barr virus (EBV), cytomegalovirus (CMV), herpes simplex virus (HSV), and HIV may also be involved. In the neonatal period, infections associated with petechiae include bacterial sepsis, congenital CMV infection, syphilis, HSV infection, toxoplasmosis, rubella, and HIV infection.

(6) DIC is a generalized consumption of clotting factors, anticoagulant proteins, and platelets. It is usually triggered by a severe illness, hypoxia, acidosis, tissue necrosis, or endothelial damage and may be accompanied by shock. It may occur as a hemorrhagic or thrombotic disorder, or both. Fibrinogen is decreased. There is an increase in fibrin degradation products (FDPs). PT and PTT are both prolonged.

(7) HUS usually follows diarrheal infection (*Escherichia coli* O157:H7). Features include hemolytic anemia, thrombocytopenia, and acute renal insufficiency. Thrombotic thrombocytopenic purpura is similar to HUS with thrombocytopenia and microangiopathic hemolytic anemia.

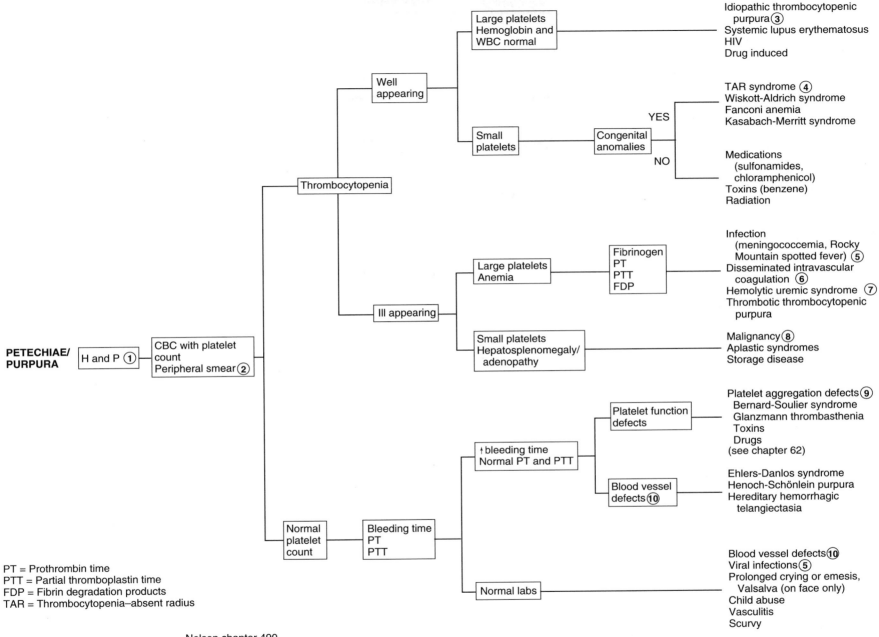

PETECHIAE/ PURPURA — H and P ①

CBC with platelet count Peripheral smear ②

Thrombocytopenia

Well appearing

- Large platelets Hemoglobin and WBC normal
  - Idiopathic thrombocytopenic purpura ③
  - Systemic lupus erythematosus
  - HIV
  - Drug induced

- Small platelets — Congenital anomalies
  - YES
    - TAR syndrome ④
    - Wiskott-Aldrich syndrome
    - Fanconi anemia
    - Kasabach-Merritt syndrome
  - NO
    - Medications (sulfonamides, chloramphenicol)
    - Toxins (benzene)
    - Radiation

Ill appearing

- Large platelets Anemia — Fibrinogen PT PTT FDP
  - Infection (meningococcemia, Rocky Mountain spotted fever) ⑤
  - Disseminated intravascular coagulation ⑥
  - Hemolytic uremic syndrome ⑦
  - Thrombotic thrombocytopenic purpura

- Small platelets Hepatosplenomegaly/ adenopathy
  - Malignancy ⑧
  - Aplastic syndromes
  - Storage disease

Normal platelet count — Bleeding time PT PTT

- ↑bleeding time Normal PT and PTT
  - Platelet function defects
    - Platelet aggregation defects ⑨
    - Bernard-Soulier syndrome
    - Glanzmann thrombasthenia
    - Toxins
    - Drugs (see chapter 62)
  - Blood vessel defects ⑩
    - Ehlers-Danlos syndrome
    - Henoch-Schönlein purpura
    - Hereditary hemorrhagic telangiectasia

- Normal labs
  - Blood vessel defects ⑩
  - Viral infections ⑤
  - Prolonged crying or emesis, Valsalva (on face only)
  - Child abuse
  - Vasculitis
  - Scurvy

PT = Prothrombin time
PTT = Partial thromboplastin time
FDP = Fibrin degradation products
TAR = Thrombocytopenia–absent radius

Nelson chapter 490
Practical Strategies chapter 51

Petechiae/Purpura *(continued)*

(8) With aplastic syndromes (congenital and acquired aplastic anemias) there is thrombocytopenia with small platelets, leukopenia, and anemia. Infiltration of the marrow by malignant cells or due to storage disorders interferes with platelet production. Malignancies may include acute lymphoblastic leukemia, lymphomas, histiocytosis X, as well as metastatic tumors (e.g., neuroblastoma). Other findings may include adenopathy, hepatosplenomegaly, masses, as well as other abnormalities of the peripheral smear. A bone marrow is diagnostic.

(9) Platelet function defects may be congenital and include Glanzmann thrombasthenia (deficiency of a fibrinogen receptor) with normal platelet counts and Bernard-Soulier syndrome (deficiency of the von Willebrand receptor) with mild thrombocytopenia. Platelet function defects may be acquired secondary to medications (aspirin, nonsteroidal antiinflammatory drugs, alcohol, high doses of penicillin, valproate, and others).

(10) Vasculitic disorders occur as hemorrhagic lesions of skin and mucous membranes and symptoms relating to involved organ systems. Coagulation studies are usually normal. Henoch-Schönlein purpura (HSP) appears as petechiae, palpable purpura over the buttocks and lower extremities, as well as arthritis, abdominal pain, and glomerulonephritis. In Ehlers-Danlos syndrome features include joint laxity, hyperelastic skin and poor wound healing, often ecchymoses, and occasionally petechiae. Bleeding time may be prolonged. Petechiae may be present with non–life-threatening viral infections, particularly enterovirus.

BIBLIOGRAPHY

Murphy S, Nepo A, Sills R: Thrombocytopenia. Pediatr Rev 20(2):64–68, 1999.

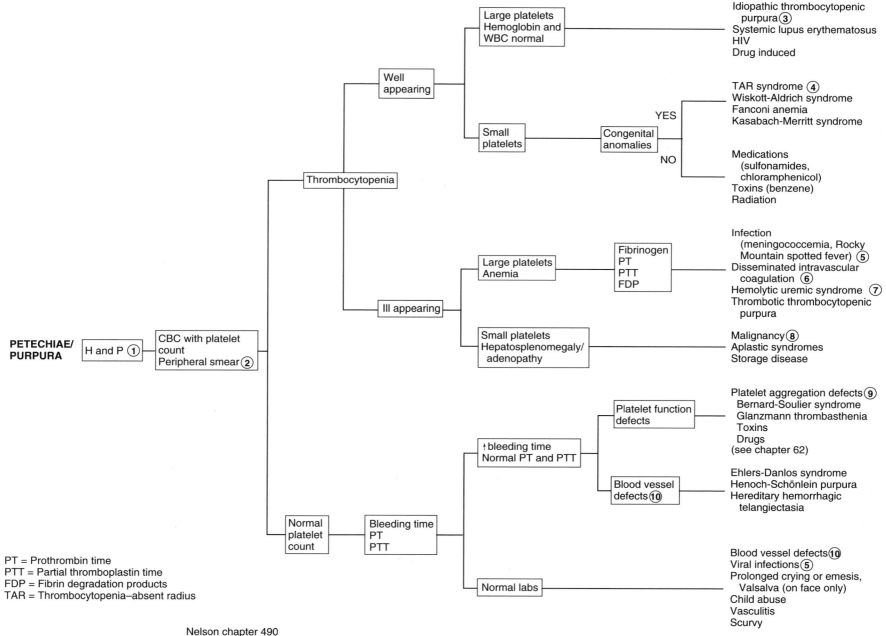

PETECHIAE/ PURPURA — H and P ① — CBC with platelet count / Peripheral smear ②

Thrombocytopenia

Well appearing

- Large platelets / Hemoglobin and WBC normal
  - Idiopathic thrombocytopenic purpura ③
  - Systemic lupus erythematosus
  - HIV
  - Drug induced

- Small platelets — Congenital anomalies
  - YES
    - TAR syndrome ④
    - Wiskott-Aldrich syndrome
    - Fanconi anemia
    - Kasabach-Merritt syndrome
  - NO
    - Medications (sulfonamides, chloramphenicol)
    - Toxins (benzene)
    - Radiation

Ill appearing

- Large platelets / Anemia — Fibrinogen / PT / PTT / FDP
  - Infection (meningococcemia, Rocky Mountain spotted fever) ⑤
  - Disseminated intravascular coagulation ⑥
  - Hemolytic uremic syndrome ⑦
  - Thrombotic thrombocytopenic purpura

- Small platelets / Hepatosplenomegaly/ adenopathy
  - Malignancy ⑧
  - Aplastic syndromes
  - Storage disease

Normal platelet count — Bleeding time / PT / PTT

- ↑ bleeding time / Normal PT and PTT
  - Platelet function defects
    - Platelet aggregation defects ⑨
      - Bernard-Soulier syndrome
      - Glanzmann thrombasthenia
      - Toxins
      - Drugs (see chapter 62)
  - Blood vessel defects ⑩
    - Ehlers-Danlos syndrome
    - Henoch-Schönlein purpura
    - Hereditary hemorrhagic telangiectasia

- Normal labs
  - Blood vessel defects ⑩
  - Viral infections ⑤
  - Prolonged crying or emesis, Valsalva (on face only)
  - Child abuse
  - Vasculitis
  - Scurvy

PT = Prothrombin time
PTT = Partial thromboplastin time
FDP = Fibrin degradation products
TAR = Thrombocytopenia–absent radius

Nelson chapter 490
Practical Strategies chapter 51

Chapter 64 **Neutropenia**

Neutropenia is an absolute decrease in the number of circulating neutrophils in the blood. It varies with age and race. In whites, the lower limit for normal absolute neutrophil counts (ANC = neutrophils + bands) is 1000 cells/μl in infants between 2 weeks and 1 year of age, and 1500 cells/μl in children older than 1 year. In blacks, the lower limits may be 200 to 600 cells/μl less than whites. The severity of neutropenia is helpful in predicting an increased likelihood of pyogenic infection. Mild neutropenia ranges from 1000 to 1500 cells/μl; moderate neutropenia ranges from 500 to 1000 cells/μl.

1 History of any recent or recurrent infections and drug exposure should be obtained. This history should include fever, which may be a sign of infection. Infections may be both a cause and a consequence of neutropenia. The duration and severity of the neutropenia is important in determining infection risk. Severe neutropenia with counts < 500 cells/μl is associated with the greatest risk of pyogenic infections, including cellulitis, abscesses including perirectal, furuncles, pneumonia, septicemia, as well as oral infections such as stomatitis, gingivitis, and periodontitis. A careful physical examination is important in locating any sites of occult infection. The usual signs of infection (erythema, warmth) may not be present because of the neutropenia. Examination should also include evaluation for lymphadenopathy, hepatosplenomegaly, and any other signs of underlying disease.

2 There are many drugs that cause neutropenia, including chemotherapeutic drugs. A partial list is presented in the algorithm. An idiosyncratic reaction generally affects only neutrophils; other cell lines are usually unaffected.

3 In patients with fever and neutropenia, particularly if the child is ill appearing, cultures of blood, urine, and any suspected sites of infection should be done. Antibody responses, antigen detection tests, and polymerase chain reaction (PCR) methods may also be useful. In patients undergoing chemotherapy, cultures should also be obtained from central venous lines. These should include aerobic and anaerobic bacteria as well as fungi. In chronically infected sites, mycobacterial and anaerobic cultures are recommended. If diarrhea is present, obtain cultures for bacteria, viruses, and parasites. *Clostridium difficile* toxin should be sought . Viral cultures may be considered in specific instances, for example, herpes culture and Tzanck preparation from vesicular skin lesions or respiratory viruses in children with respiratory symptoms. Mild neutropenia in a child with a febrile viral-appearing illness and without a history of recurrent significant infections may not need further evaluation.

4 The most common cause of transient neutropenia in children is viral infection. Viruses commonly causing neutropenia include hepatitis A and B, respiratory syncytial virus, influenza virus types A and B, measles, rubella, and varicella. It may also occur in early stages of infectious mononucleosis. Leukopenia may be seen in patients with HIV infection. This may be due to the virus or due to antiviral drugs.

5 There may be neutropenia associated with typhoid, paratyphoid, tuberculosis, brucellosis, tularemia, and rickettsial infections. In patients with an immunodeficiency, commonly cultured organisms include *Staphylococcus aureus*, coagulase-negative staphylococci, and gram-negative organisms, including *E. coli* and *Klebsiella pneumoniae*. *Candida* may also be cultured. Although any severe infection may result in neutropenia, cyclic neutropenia and chronic neutropenia need to be excluded with twice weekly WBC counts for 6 to 8 weeks. Reticulocyte, platelet, and other leukocyte counts may also cycle.

6 Cyclic neutropenia is a congenital condition with regular fluctuation in neutrophil counts. The nadir occurs approximately every 21 days, often to an absolute neutrophil count of < 200 cells/μl. During the neutropenic period there may be fever, oral ulcers, gingivitis, periodontitis, and pharyngitis with lymphadenopathy. More serious infections such as mastoiditis or pneumonia may also occur.

7 Congenital neutropenias include those associated with phenotypic abnormalities. Chédiak-Higashi syndrome is characterized by oculocutaneous albinism. There is an increased susceptibility to infection due to neutropenia, as well as defective function of the remaining neutrophils. Dyskeratosis congenita is associated with nail dystrophy, leukoplakia, and reticulated hyperpigmentation of the skin. Shwachman syndrome is characterized by dwarfism, growth failure, skeletal abnormalities, and exocrine pancreatic insufficiency, causing diarrhea, weight loss, and failure to thrive. Cartilage-hair hypoplasia features neutropenia with short-limbed dwarfism and fine hair.

8 Autoimmune neutropenia may be associated with other autoimmune diseases (e.g., systemic lupus erythematosus, autoimmune hemolytic anemia, and thrombocytopenia). It may also be associated with infection (e.g., infectious mononucleosis, HIV infection), malignancy (e.g., leukemia, lymphoma), and drugs. Antineutrophil antibodies may be present on testing; Coombs testing may identify associated hemolytic conditions.

9 Chronic benign neutropenia is believed to be a form of autoimmune neutropenia. It occurs in children younger than age 3 years. Antineutrophil antibodies may be present.

10 Immune neonatal neutropenia is similar to Rh-hemolytic anemia. It occurs due to maternal sensitization caused by fetal neutrophil antigens. The neutropenia may last for weeks and as long as 6 months. Antineutrophil antibodies are found in maternal and infant serum. It can also occur in infants whose mothers have autoimmune neutropenia.

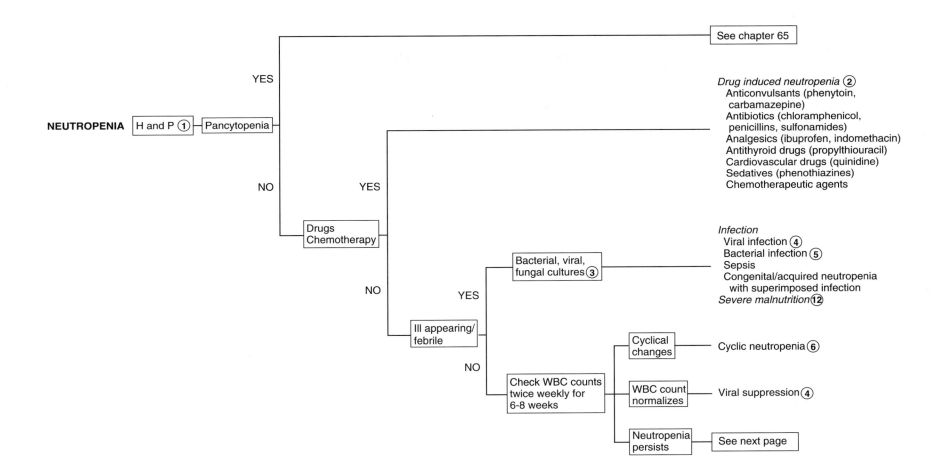

NEUTROPENIA — H and P ① — Pancytopenia

YES — See chapter 65

NO

Drugs Chemotherapy

YES — *Drug induced neutropenia* ②
  Anticonvulsants (phenytoin, carbamazepine)
  Antibiotics (chloramphenicol, penicillins, sulfonamides)
  Analgesics (ibuprofen, indomethacin)
  Antithyroid drugs (propylthiouracil)
  Cardiovascular drugs (quinidine)
  Sedatives (phenothiazines)
  Chemotherapeutic agents

NO

Ill appearing/ febrile

YES — Bacterial, viral, fungal cultures ③ — *Infection*
  Viral infection ④
  Bacterial infection ⑤
  Sepsis
  Congenital/acquired neutropenia with superimposed infection
  Severe malnutrition ⑫

NO — Check WBC counts twice weekly for 6-8 weeks

Cyclical changes — Cyclic neutropenia ⑥

WBC count normalizes — Viral suppression ④

Neutropenia persists — See next page

Nelson chapter 131
Practical Strategies chapter 60

(11) Neutropenia may be associated with disorders of immune dysfunction; these conditions include X-linked agammaglobulinemia, hyper-IgM syndrome, cartilage-hair hypoplasia, as well as HIV infection.

(12) Nutritional deficiencies including those of vitamin B_{12}, folate, and copper may be associated with neutropenia. Severe malnutrition seen in anorexia nervosa and marasmus may also cause neutropenia. Reticuloendothelial sequestration secondary to splenic enlargement can lead to neutropenia. Causes include portal hypertension, splenic disease, and splenic hyperplasia. Many metabolic diseases are associated with neutropenia. Some of these include hyperglycinemia, isovalericacidemia, propionicacidemia, methylmalonicacidemia, and tyrosinemia. Neutropenia may also be noted in some glycogen storage disorders. Other congenital causes of neutropenia include reticular dysgenesis, which is characterized by neutropenia and lymphopenia. Lymphoid tissue (e.g., tonsils, lymph nodes, Peyer patches, and lymphoid follicles) is absent. Severe congenital neutropenia (Kostmann disease) is a severe disease with an absolute neutrophil count of < 200 cells/μl. The disease occurs in early infancy with recurrent severe pyogenic infections. Familial benign neutropenia is mild with no increased tendency for infection.

BIBLIOGRAPHY

Nathan DG, Orkin SH (eds): Nathan and Oski's Hematology of Infancy and Childhood, 5th ed. Philadelphia: WB Saunders Company, 1998.

NEUTROPENIA (continued)

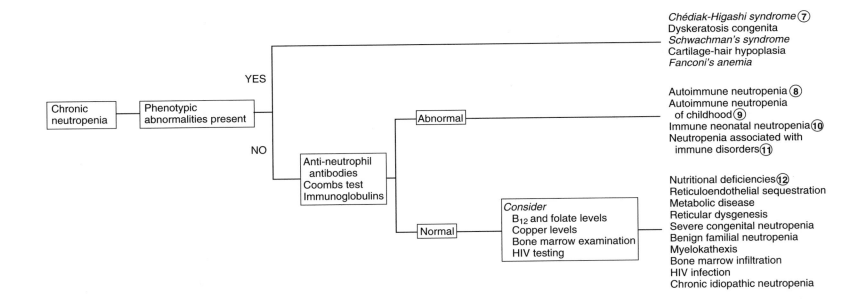

Chapter 65 *Pancytopenia*

Pancytopenia is caused by a decrease in production of erythrocytes, granulocytes, and platelets by the bone marrow. Clinically, this results in anemia, hemorrhage, and decreased resistance to infection. Severe aplastic anemia is diagnosed when at least two of the following are present: granulocyte count < 500/μl, platelet count < 20,000 μl, and corrected reticulocyte count < 1%. The bone marrow contains < 25% of the normal cellularity. Mild or moderate aplastic anemia (i.e., hypoplastic anemia) has a mild or moderate decrease in granulocytes, platelets, and erythrocytes. There may be normal or increased bone marrow cellularity.

(1) History should include exposure to agents that are potentially myelosuppressive. These include radiation and chemotherapy (e.g., 6-mercaptopurine, methotrexate, nitrogen mustard). Other drugs include chloramphenicol, sulfonamides, phenylbutazone, and anticonvulsants. Chemicals and toxins include benzene and other aromatic hydrocarbons present in insecticides and herbicides. A history and physical examination compatible with certain viral infections should be sought. A susceptibility to infection above and beyond that expected may suggest an immunodeficiency syndrome. A family history of congenital anomalies, aplastic syndromes, and leukemias may indicate syndromes associated with constitutional aplastic pancytopenias.

Physical examination may reveal the effects of the cytopenias: anemia results in tachycardia and pallor; thrombocytopenia may cause bleeding, bruising, epistaxis, petechiae, or ecchymoses; and neutropenia may be associated with oral ulcerations and fevers. Examination should include identification of congenital anomalies associated with Fanconi and other syndromes (i.e., Down syndrome).

(2) Patients with hemolytic anemia who have shortened red blood cell survival time are at risk of transient aplastic crisis. This is most commonly associated with parvovirus and may occur in children with sickle cell disease, thalassemia, hereditary spherocytosis, and other types of erythroid stress.

(3) When severe aplastic anemia is present a bone marrow examination by a hematologist is recommended. On peripheral smear the RBCs are often macrocytic. There may be an increase in hemoglobin F. The bone marrow is usually hypocellular. In some conditions there may be replacement of the bone marrow by nonhematopoietic cells (e.g., metastatic cells).

(4) Fanconi anemia is an autosomal recessive condition. Two thirds of affected children have congenital anomalies. These include microcephaly, microphthalmia, absent radii and thumbs, as well as heart and kidney abnormalities. There may be hypopigmentation of the skin and short stature. Chromosomal breakage studies are needed for diagnosis.

(5) Dyskeratosis congenita is a rare form of ectodermal dysplasia associated with pancytopenia. Dermatologic manifestations include hyperpigmented skin, dystrophic nails, and mucous membrane leukoplakia.

(6) Schwachman-Diamond syndrome is characterized by neutropenia with exocrine pancreatic insufficiency (e.g., malabsorption, steatorrhea, failure to thrive). About 25% develop aplastic anemia.

(7) Pregnancy may be associated with aplastic anemia; estrogens may play a role.

(8) Paroxysmal nocturnal hemoglobinuria is characterized by intravascular hemolysis and hemoglobinuria as well as venous thrombosis. There is a strong association with aplastic anemia.

(9) Systemic diseases may be associated with pancytopenias. These may include systemic lupus erythematosus, metabolic diseases, brucellosis, sarcoidosis, and tuberculosis.

(10) Replacement of the marrow by nonhematopoietic cells may cause pancytopenias. Neuroblastomas metastasize to the bone marrow. Osteopetrosis may cause obliteration of the marrow. Myelofibrosis may also be a cause.

(11) The most common cause of mild or moderate pancytopenias in healthy patients is suppression due to infectious agents. Specific viruses include human parvovirus B19, hepatitis viruses B and C, dengue virus, cytomegalovirus, human herpesvirus 6, and Ebstein-Barr virus. Patients with HIV may have pancytopenia for a number of reasons, including opportunistic infections, drugs used in treatment, and neoplasms associated with the disease. Other viruses that may cause cytopenias include measles, mumps, rubella, varicella, and influenza A. If a viral etiology is suggested, it is reasonable to recheck the CBC in a few weeks. If the pancytopenia persists or becomes more severe, referral to a hematologist for further evaluation is recommended.

BIBLIOGRAPHY

Alter BP, Young NS: The bone marrow failure syndromes. In Nathan DG, Orkin SH (eds): Nathan and Oski's Hematology of Infancy and Childhood, 5th ed, pp 237–335. Philadelphia: WB Saunders Company, 1998.

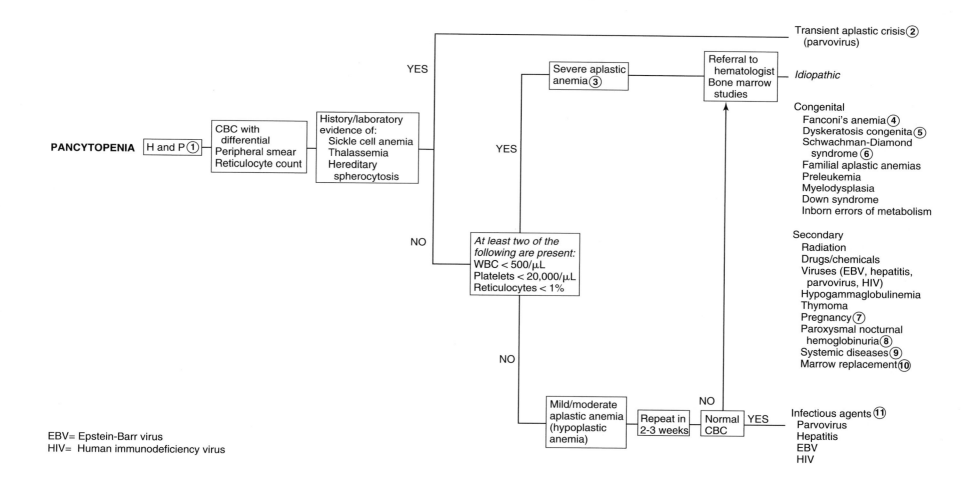

PANCYTOPENIA — H and P ① → CBC with differential / Peripheral smear / Reticulocyte count → History/laboratory evidence of: Sickle cell anemia / Thalassemia / Hereditary spherocytosis

YES → Transient aplastic crisis ② (parvovirus)

At least two of the following are present: WBC < 500/μL / Platelets < 20,000/μL / Reticulocytes < 1%

YES → Severe aplastic anemia ③ → Referral to hematologist / Bone marrow studies

Idiopathic

Congenital
  Fanconi's anemia ④
  Dyskeratosis congenita ⑤
  Schwachman-Diamond syndrome ⑥
  Familial aplastic anemias
  Preleukemia
  Myelodysplasia
  Down syndrome
  Inborn errors of metabolism

Secondary
  Radiation
  Drugs/chemicals
  Viruses (EBV, hepatitis, parvovirus, HIV)
  Hypogammaglobulinemia
  Thymoma
  Pregnancy ⑦
  Paroxysmal nocturnal hemoglobinuria ⑧
  Systemic diseases ⑨
  Marrow replacement ⑩

NO → Mild/moderate aplastic anemia (hypoplastic anemia) → Repeat in 2-3 weeks → Normal CBC

NO → Referral to hematologist / Bone marrow studies

YES → Infectious agents ⑪
  Parvovirus
  Hepatitis
  EBV
  HIV

EBV = Epstein-Barr virus
HIV = Human immunodeficiency virus

Nelson chapters 474, 475

Eosinophilia is most commonly associated with exposure to an antigen. Normal eosinophil counts range from 250 to 700 cells/mm³.

(1) History should include exposure to drugs that may cause hypersensitivity. Many rashes are associated with eosinophilia. These may be infectious or allergic. Travel history, particularly to tropical countries, is helpful in the diagnosis of parasitic infections. Exposure to cats and dogs may also be associated with parasites. Respiratory signs and symptoms (e.g., wheezing, cough, rales, and rhonchi) may indicate the presence of asthma or allergic rhinitis. If atopic disease is not suggested, a careful search for other causes is indicated. Gastrointestinal signs and symptoms such as weight loss, diarrhea, and failure to thrive may suggest either parasite infestation or chronic gastrointestinal disease associated with eosinophilia. Hematologic and oncologic conditions may also be associated with eosinophilia, as well as many chronic diseases. A family history of atopic disease (e.g., asthma, allergic rhinitis, and atopic dermatitis) should be obtained. Eosinophilia may be a familial condition. Because eosinophilia is associated with so many conditions, the algorithm focuses on more common pediatric causes.

(2) If respiratory symptoms are present and asthma is not suggested, a chest X-ray should be obtained. Serologic tests for *Toxocara* may be done in children with exposure to pets (cats or dogs). Stool studies for cysts and ova may reveal parasite infestation. Serologic and skin tests for aspergillosis and coccidioidomycosis may be considered in specific cases.

(3) Löffler syndrome is a transient allergic response to antigens, usually parasites or drugs. It is characterized by pulmonary infiltrates, which may resemble miliary tuberculosis, as well as by paroxysmal episodes of coughing, dyspnea, and pleurisy, usually without fever. Eosinophilia may be as high as 70%. The most common parasites causing Löffler syndrome are *Toxocara (T. canis* and *T. cati), Ascaris lumbricoides, Strongyloides stercoralis,* and hookworms. *Echinococcus granulosus* may produce dyspnea, cough, and hemoptysis due to hydatid cysts in the lungs. Drugs that may cause Löffler syndrome include aspirin, penicillin, sulfonamides, and imipramine. This syndrome is part of a spectrum of hypereosinophilic syndromes (HES), ranging in severity from mild and self-resolving to severe, chronic, and fatal conditions.

(4) Allergic bronchopulmonary aspergillosis (ABPA) is a hypersensitivity reaction characterized by recurrent bronchospasm, transient pulmonary infiltrates, and bronchiectasis. It occurs in children with chronic pulmonary disease (e.g., asthma, cystic fibrosis). Skin testing as well as testing for antibodies to *Aspergillus* antigen may aid in the diagnosis.

(5) Sarcoidosis is a chronic granulomatous disease affecting primarily the lungs; however, it may affect any organ system. Pulmonary involvement includes parenchymal infiltrates, miliary nodules, and hilar and paratracheal lymphadenopathy. Pulmonary function test findings show a restrictive pattern.

(6) Coccidioidomycosis is caused by *Coccidioides immitis*; it is endemic in California (San Joaquin valley), central and southern Arizona, and southwestern Texas. It may occur as a primary infection. Symptoms may include fever, rash, cough, chest pain, anorexia, malaise, and, occasionally, hemoptysis. A majority of cases are asymptomatic. Results of a chest examination are usually normal; however, on chest X-ray there may be significant findings, including consolidation or pleural effusion. A residual cavity may develop in an area of consolidation. Diagnosis of coccidioidomycosis may be done using skin tests or serology. Negative skin test results do not exclude coccidioidal infection. Skin tests cannot distinguish recent from old infections.

(7) Tropical pulmonary eosinophilia is caused by filarial infection of the lymph nodes and lungs. Signs and symptoms include cough, dyspnea, fever, weight loss, and fatigue; there may be rales and rhonchi on chest examination. Chest X-ray shows increased bronchovascular markings, discrete opacities, or diffuse miliary lesions. Hepatosplenomegaly and generalized lymphadenopathy may be present. Laboratory findings include eosinophilia (> 2000/mm³), increased IgE levels, and high titers of antifilarial antibodies.

(8) Eosinophilic gastroenteritis is a rare condition involving infiltration of the stomach and intestine with eosinophils. Signs and symptoms include abdominal pain, vomiting, and diarrhea. There may be hypoalbuminemia due to protein-losing enteropathy.

(9) Eosinophilia is seen with many immunodeficiency syndromes. Wiskott-Aldrich syndrome is an X-linked recessive syndrome presenting as eczema, thrombocytopenia, and susceptibility to infections. Hyperimmunoglobulinemia E (hyper-IgE) syndrome is characterized by recurrent staphylococcal abscesses involving the skin, lungs, and joints.

(10) Hypereosinophilic syndrome is an idiopathic disease characterized by sustained overproduction of eosinophils and signs and symptoms of organ involvement, including the heart, skin, liver, spleen, gastrointestinal tract, brain, and lungs.

(11) Familial eosinophilia is usually benign, with no associated symptoms. Episodic angioedema is a familial syndrome associated with eosinophilia. Features include recurrent episodes of fever, urticaria, and angioedema.

BIBLIOGRAPHY

Nathan DG, Orkin SH (eds): Nathan and Oski's Hematology of Infancy and Childhood, 5th ed. Philadelphia: WB Saunders Company, 1998.

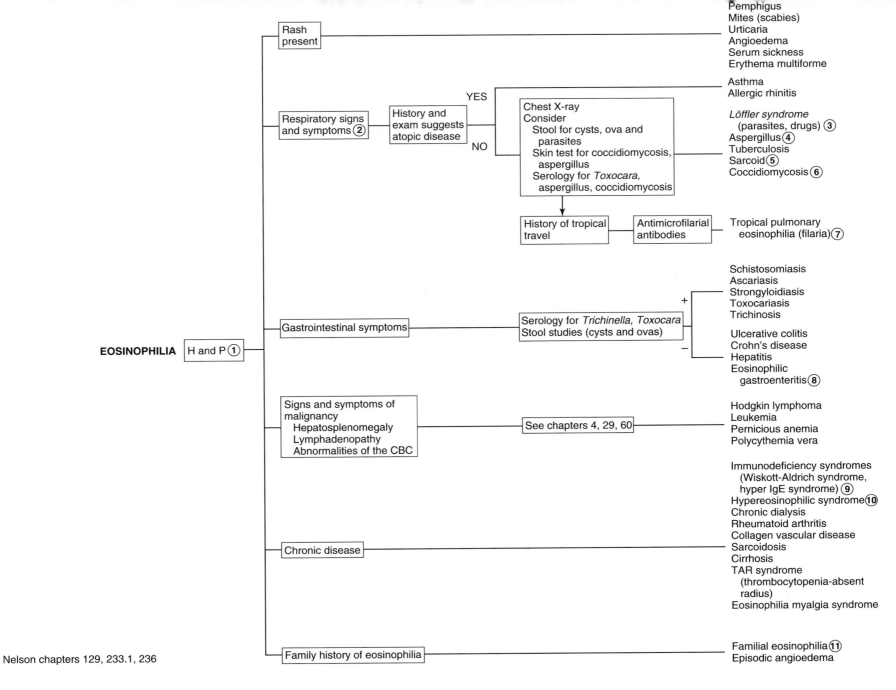

EOSINOPHILIA   H and P ①

Rash present
- Pemphigus
- Mites (scabies)
- Urticaria
- Angioedema
- Serum sickness
- Erythema multiforme

Respiratory signs and symptoms ②
→ History and exam suggests atopic disease

YES
- Asthma
- Allergic rhinitis

NO → Chest X-ray
Consider
- Stool for cysts, ova and parasites
- Skin test for coccidiomycosis, aspergillus
- Serology for *Toxocara*, aspergillus, coccidiomycosis

- *Löffler syndrome* (parasites, drugs) ③
- Aspergillus ④
- Tuberculosis
- Sarcoid ⑤
- Coccidiomycosis ⑥

→ History of tropical travel — Antimicrofilarial antibodies
- Tropical pulmonary eosinophilia (filaria) ⑦

Gastrointestinal symptoms → Serology for *Trichinella, Toxocara*
Stool studies (cysts and ovas)

+
- Schistosomiasis
- Ascariasis
- Strongyloidiasis
- Toxocariasis
- Trichinosis

−
- Ulcerative colitis
- Crohn's disease
- Hepatitis
- Eosinophilic gastroenteritis ⑧

Signs and symptoms of malignancy
- Hepatosplenomegaly
- Lymphadenopathy
- Abnormalities of the CBC
→ See chapters 4, 29, 60
- Hodgkin lymphoma
- Leukemia
- Pernicious anemia
- Polycythemia vera

Chronic disease
- Immunodeficiency syndromes (Wiskott-Aldrich syndrome, hyper IgE syndrome) ⑨
- Hypereosinophilic syndrome ⑩
- Chronic dialysis
- Rheumatoid arthritis
- Collagen vascular disease
- Sarcoidosis
- Cirrhosis
- TAR syndrome (thrombocytopenia-absent radius)
- Eosinophilia myalgia syndrome

Family history of eosinophilia
- Familial eosinophilia ⑪
- Episodic angioedema

Nelson chapters 129, 233.1, 236

255

ENDOCRINE SYSTEM

Short stature is defined as height less than 2 to 2.5 standard deviations (SD) below the mean for age. It is important to distinguish normal short stature from that due to a medical problem. Short stature must also be distinguished from failure to thrive, with associated poor weight gain. Because of the importance our culture places on height for males, boys are more likely to be brought to medical attention for this complaint. Many factors such as parental height and growth patterns, ethnicity, nutritional status, chronic illnesses, and emotional and psychological effects may influence stature. Infants of very low birth weight and small for gestational age (SGA) for various reasons (chromosomal disorders or syndromes, infections, or maternal alcohol use) are more likely to be of shorter stature.

(1) History and physical examination should rule out any obvious dysmorphisms, syndromes, or diseases that may be associated with short stature. Birth history should include height and weight, prenatal exposures and illnesses, as well as perinatal problems. Prolonged jaundice, hypoglycemia, and small phallus suggest growth hormone deficiency; puffy extremities suggest Turner syndrome. Growth velocity and growth patterns must be plotted. A short child who remains along the growth percentile may have familial or constitutional delay. Progressive deviation below the curve suggests a congenital disorder (Turner syndrome, growth hormone deficiency). Developmental delay is associated with syndromes such as Prader-Willi syndrome. Weight for age that is less than height for age suggests malnutrition or chronic illness. A history of cranial irradiation for CNS malignancies suggests growth hormone deficiency. Midline defects may be present in hypopituitarism.

(2) A child with moderate short stature (1.5–2 SD), with a family history of short stature or pubertal delay who is staying along his or her growth curve, may be followed clinically.

(3) A child with familial short stature follows parallel to the normal growth curve and has normal pubertal development. Bone age may be considered and is normal. If there is deviation from the growth curve, further evaluation is needed.

(4) Constitutional delay is a normal variation, recognized more commonly in boys. There is pubertal delay, delayed bone age, and delayed growth spurt, with subsequent attainment of normal adult height. There is also a family history of delayed puberty. Laboratory test results are normal. It may be difficult to distinguish these children from those with mild growth hormone defects, chronic disease, or central hypogonadism.

(5) If the child has decelerating growth patterns or is significantly short (<2–2.5 SD), further evaluation should be guided by the clinical findings. A chronic illness may be suggested by the results of a complete blood cell count (CBC), erythrocyte sedimentation rate (ESR), chemistry profile, and urinalysis. Hypothyroidism can be detected by obtaining free-thyroxine (T_4) and thyroid-simulating hormone (TSH) levels. Suspicion of Turner syndrome in girls with unexplained short stature requires a karyotype. Growth hormone deficiency may be screened for by obtaining an insulin-like growth factor-1 (IGF-1); however, the definitive test involves growth hormone (GH) levels in response to pharmacologic stimulation. Further evaluation by an endocrinologist is required.

(6) We suggest using a weight:height ratio to organize a differential diagnosis for a child with short stature. This is an inexact method, and it is not a formal means of classification. The specific laboratory tests ordered should be based on the findings of the history and physical examination. In general, however, weight for age < height for age may indicate chronic illness or malnutrition, weight for age > height for age may indicate endocrinopathies or syndromes, and weight proportional to height may indicate emotional deprivation.

(7) Children with weight disproportionately lower than height may be malnourished or have specific deficiencies (e.g., rickets). Chronic illness may be a cause, including gastrointestinal disease (inflammatory bowel disease, celiac disease), renal disease (renal tubular acidosis), pulmonary disease (asthma, cystic fibrosis), hematologic disease (sickle cell, thalassemia), immunologic disease (juvenile rheumatoid arthritis, connective tissue disease, AIDS), and cardiac disorders (left-to-right shunts, congestive heart failure). Screening laboratory tests (e.g., ESR, CBC, urinalysis, and chemistry profile) may indicate the diagnosis. Specific tests such as sweat chloride may be required. Renal tubular acidosis (RTA) may result in failure to thrive (FTT) and short stature. A low serum bicarbonate on the chemistry profile may be the clue. Further evaluation reveals a normal anion gap metabolic acidosis. (See Ch. 82.)

(8) Hypothyroidism may be congenital or acquired. Children with Turner syndrome, Down syndrome, Klinefelter syndrome, or diabetes mellitus are at risk for autoimmune hypothyroidism. Free T_4 is decreased; TSH is increased with acquired hypothyroidism. Low TSH and free T_4 suggest a hypothalamic/pituitary defect.

(9) Growth hormone (GH) deficiency is congenital or acquired. There may be isolated GH deficiency or panhypopituitarism. Congenital deficiencies are idiopathic, associated with midline defects (e.g., septooptic dysplasia, cleft palate, single central incisor), or inherited. The infants tend to be slightly smaller at birth (most are appropriate for gestational age); have hypoglycemia, jaundice, and micropenis; and show poor postnatal linear growth. Acquired GH deficiency may be due to injury, irradiation, or tumor. Bone age is delayed, and insulin-like growth factor-1 (IGF-1) levels are often low. Levels are influenced by age, puberty, and nutrition. Further evaluation requires referral to an endocrinologist for GH testing and testing for other pituitary hormones. Laron dwarfism features end-organ resistance to GH with elevated GH levels and low levels of IGF-1.

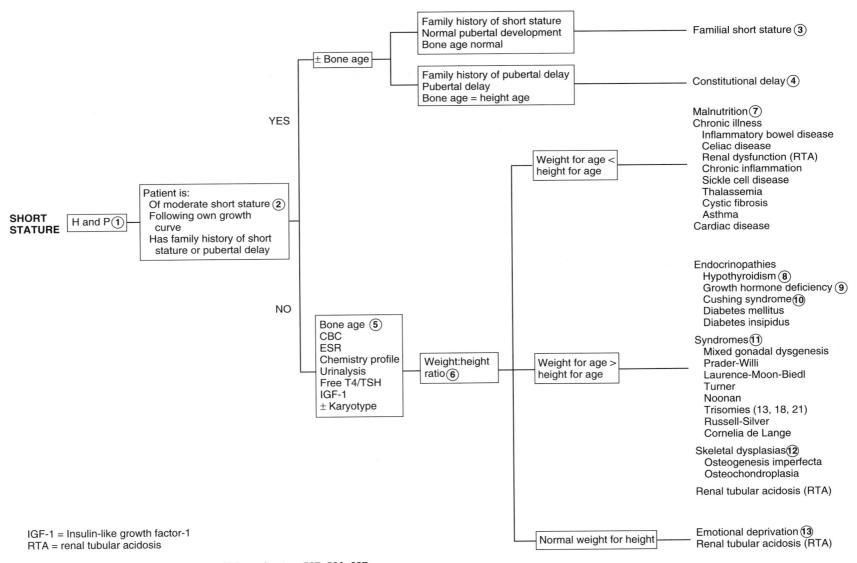

SHORT STATURE — H and P ①

Patient is:
Of moderate short stature ②
Following own growth curve
Has family history of short stature or pubertal delay

YES

± Bone age

Family history of short stature
Normal pubertal development
Bone age normal — Familial short stature ③

Family history of pubertal delay
Pubertal delay
Bone age = height age — Constitutional delay ④

NO

Bone age ⑤
CBC
ESR
Chemistry profile
Urinalysis
Free T4/TSH
IGF-1
± Karyotype

Weight:height ratio ⑥

Weight for age < height for age

Malnutrition ⑦
Chronic illness
    Inflammatory bowel disease
    Celiac disease
    Renal dysfunction (RTA)
    Chronic inflammation
    Sickle cell disease
    Thalassemia
    Cystic fibrosis
    Asthma
Cardiac disease

Weight for age > height for age

Endocrinopathies
    Hypothyroidism ⑧
    Growth hormone deficiency ⑨
    Cushing syndrome ⑩
    Diabetes mellitus
    Diabetes insipidus

Syndromes ⑪
    Mixed gonadal dysgenesis
    Prader-Willi
    Laurence-Moon-Biedl
    Turner
    Noonan
    Trisomies (13, 18, 21)
    Russell-Silver
    Cornelia de Lange

Skeletal dysplasias ⑫
    Osteogenesis imperfecta
    Osteochondroplasia

Renal tubular acidosis (RTA)

Normal weight for height

Emotional deprivation ⑬
Renal tubular acidosis (RTA)

IGF-1 = Insulin-like growth factor-1
RTA = renal tubular acidosis

Nelson chapters 567, 596, 697
Practical Strategies chapter 62

10 Cushing syndrome is due to excessive levels of glucocorticoids, which may be exogenous (i.e., high doses of oral/topical corticosteroids) or endogenous due to excess adrenocorticotropic hormone (ACTH) from pituitary tumors or ectopic production. Examination reveals an obese child who often has plethora, moon facies, buffalo hump, striae, acne, and hypertension. Hyperpigmentation occurs when excess ACTH is present. Significant virilization may indicate an adrenal tumor.

11 Syndromes or chromosomal abnormalities may be associated with short stature. The more common syndromes include Turner syndrome, mixed gonadal dysgenesis, Down syndrome, and other trisomies. Syndromes such as Prader-Willi and Laurence-Moon-Biedl syndromes may present as hypogonadism, obesity, and mental retardation.

12 Bone dysplasias usually appear as abnormal body proportions, including achondroplasia and hypochondroplasia. Genetic consultation may be helpful.

13 Emotional deprivation may cause short stature even without malnutrition. There may be clinical features of GH deficiency and evidence of hypopituitarism, which normalize in an improved environment.

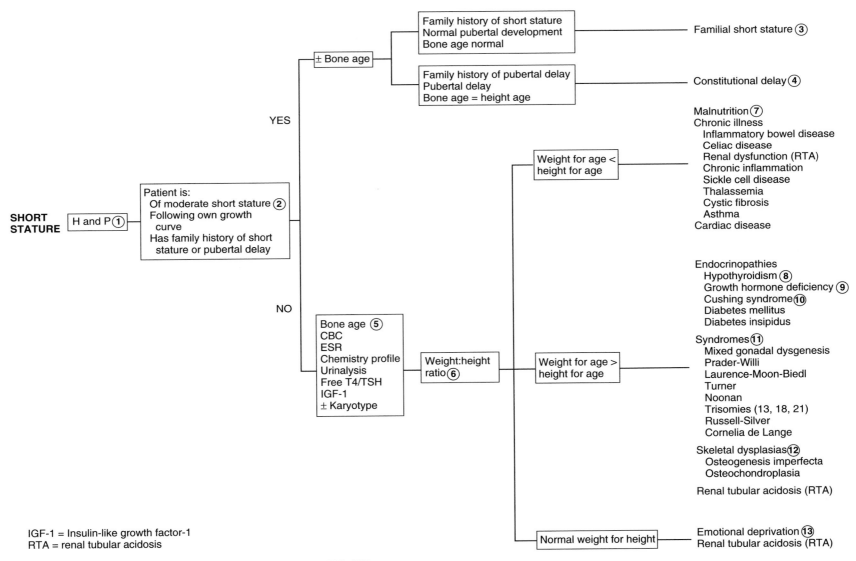

SHORT STATURE — H and P ①

Patient is:
Of moderate short stature ②
Following own growth curve
Has family history of short stature or pubertal delay

YES

± Bone age

Family history of short stature
Normal pubertal development
Bone age normal → Familial short stature ③

Family history of pubertal delay
Pubertal delay
Bone age = height age → Constitutional delay ④

NO

Bone age ⑤
CBC
ESR
Chemistry profile
Urinalysis
Free T4/TSH
IGF-1
± Karyotype

Weight:height ratio ⑥

Weight for age < height for age →
Malnutrition ⑦
Chronic illness
  Inflammatory bowel disease
  Celiac disease
  Renal dysfunction (RTA)
  Chronic inflammation
  Sickle cell disease
  Thalassemia
  Cystic fibrosis
  Asthma
Cardiac disease

Weight for age > height for age →
Endocrinopathies
  Hypothyroidism ⑧
  Growth hormone deficiency ⑨
  Cushing syndrome ⑩
  Diabetes mellitus
  Diabetes insipidus

Syndromes ⑪
  Mixed gonadal dysgenesis
  Prader-Willi
  Laurence-Moon-Biedl
  Turner
  Noonan
  Trisomies (13, 18, 21)
  Russell-Silver
  Cornelia de Lange

Skeletal dysplasias ⑫
  Osteogenesis imperfecta
  Osteochondroplasia

Renal tubular acidosis (RTA)

Normal weight for height →
Emotional deprivation ⑬
Renal tubular acidosis (RTA)

IGF-1 = Insulin-like growth factor-1
RTA = renal tubular acidosis

Nelson chapters 567, 596, 697
Practical Strategies chapter 62

Chapter 68 *Pubertal Delay*

Pubertal delay is defined as absence of development of secondary sexual characteristics (breast budding in girls, testicular enlargement in boys) by age 13 in girls and by age 14 in boys. For discussion of girls with some sexual maturation but with primary amenorrhea, please see Chapter 39.

(1) History must include infections, chronic illness, endocrinopathies, trauma, chemotherapy, irradiation, CNS disorders, and syndromes. Growth patterns and growth velocity should be evaluated. Severe growth retardation may indicate growth hormone (GH) deficiency. A family history of pubertal onset should be obtained.

Examination includes careful measurements of height, weight, arm span, and head circumference. Body proportions may be helpful; with GH deficiency height age is less than weight age. Eunuchoidal proportions (arm span > height, long legs) are noted with hypogonadism. Androgen effects include phallic growth, increased testicular size, sexual hair, voice change, increased stature and muscle mass, hairline recession, and body odor. Estrogen effects include vaginal cornification/discharge, breast development, uterine size, and onset of menarche 2 to 2.5 years after breast budding. A careful CNS examination should include tests for olfaction (i.e., anosmia/hyposmia in Kallmann syndrome) as well as visual acuity. Pubertal staging and the presence of gynecomastia and galactorrhea should be noted. Skin examination includes café-au-lait spots (neurofibromatosis), tanning (adrenal insufficiency), and ichthyosis (congenital ichthyosis, Kallmann syndrome).

(2) Plasma follicle-stimulating hormone (FSH) and luteinizing hormone (LH) levels can be used to classify the causes of pubertal delay into hypogonadotropic ($\downarrow$ FSH/LH) or hypergonadotropic ($\uparrow$ FSH/LH) hypogonadism. Bone age assessment, estradiol or testosterone levels, and prolactin and thyroid studies may be considered.

(3) Stigmata of gonadal dysgenesis syndromes (Turner syndrome) include short stature, pigmented nevi, high arched palate, low hairline, shield chest, ptosis, cutis laxa, pterygium coli, shortened fourth metacarpals, cubitus valgus, heart murmurs, nail changes, and deformed ears.

(4) Mixed gonadal dysgenesis is a common cause of ambiguous genitalia in newborns. The karyotype usually shows mosaicism (45,XO/46,XY). Patients often have a female phenotype and features of Turner syndrome. Some patients have no signs of masculinization, whereas in others there may be prepubertal clitoromegaly with further virilization occurring at puberty.

(5) Klinefelter syndrome is the most common cause of testicular failure; the karyotype is 47,XXY. Testes are small, there is mild mental retardation, and gynecomastia may be present.

(6) In pure gonadal dysgenesis, variants include XX or XY karyotype with normal stature and streak gonads.

(7) Noonan syndrome has similar features to Turner syndrome but a normal karyotype.

(8) Primary ovarian failure may be due to autoimmune oophoritis, often associated with other endocrinopathies, and may be screened for with antiovarian antibodies. Resistant ovary syndrome is due to defects in the FSH or LH receptors.

(9) Anorchia is the absence of testes and must be distinguished from bilateral cryptorchidism in which normal puberty may occur; however, due to compromised Leydig cell function normal testosterone levels may only be achieved with elevated FSH and LH levels. Irradiation or chemotherapy may cause gonadal injury. Enzyme defects include 17 α-hydroxylase deficiency and 17-ketosteroid reductase deficiency.

(10) The genetic male with androgen insensitivity (i.e., testicular feminization) appears phenotypically female, with primary amenorrhea, breast development, and absence of pubic hair. There is wide variation in the degree of androgen resistance. Levels of LH are usually elevated but FSH levels may be normal because estrogen from the testes may suppress it.

(11) Constitutional delay is the most common cause of delayed puberty and is brought to medical attention more often in boys. There is a family history of delayed puberty, a consistent growth velocity, and a normal examination. The bone age = height age, which is less than the chronologic age.

(12) Specific stigmata may be indicative of certain syndromes. In Prader-Willi syndrome there is obesity, hyperphagia, short stature, and mild mental retardation. The hypogonadism is hypothalamic. Laurence-Moon-Biedl syndrome is associated with mild mental retardation, retinitis pigmentosa, syndactyly, polydactyly, and obesity. Pubertal delay is due to deficient gonadotropin-releasing hormone (GnRH), resulting in decreased FSH and LH. Kallmann syndrome (GnRH deficiency) is associated with midline defects (cleft lip/palate), congenital deafness, deficient sense of smell, and sometimes ichthyosis. Multiple lentigines syndrome includes cardiac defects, urologic abnormalities, short stature, and deafness. Other syndromes with hypogonadism include Möbius syndrome and congenital ichthyosis.

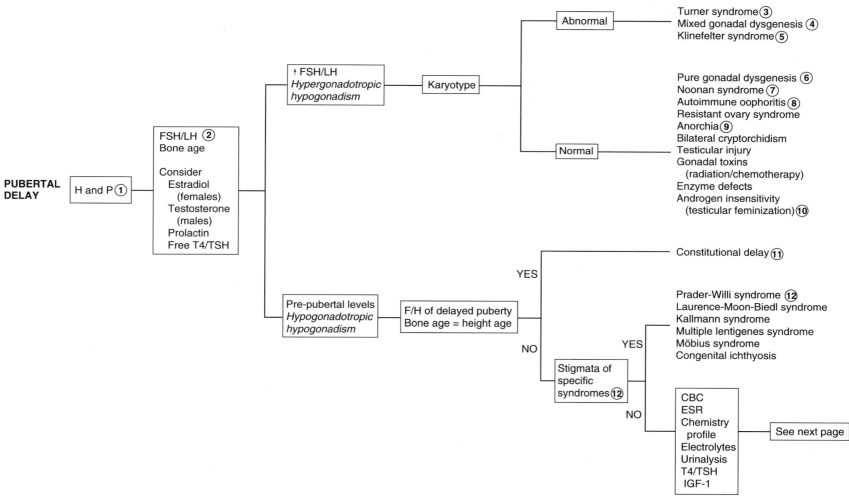

PUBERTAL DELAY → H and P ①

FSH/LH ②
Bone age

Consider
Estradiol
(females)
Testosterone
(males)
Prolactin
Free T4/TSH

↑ FSH/LH
Hypergonadotropic hypogonadism → Karyotype

Abnormal →
Turner syndrome ③
Mixed gonadal dysgenesis ④
Klinefelter syndrome ⑤

Normal →
Pure gonadal dysgenesis ⑥
Noonan syndrome ⑦
Autoimmune oophoritis ⑧
Resistant ovary syndrome
Anorchia ⑨
Bilateral cryptorchidism
Testicular injury
Gonadal toxins
(radiation/chemotherapy)
Enzyme defects
Androgen insensitivity
(testicular feminization) ⑩

Pre-pubertal levels
Hypogonadotropic hypogonadism → F/H of delayed puberty
Bone age = height age

YES → Constitutional delay ⑪

NO → Stigmata of specific syndromes ⑫

YES →
Prader-Willi syndrome ⑫
Laurence-Moon-Biedl syndrome
Kallmann syndrome
Multiple lentigenes syndrome
Möbius syndrome
Congenital ichthyosis

NO →
CBC
ESR
Chemistry
profile
Electrolytes
Urinalysis
T4/TSH
IGF-1
→ See next page

F/H= Family history
IGF-1= Insulin-like growth factor-1

Nelson chapters 567, 593, 596
Practical Strategies chapter 61

(13) Hypopituitarism with multiple tropic hormone deficiencies is usually idiopathic. However, it may be due to a tumor, trauma, congenital malformation (septo-optic dysplasia), infiltrative diseases (tuberculosis, sarcoidosis, histiocytosis X), and cranial irradiation. Neuroimaging (MRI) should be considered to exclude these conditions. Patients with isolated GH deficiency usually have pubertal delay. Isolated gonadotropin deficiency is associated with a number of genetic disorders, including a subset with anosmia/hyposmia (Kallmann syndrome).

(14) Systemic illness may affect both growth and pubertal development by GnRH suppression. Malnutrition, chronic illness such as renal failure, inflammatory bowel disease, celiac disease, recurrent infections, sickle cell disease, and malignancies may be causes.

(15) Endocrinopathies include hypothyroidism, diabetes insipidus, Cushing disease, and diabetes mellitus. In prolonged hypothyroidism FSH and LH may be paradoxically increased. Hyperprolactinemia is rare in boys; it may be primary (idiopathic, pituitary adenoma) or secondary to disruption of pituitary stalk or to hypothyroidism. Galactorrhea is present in 50%.

BIBLIOGRAPHY

Emans SJ, Goldstein DP (eds): Delayed puberty and menstrual irregularities. In: Pediatric and Adolescent Gynecology, 3rd ed. Boston, Little, Brown & Co, 1999.

Miller WL, Styne DM: Female puberty and its disorders. In Yen SSC, Jaffe RB, Barbieri R (eds): Reproductive Endocrinology: Physiology, Pathophysiology and Clinical Management, 4th ed. Philadelphia, WB Saunders Company, 1990.

Sanfilippo JS, Finkelstein JW, Styne DM (eds): Medical and Gynecologic Endocrinology. Philadelphia, Hanley & Belfus, 1994.

PUBERTAL DELAY (continued)

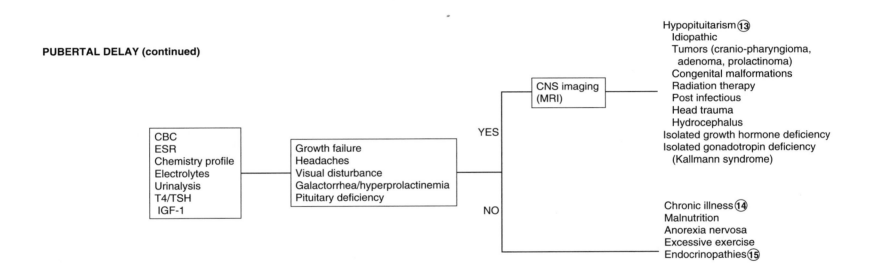

CBC
ESR
Chemistry profile
Electrolytes
Urinalysis
T4/TSH
IGF-1

Growth failure
Headaches
Visual disturbance
Galactorrhea/hyperprolactinemia
Pituitary deficiency

YES

CNS imaging
(MRI)

Hypopituitarism⑬
  Idiopathic
  Tumors (cranio-pharyngioma,
    adenoma, prolactinoma)
  Congenital malformations
  Radiation therapy
  Post infectious
  Head trauma
  Hydrocephalus
Isolated growth hormone deficiency
Isolated gonadotropin deficiency
  (Kallmann syndrome)

NO

Chronic illness⑭
Malnutrition
Anorexia nervosa
Excessive exercise
Endocrinopathies⑮

Chapter 69 *Precocious Puberty in the Male*

Precocious puberty in the male is defined as the beginning of secondary sexual characteristics before the age of 9 years. Isosexual puberty, with characteristic male sexual features, occurs due to normal male sex steroids. Heterosexual development with female characteristics (i.e., gynecomastia) occurs due to female sex steroids. Early pubarche is the isolated development of pubic or axillary hair, usually due to precocious adrenarche.

(1) History of growth patterns, chronologic development of secondary sex characteristics, exposure to exogenous sex steroids (e.g., creams, lotions, meats, anabolic steroids), possible ambiguous genitalia, and family history of early pubertal development may be helpful. Evidence of CNS disease, such as behavioral or emotional changes, head trauma, hydrocephalus, headache, and vision problems, should be assessed. Skin changes such as café-au lait spots may indicate neurofibromatosis. Genital examination includes penile length and diameter and testicular volume, which is measured by orchidometer. Pubertal testes are more than 8 ml in volume or greater than 2.5 cm in longest diameter. Tanner staging of pubic hair, and breasts in the case of gynecomastia, should be done.

(2) Central or gonadotropin-dependent precocious puberty is due to early activation of the normal physiologic pubertal development. There is increased follicle-stimulating hormone (FSH) and luteinizing hormone (LH), acceleration of growth, testicular enlargement, and pubertal levels of testosterone. The bone age is advanced beyond the height age and chronologic age.

Precocious puberty in males may be idiopathic, but approximately 40% have a CNS lesion; therefore, imaging of the head, preferably by MRI, is imperative, in addition to a careful neurologic and visual examination. Prolonged untreated hypothyroidism may cause precocious puberty, in which case the bone age is delayed. Late treatment of congenital adrenal hyperplasia may also cause precocious puberty.

(3) If the FSH and LH levels are prepubertal and testosterone levels are elevated to pubertal levels, β-human chorionic gonadotropin (β-hCG) levels should be checked. This hormone acts like LH, stimulating the testes to produce testosterone. Tumors producing β-hCG may be hepatomas, hepatoblastomas, teratomas, and chorioepitheliomas.

(4) If β-hCG levels are normal, the diagnosis is testotoxicosis, a familial condition with autonomous production of testosterone and enlarged testes.

(5) Elevated testosterone levels, particularly with asymmetric enlargement of one testis, may indicate a Leydig cell adenoma. Another source of androgens is an adrenal tumor. Elevation of dehydroepiandrosterone sulfate (DHAS) > 700 Mcg/dl or testosterone > 200 ng/dl warrants imaging for adrenal tumors. Adrenal tumors are also associated with increased dehydroepiandrosterone (DHA) and androstenedione. Testosterone may be increased owing to production by the tumor or by peripheral conversion.

(6) Congenital adrenal hyperplasia is screened for by an early morning 17-hydroxyprogesterone level. Levels < 200 ng/dl are normal; levels > 800 ng/dl are diagnostic of 21-hydroxylase deficiency, which is the most common form of CAH. Deficiency of 3β-hydroxysteroid dehydrogenase may result in precocious pubarche.

(7) Premature pubarche is most commonly due to premature adrenarche, when there is an early increase in adrenal androgens. Testosterone and gonadotropin levels are prepubertal, and DHAS may be moderately elevated but appropriate for stage 2 pubic hair. A 17-hydroxyprogesterone level may be considered to rule out late-onset congenital adrenal hyperplasia. Significantly elevated DHAS or testosterone levels may require imaging studies to exclude a testicular or adrenal tumor. Clinical follow-up of premature adrenarche at 3-month intervals is usually adequate. Bone age is usually consistent with chronologic age. If it is advanced, additional laboratory tests may be indicated.

BIBLIOGRAPHY

Ghai K, Rosenfield RL: Disorders of pubertal development. In Sanfilippo JS, Finkelstein JW, Styne DM (eds): Adolescent Medicine: State of the Art Reviews. Med Gynecol Endocrinol 5(1), 1994.

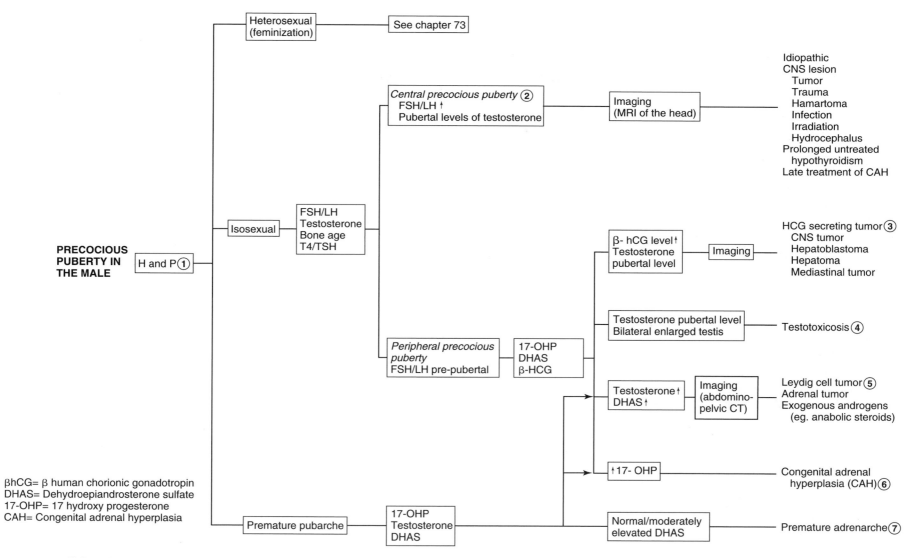

PRECOCIOUS PUBERTY IN THE MALE — H and P ①

- Heterosexual (feminization) → See chapter 73
- Isosexual → FSH/LH, Testosterone, Bone age, T4/TSH
  - Central precocious puberty ② — FSH/LH ↑, Pubertal levels of testosterone → Imaging (MRI of the head) →
    - Idiopathic
    - CNS lesion
      - Tumor
      - Trauma
      - Hamartoma
      - Infection
      - Irradiation
      - Hydrocephalus
    - Prolonged untreated hypothyroidism
    - Late treatment of CAH
  - Peripheral precocious puberty — FSH/LH pre-pubertal → 17-OHP, DHAS, β-HCG
    - β- hCG level ↑, Testosterone pubertal level → Imaging →
      - HCG secreting tumor ③
        - CNS tumor
        - Hepatoblastoma
        - Hepatoma
        - Mediastinal tumor
    - Testosterone pubertal level, Bilateral enlarged testis → Testotoxicosis ④
    - Testosterone ↑, DHAS ↑ → Imaging (abdomino-pelvic CT) →
      - Leydig cell tumor ⑤
      - Adrenal tumor
      - Exogenous androgens (eg. anabolic steroids)
    - ↑17- OHP → Congenital adrenal hyperplasia (CAH) ⑥
- Premature pubarche → 17-OHP, Testosterone, DHAS
  - Normal/moderately elevated DHAS → Premature adrenarche ⑦

βhCG= β human chorionic gonadotropin
DHAS= Dehydroepiandrosterone sulfate
17-OHP= 17 hydroxy progesterone
CAH= Congenital adrenal hyperplasia

Nelson chapters 560, 572, 586
Practical Strategies chapter 61

Chapter 70 *Precocious Puberty in the Female*

Precocious puberty has been redefined for girls as the presence of either pubic hair or breast development before age 6 for blacks and age 7 for whites. Isosexual puberty occurs because of normal female sex steroids. Heterosexual development is due to male sex steroids. Early pubarche is the isolated development of pubic or axillary hair. Premature thelarche is the isolated development of the breasts, with no other secondary sexual development.

1 History of growth patterns, chronologic development of secondary sex characteristics, exposure to exogenous sex steroids (e.g., creams, lotions, meats, anabolic steroids), possible ambiguous genitalia, and family history of early pubertal development may be helpful. Evidence of CNS disease such as behavioral or emotional changes, head trauma, hydrocephalus, headache, and vision problems should be assessed. Skin changes such as café-au-lait spots may indicate McCune-Albright syndrome or neurofibromatosis.

Vaginal mucosal changes, enlargement of labia minora, and Tanner staging of pubic hair and breasts should be assessed. Rectoabdominal examination may indicate ovarian or abdominal masses. Virilization is indicated by excessive hirsutism, clitoromegaly, deepening voice, acne, and muscle development.

2 Central or gonadotropin-dependent precocious puberty is due to early activation of the normal physiologic pubertal development. There is increased follicle-stimulating hormone (FSH) and luteinizing hormone (LH), acceleration of growth, breast development, enlargement of the labia minora, vaginal mucosal change with enlargement of the ovaries and uterus, and pubertal levels of estradiol. The bone age is advanced beyond the height age and chronologic age.

3 Precocious puberty in females is often idiopathic, but a CNS lesion should be considered. Imaging of the head, preferably using MRI, is imperative in addition to a careful neurologic and visual examination. Late treatment of congenital adrenal hyperplasia (CAH) and prolonged untreated hypothyroidism may cause precocious puberty.

4 If the FSH and LH levels are prepubertal and estradiol levels are elevated to pubertal levels, then abdominopelvic imaging should be considered to exclude estrogen-secreting ovarian or adrenal tumors. Autonomous ovarian follicular cysts are the most common estrogen-secreting masses. Plasma estradiol levels fluctuate with the size of the cyst. In McCune-Albright syndrome, there are café-au-lait spots, polyostotic fibrous dysplasia of the bones, and autonomously functioning follicular cysts. Skeletal imaging should be considered. Exogenous sources of estrogens include oral contraceptive pills and estrogen-containing tonics, lotions, and creams. Contamination of meat has been reported.

5 Benign premature thelarche is unilateral or bilateral breast enlargement, usually before age 2 years and resolving within 6 months to 6 years. No other signs of estrogenization are present. Plasma estrogen levels may be normal to slightly elevated. Laboratory studies are usually not indicated for premature thelarche. Clinical follow-up is adequate to detect progression to precocious puberty or onset of virilization. Occurrence in children older than 3 years should prompt further evaluation.

6 Premature adrenarche is the most common form of isolated precocious puberty, with an early increase in adrenal androgens. In addition to bone age, it is reasonable to obtain a 17-hydroxy-progesterone level to detect mild CAH due to 21-hydroxylase deficiency. Bone age is usually consistent with chronologic age in premature adrenarche. Estradiol and gonadotropin levels are prepubertal, and dehydroepiandrosterone sulfate (DHAS) may be moderately elevated (appropriate for stage 2 pubic hair). If bone age is advanced or signs of virilization are present, further testing is needed.

7 Virilization requires evaluation for androgen-producing adrenal or ovarian tumors, CAH, or exogenous androgen exposure in female athletes. CAH is screened for by an early morning 17-hydroxyprogesterone level. Levels < 200 ng/dl are normal; levels > 800 ng/dl are diagnostic of 21-hydroxylase deficiency, which is the most common form of CAH. Bone age is greater than the chronologic age. Deficiency of 3β-hydroxysteroid dehydrogenase may also result in precocious pubarche.

8 Elevation of DHAS > 700 Mcg/dl or testosterone > 200 ng/dl warrants imaging for adrenal or ovarian tumors. Bone age is usually greater than chronologic age.

BIBLIOGRAPHY

Ghai K, Rosenfield RL: Disorders of pubertal development. In Sanfilippo JS, Finkelstein JW, Styne DM (eds): Adolescent Medicine: State of the Art Reviews. Med Gynecol Endocrinol 5(1), 1994.

Kaplowitz PB, Oberfield SE: Reexamination of the age limit for defining when puberty is precocious in girls in the United States: Implications for evaluation and treatment. Pediatrics 104:936–941, 1999.

Miller WL, Styne DM: Female puberty and its disorders. In Yen SSC, Jaffe RB, Barbieri R (eds): Reproductive Endocrinology: Physiology, Pathophysiology and Clinical Management, 4th ed. Philadelphia: WB Saunders Company, 1999.

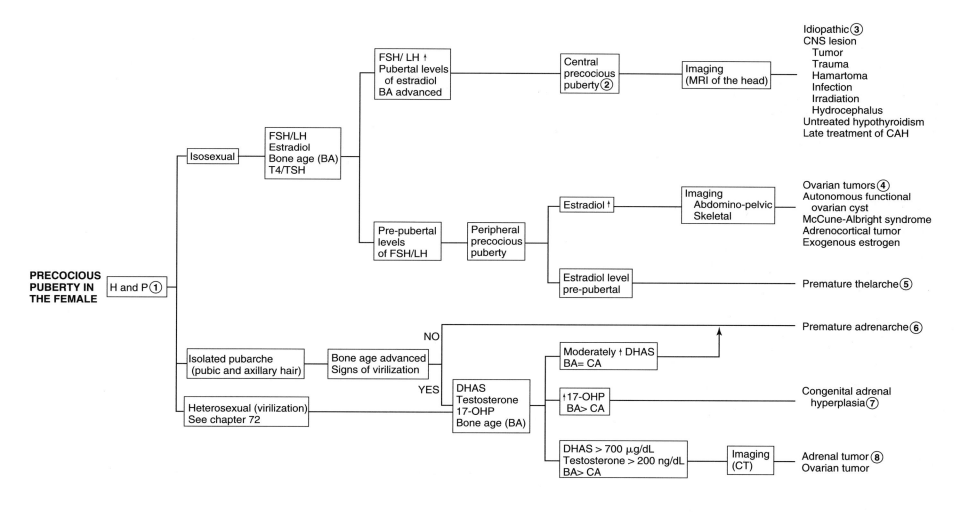

PRECOCIOUS PUBERTY IN THE FEMALE

H and P ①

Isosexual

FSH/LH
Estradiol
Bone age (BA)
T4/TSH

FSH/ LH ↑
Pubertal levels
of estradiol
BA advanced

Central
precocious
puberty ②

Imaging
(MRI of the head)

Idiopathic ③
CNS lesion
    Tumor
    Trauma
    Hamartoma
    Infection
    Irradiation
    Hydrocephalus
Untreated hypothyroidism
Late treatment of CAH

Pre-pubertal
levels
of FSH/LH

Peripheral
precocious
puberty

Estradiol ↑

Imaging
Abdomino-pelvic
Skeletal

Ovarian tumors ④
Autonomous functional
    ovarian cyst
McCune-Albright syndrome
Adrenocortical tumor
Exogenous estrogen

Estradiol level
pre-pubertal

Premature thelarche ⑤

Isolated pubarche
(pubic and axillary hair)

Bone age advanced
Signs of virilization

NO

Premature adrenarche ⑥

YES

Heterosexual (virilization)
See chapter 72

DHAS
Testosterone
17-OHP
Bone age (BA)

Moderately ↑ DHAS
BA= CA

↑17-OHP
BA> CA

Congenital adrenal
hyperplasia ⑦

DHAS > 700 μg/dL
Testosterone > 200 ng/dL
BA> CA

Imaging
(CT)

Adrenal tumor ⑧
Ovarian tumor

CAH= Congenital adrenal hyperplasia
BA= Bone age
CA= Chronological age
DHAS= Dehydroepiandrosterone sulfate
17-OHP= 17 hydroxy progesterone

Nelson chapters 560, 572, 586
Practical Strategies chapter 61

Chapter 71 Ambiguous Genitalia

Evaluation of ambiguous genitalia in an infant requires a great deal of sensitivity. A geneticist, an endocrinologist, and a urologist should all be included. Bilateral cryptorchidism, unilateral cryptorchidism with incomplete scrotal fusion, subcoronal hypospadias, labial fusion, or clitoromegaly should prompt evaluation for ambiguous genitalia.

(1) A careful history includes family history of male infants with increased scrotal pigmentation or rugae, infant deaths due to vomiting and dehydration, female relatives with amenorrhea or infertility (i.e., possible male pseudohermaphroditism), and any variant sexual development. History of maternal drug ingestion (hormones), virilization, or congenital adrenal hyperplasia (CAH) should be obtained. Vomiting, dehydration, or failure to thrive may suggest CAH.

Physical examination includes measurement of clitoris/penis; a stretched penile length < 2.5 cm at term, or a clitoris > 1 cm is abnormal at term. The urethral site, whether perineal or penile, should be determined. The presence of labioscrotal fusion and whether the gonad (almost always a testis) is palpable in the scrotum or inguinal rings should be assessed. Hyperpigmentation of areola and labioscrotal folds suggests CAH. A rectal examination is done to assess for the presence of a uterus. Often the cervix can be felt. Stigmata of other congenital syndromes should be noted.

(2) In addition to ultrasonography, other imaging may include voiding cystourethrography and retrograde genitography. Endoscopy, laparotomy, and gonadal biopsy may be required for complete examination of genitalia with true hermaphroditism.

(3) Mixed gonadal dysgenesis is the second most common cause of ambiguous genitalia. The karyotype is 45,XO/46,XY. There is mosaicism involving the Y chromosome—usually a streak gonad on one side and a dysgenetic or normal-appearing testis on the other. Müllerian and wolffian duct development corresponds to the ipsilateral gonad. There is wide phenotypic variation.

Stigmata of Turner syndrome are present in one third of patients.

(4) True hermaphroditism is rare. Gonads contain both ovarian and testicular tissue. Both tissue types may be present in one gonad (ovotestis), or there may be a testis on one side and ovary on the other. If the karyotype is XY, then further testing is needed to differentiate true hermaphroditism from male pseudohermaphroditism.

(5) Male pseudohermaphroditism occurs when a chromosomal male (46,XY) undergoes incomplete virilization. It may be due to defects in testicular differentiation. These include the Denys-Drash syndrome characterized by nephropathy with ambiguous genitalia or Wilms tumor. WAGR syndrome consists of Wilms tumor, aniridia, genitourinary malformations, and retardation. Camptomelic syndrome is a short-limbed dysplasia with anterior bowing of the femurs and tibia and organ malformations. In Swyer syndrome (XY pure gonadal dysgenesis) patients have female phenotype and normal stature but do not have pubertal development. Testicular regression syndrome (XY gonadal agenesis syndrome) is a rare condition with female appearance of the external genitalia but absent uterus and vagina. Regression of the testis is believed to occur between the 8th and 12th weeks of gestation. Thus, the testicular tissue secretes müllerian inhibiting substance long enough to inhibit müllerian duct development but not long enough for virilization. If this occurs before 8 weeks of gestation, it results in Swyer syndrome and female genitalia develop. It may also occur later, owing to testicular torsion. Testosterone levels are low, and gonadotropin levels are elevated.

(6) Enzymatic disorders in testosterone synthesis also cause incomplete virilization. Deficiency of 20,22-desmolase causes adrenal and gonadal insufficiency. With 3β-dehydrogenase deficiency there is decreased testosterone and increased dehydroepiandrosterone (DHA), resulting in some virilization. In the complete form, patients present with salt loss and increased DHA, 17-hydroxy-

pregnenolone, and pregnenolone. Deficiency of 17α-hydroxylase causes impaired cortisol and sex steroid synthesis, resulting in hypertension, hypokalemia, and alkalosis. Defects in 17,20-desmolase activity or 17β-hydroxysteroid dehydrogenase activity cause decreased testosterone synthesis and ambiguous genitalia.

(7) Other causes of male pseudohermaphroditism include defects in androgen action. In testicular feminization (i.e., androgen resistance) there is a defect in androgen receptors. Although testes are present, and testosterone levels are high, external genitalia are female, with a blind-ending vagina. Diagnosis is usually at the time of puberty, when the phenotypic female presents with amenorrhea. In 5α reductase deficiency, inadequate conversion of testosterone to dihydrotestosterone (DHT) occurs, which is necessary for fetal masculinization. Consequently, the newborn is characterized by a small phallus/ambiguous genitalia, hypospadias, bifid scrotum, and, on occasion, scrotal/labial testes. A high testosterone to DHT ratio is diagnostic.

(8) Smith-Lemli-Opitz syndrome is an autosomal recessive disorder characterized by growth retardation, microcephaly, ptosis, syndactyly, mental retardation, and genital ambiguity in males.

(9) Elevated maternal androgens may be due to maternal ingestion of medications or hormones or to a virilizing adrenal or ovarian tumor in the mother or may be idiopathic. The degree of virilization depends on the timing of the exposure to the fetus.

(10) Female pseudohermaphroditism is the most common intersex disorder and is usually due to CAH. Normal ovaries and müllerian structures are present. External genitalia changes depend on time of intrauterine exposure and can range from complete labioscrotal fusion to clitoral hypertrophy.

AMBIGUOUS GENITALIA

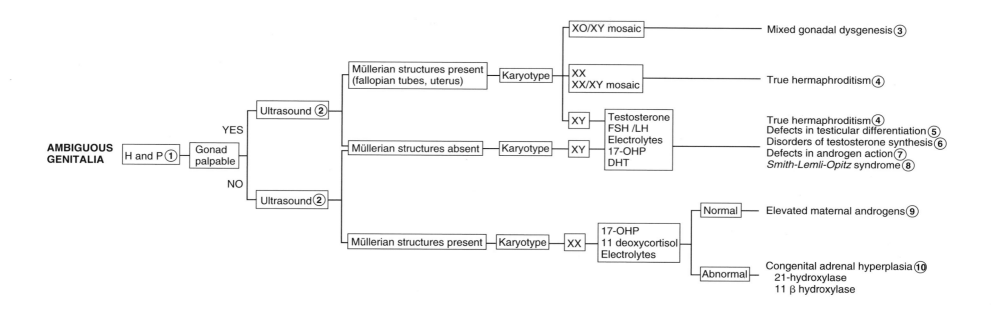

17-OHP= 17 hydroxy progesterone
DHT= Dihydrotestosterone

Nelson chapters 586, 598
Practical Strategies chapter 33

CAH is usually due to 21-hydroxylase deficiency, with increased 17-hydroxyprogesterone and adrenal androgens (e.g., dehydroepiandrosterone, androstenedione, and androstenediol). The severe form may occur as salt wasting (hyponatremia, hyperkalemia, and acidosis), vomiting, dehydration, and circulatory collapse. In 11β-hydroxylase deficiency, 11-deoxycortisol and deoxycorticosterone levels are high, producing hypertension in infancy.

BIBLIOGRAPHY

Emans SJ, Goldstein DP (eds): Ambiguous genitalia in the newborn. In: Pediatric and Adolescent Gynecology, 3rd ed. Boston: Little, Brown & Co, 1990.

Speroff L, Glass RH, Kase NG (eds): Normal and abnormal sexual development. In: Clinical Gynecologic Endocrinology and Infertility, 5th ed. Baltimore: Williams & Wilkins, 1994.

AMBIGUOUS GENITALIA

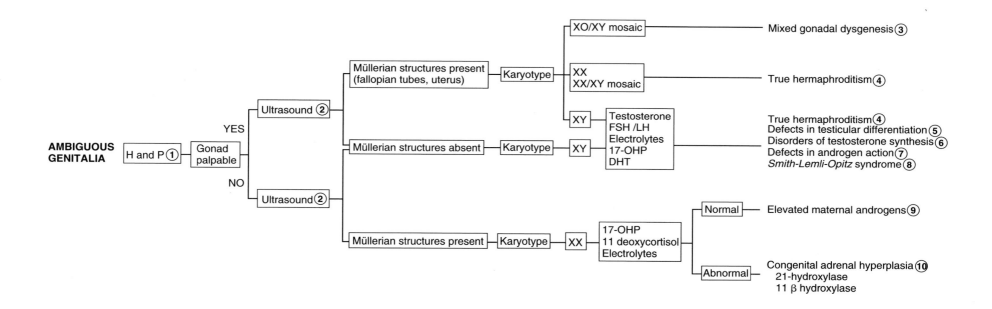

17-OHP= 17 hydroxy progesterone
DHT= Dihydrotestosterone

Nelson chapters 586, 598
Practical Strategies chapter 33

Chapter 72 **Hirsutism**

Hirsutism implies an excessive growth of body hair in women and children in an adult male pattern. It is often due to androgen excess. Hirsutism is increased density of terminal hair (coarse, adult type) and must be differentiated from hypertrichosis. Hypertrichosis is an increase in vellus hair (i.e., the downy hair seen in prepubertal years) and is often associated with drugs, malignancy, and anorexia. Sexual hair grows in response to sex steroids. It grows on the face, lower abdomen, anterior thighs, chest, breasts, pubic area, and axilla. Androgens, especially testosterone, stimulate growth of sexual hair, whereas estrogens have an opposite effect. Other hormones also affect hair growth, such as thyroxine and prolactin.

1 Increased androgen production usually causes hirsutism, acne, and increased oiliness of the skin. In extreme cases it causes virilization or masculinization with male baldness patterns, clitoromegaly, deepening voice, increased muscle mass, and male body habitus. The age and rapidity of onset may indicate the etiology of the hirsutism. Rapid onset of virilization may indicate a tumor. Early onset of hirsutism is often seen with congenital adrenal hyperplasia (CAH). Amenorrhea or galactorrhea may indicate hyperprolactinemia. A history of CNS problems such as head trauma or encephalitis should be sought. Medications may at times be responsible and should be reviewed. A family history of hirsutism, polycystic ovary syndrome, CAH, diabetes, hyperinsulinism, and infertility should be obtained. Careful examination should include the degree of virilization, and a search for thyromegaly, abdominal or pelvic masses, and skin changes (e.g., acanthosis nigri-

cans or any chronic skin irritation such as from a cast). Presence of striae and a buffalo hump may indicate Cushing syndrome.

2 Polycystic ovary syndrome is the most common cause of hirsutism in adolescents. This is a spectrum of clinical disease that is ill defined, especially in adolescents. Features include persistent anovulation, irregular menstrual cycles, hirsutism, and obesity. On ultrasound evaluation the ovaries may appear normal or have a number of small cysts (25%). There is an increased sensitivity to gonadotropin-releasing hormones, resulting in an increase in luteinizing hormone (LH) levels and in the ratio of LH to follicle-stimulating hormone (FSH). The elevated LH causes an increase in ovarian androgen production and a decrease in sex hormone–binding globulin (SHBG), resulting in an overall increase in free androgen, including testosterone and DHAS. If anovulation or galactorrhea is present, consider a prolactin level and thyroid function tests to exclude hyperprolactinemia and hypothyroidism.

3 Hyperandrogenism (HA) is often associated with insulin resistance (IR) and acanthosis nigricans (AN), otherwise known as the HAIR-AN syndrome. The mechanism of this syndrome is unknown; however, there is a defect in membrane insulin receptors. Testing for hyperinsulinism is therefore indicated in women with persistent anovulation, android obesity, and acanthosis nigricans.

4 Late-onset adrenal hyperplasia is screened for by an early morning 17-hydroxyprogesterone level. Levels < 200 ng/dl are normal; lev-

els > 800 ng/dl are diagnostic of 21-hydroxylase deficiency, which is the most common form of CAH. Levels > 200 ng/dl require adrenocorticotropic hormone testing for 3β-hydroxysteroid dehydrogenase and 11β-hydroxylase deficiency.

5 Elevation of DHAS > 700 Mcg/dl, testosterone > 200 ng/dl, or history of rapid onset of virilizing symptoms warrants imaging for adrenal or ovarian tumors.

6 Idiopathic or familial hirsutism is seen in certain geographic areas or ethnic groups. It is probably due to increased sensitivity of the skin's hair apparatus to normal levels of androgens. These women ovulate regularly.

7 Consider karyotype testing if there is a history of ambiguous genitalia to identify incomplete androgen insensitivity and mixed gonadal dysgenesis. Females with mixed gonadal dysgenesis with Y-containing mosaics or males with partial androgen insensitivity who are phenotypically female may develop signs of androgen stimulation at puberty.

8 Virilization during pregnancy may indicate a luteoma, which is an exaggerated response of ovarian stroma to chorionic gonadotropin; this regresses postpartum.

BIBLIOGRAPHY

Emans SJ, Goldstein DP (eds): Hirsutism. In: Pediatric and Adolescent Gynecology, 3rd ed. Boston: Little, Brown & Co, 1990.
Speroff L, Glass RG, Kase NG (eds): Hirsutism. In: Clinical Gynecologic Endocrinology and Infertility, 5th ed. Baltimore: Williams & Wilkins, 1994.

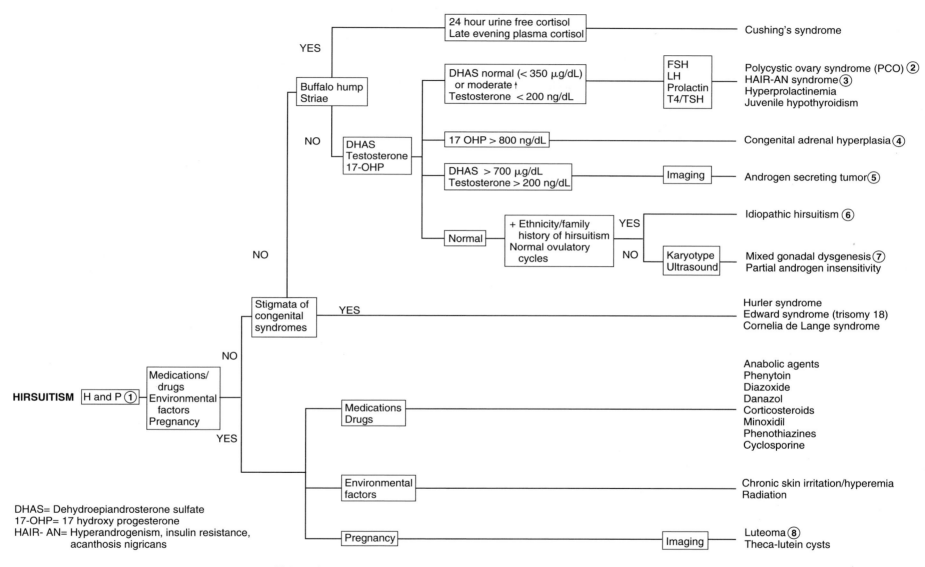

HIRSUITISM — H and P ①

Medications/drugs, Environmental factors, Pregnancy

NO → Stigmata of congenital syndromes

NO → Buffalo hump / Striae

YES → 24 hour urine free cortisol / Late evening plasma cortisol → Cushing's syndrome

NO → DHAS, Testosterone, 17-OHP

- DHAS normal (< 350 μg/dL) or moderate ↑ / Testosterone < 200 ng/dL → FSH, LH, Prolactin, T4/TSH → Polycystic ovary syndrome (PCO) ② / HAIR-AN syndrome ③ / Hyperprolactinemia / Juvenile hypothyroidism
- 17 OHP > 800 ng/dL → Congenital adrenal hyperplasia ④
- DHAS > 700 μg/dL / Testosterone > 200 ng/dL → Imaging → Androgen secreting tumor ⑤
- Normal → + Ethnicity/family history of hirsuitism / Normal ovulatory cycles
  - **YES →** Idiopathic hirsuitism ⑥
  - **NO →** Karyotype / Ultrasound → Mixed gonadal dysgenesis ⑦ / Partial androgen insensitivity

Stigmata of congenital syndromes **YES →** Hurler syndrome / Edward syndrome (trisomy 18) / Cornelia de Lange syndrome

Medications/drugs Environmental factors Pregnancy **YES →**

- Medications / Drugs → Anabolic agents / Phenytoin / Diazoxide / Danazol / Corticosteroids / Minoxidil / Phenothiazines / Cyclosporine
- Environmental factors → Chronic skin irritation/hyperemia / Radiation
- Pregnancy → Imaging → Luteoma ⑧ / Theca-lutein cysts

DHAS= Dehydroepiandrosterone sulfate
17-OHP= 17 hydroxy progesterone
HAIR- AN= Hyperandrogenism, insulin resistance, acanthosis nigricans

Nelson chapter 560

Gynecomastia is enlargement of the male breast tissue due to a decrease in the ratio of androgens to estrogens. Testosterone weakly inhibits and estrogen strongly stimulates breast tissue development. In males, estrogen is usually produced by the aromatization of androgens in peripheral tissues. Macrogynecomastia is when the breast tissue is greater than 5 cm in diameter. It is similar to middle and late stages of female breast development and is less likely to resolve spontaneously. Asymmetry of breasts is common; however, any hardness of breast tissue or asymmetric placement of the nipple requires evaluation. Lipomastia, the fatty tissue in overweight boys, may cause pseudogynecomastia.

(1) History should include a family history of permanent gynecomastia as well as history of systemic or chronic illness, including endocrinopathies, renal failure, liver disease, and malnutrition. A careful history of drug or medication intake, including hormone-containing lotion, creams, foods, and other products, should be obtained. History of excessive alcohol intake as well as illicit drug intake (i.e., marijuana) should be sought. Gynecomastia that develops before the onset of other pubertal changes or before age 10 years or is associated with precocious or delayed puberty or macrogynecomastia requires further evaluation. Physical examination should include a careful examination of the breast, including diameter and consistency of breast tissue and position of the nipple. Determination of pubertal staging and testicular size is also important. If testes are smaller than 3 cm in diameter or 8 ml in volume, a karyotype should be obtained.

(2) Pubertal or physiologic gynecomastia is common in adolescents. It occurs in 40% of boys aged 10 to 16 and usually resolves spontaneously (i.e., 90% within 3 years). The breast tissue is less than 4 cm in diameter and resembles breast budding in females. Signs of pubertal development usually precede gynecomastia by at least 6 months. Puberty is between Tanner stage II–IV.

(3) Obesity is commonly associated with gynecomastia, usually due to increased aromatization of androgens to estrogen. Lipomastia may also cause prominence of the breast tissue.

(4) Familial gynecomastia may be X-linked recessive or sex-linked autosomal dominant; it may occur with or without other signs of hypogonadism.

(5) Unilateral enlargement, especially with asymmetry and hard breast tissue, suggests local tumors. These are rare in adolescents. They may be caused by neurofibromas, dermoid cyst, lipoma, lymphangioma, metastatic neuroblastoma, leukemia, lymphoma, and rhabdomyosarcoma.

(6) Medications and drugs that can cause gynecomastia include hormones: estrogens in meat, milk, lotions, and oils; androgens, which are aromatized to estrogens; and human chorionic gonadotropin (hCG), which causes increased estradiol secretion from the testis. Cardiovascular agents include reserpine, methyldopa, digitalis, calcium channel blockers, amiodarone, and angiotensin-converting enzyme inhibitors. Cytotoxic agents such as busulfan, vincristine, nitrosoureas, procarbazine, methotrexate, cyclophosphamide, and chlorambucil may cause gynecomastia. Antituberculosis drugs (e.g., ethionamide, thiacetazone, and isoniazid) and psychoactive drugs (e.g., tricyclic antidepressants, diazepam, and phenothiazines) may cause gynecomastia. Ketoconazole, spironolactone, cimetidine, and phenytoin are testosterone antagonists. Other causes of gynecomastia include alcohol, heroin, methadone, amphetamines, and marijuana.

(7) Gynecomastia may be seen in some chronic diseases such as cystic fibrosis, ulcerative colitis, cirrhosis, and acquired immunodeficiency syndrome (AIDS). It may be related to hepatic dysfunction. Uremia due to renal failure may cause testicular damage and decreased testosterone. CNS injury (paraplegia) may be associated with decreased testicular function, leading to gynecomastia.

(8) If there is evidence of hypogonadism, precocious puberty, or macrogynecomastia, obtain luteinizing hormone (LH), follicle-stimulating hormone (FSH), estradiol, testosterone, dehydroepiandrosterone sulfate (DHAS), free T_4, TSH, and hCG levels. If galactorrhea is present, obtain a prolactin level. Karyotype may also be considered if there is a history of ambiguous genitalia at birth or if there is evidence of hypergonadotropic hypogonadism (testicular size < 8 ml, ↑ FSH, ↑ LH).

(9) If DHAS is increased, imaging for adrenal tumors is needed. Increased estradiol levels require ultrasound of the liver, adrenals, and testes for hormone producing tumors. Adrenal tumors usually cause feminization by conversion of androstenedione to estradiol. Imaging of the brain using MRI, as well as chest, abdomen, and testis, should be considered for evaluation for hCG-secreting tumors, which may also cause precocious puberty. Other hormone-producing tumors include LH-secreting pituitary tumors and prolactinomas, which cause galactorrhea but usually not gynecomastia.

(10) In hypogonadism, gynecomastia develops during adrenarche due to aromatization of adrenal androgens to estrogen. Patients with Klinefelter syndrome have decreased testosterone levels. In androgen resistance (XY), there is end organ resistance to testosterone. In both conditions, Leydig cell action is retained and there is secretion of estradiol in response to the increased LH. Klinefelter syndrome (47,XXY) usually occurs as delayed puberty, gynecomastia, and small testes. Enzyme defects of 17α-hydroxylase, 17/20-desmolase, and 17-ketosteroid reductase result in decreased synthesis of testosterone. Patients with these defects may also present with ambiguous genitalia at birth. Testicular damage due to orchitis, injury, or radiation and congenital anorchia due to fetal testicular regression may occur as gynecomastia at puberty.

11 Gynecomastia is seen in a third of patients with thyrotoxicosis. It is primarily due to increased androstenedione, which is aromatized to estradiol.

12 Gynecomastia may also be seen in the rare condition of hermaphroditism: karyotype XX; XY; XX/XY mosaic.

BIBLIOGRAPHY

Mahoney CP (ed): Adolescent Gynecomastia. Pediatr Clin North Am 37(6), 1990.

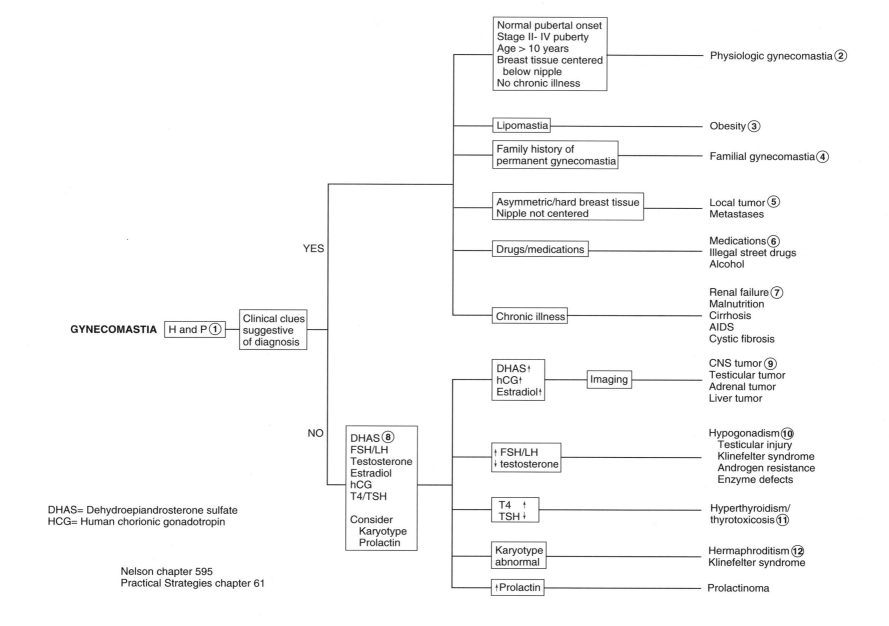

DHAS= Dehydroepiandrosterone sulfate
HCG= Human chorionic gonadotropin

Nelson chapter 595
Practical Strategies chapter 61

Obesity among children is increasing. Data from the National Center for Health Statistics (NCHS) suggest that one in five children in the United States is overweight. These children are at greater risk for obesity as adults, which is associated with an increased risk of diabetes, hypertension, and atherosclerosis.

(1) Children should be carefully evaluated for any disorder that may be associated with obesity. These disorders are rare and are usually associated with specific signs and symptoms. A drug history should be obtained because certain medications are associated with obesity. A history of headaches, visual changes, or CNS injuries or infections may indicate a hypothalamic cause. Short stature and delayed sexual development are often present. In girls, hirsutism, amenorrhea, or oligomenorrhea may suggest an underlying condition. Striae, buffalo hump, or truncal obesity, as well as acne and hypertrichosis, are present in Cushing syndrome. Dysmorphic features associated with syndromes should also be noted. Developmental delay is often a feature of these syndromes. Hyperinsulinemia should be considered in patients with hyperphagia who have an excessive increase in stature. Acanthosis nigricans is often present in obese children and has a strong association with insulin resistance. The presence of a goiter indicates thyroid disease.

(2) It is important to differentiate bigger or stockier children with larger skeletal frames from those who are obese. In younger children, the most common measurement used is weight for height measured on standard NCHS growth curves (i.e., observed weight/expected weight for height × 100). An obese child is > 120% and an overweight child > 110% weight for height. Body mass index (BMI) is a standard measurement used in assessment of obesity in adults and can be used in adolescents. BMI is the body weight in kilograms divided by the square of the height in meters (kg/m^2). A child whose BMI is > 95th percentile or > 30 in adolescents is clinically obese. A child whose BMI is between the 85th and 95th percentiles for age and sex should be carefully evaluated. Triceps skinfold thickness > 85th percentile for age may be helpful if measured by a person with experience with this method.

(3) The Diagnostic and Statistical Manual for Primary Care (DSM-PC), Child and Adolescent Version, lists criteria for eating disorders. Eating disorders are more common in females and among whites. Most patients first develop symptoms during adolescence. Bulimia nervosa and binge-eating disorders are characterized by weight gain in contrast to anorexia nervosa. In binge-eating disorders, a "distorted" body image is often present. The patient perceives herself to be less heavy than she really is. She may tend to eat alone and have feelings of guilt or disgust after binge eating. The hallmark of bulimia nervosa is binge eating followed by compensatory behavior such as purging, exercise, fasting, and laxative use.

(4) In most cases, obesity is the result of a positive energy balance, which is stored as adipose tissue. Factors associated with a positive balance include excessive intake of high-energy foods, inadequate exercise, sedentary lifestyle, low metabolic rate, and increased insulin sensitivity.

(5) Prader-Willi syndrome is associated with transient neonatal hypotonia, developmental delay, and mental retardation. There is a hypogonadotropic hypogonadism and associated short stature. Feeding problems may occur during infancy, and extreme hyperphagia may occur in childhood and adolescence. The hands and feet are small. Strabismus is often present.

(6) Turner syndrome should be suspected in short females, particularly if there is a history of pubertal delay and amenorrhea. Features of this syndrome include webbed neck, low posterior hairline, small mandible, prominent ears, epicanthal folds, high arched palate, broad chest with wide spaced nipples, cubitus valgus, and hyperconvex fingernails. Diagnosis may be made by chromosome analysis.

(7) Laurence-Moon-Biedl (Bardet-Biedl) syndrome is characterized by truncal obesity and retinal dystrophy/retinitis pigmentosa with progressive visual impairment. Other features include mental retardation, digital anomalies (polydactyly, syndactyly), hypogenitalism, and nephropathy.

(8) Alström-Hallgren syndrome is associated with nerve deafness, diabetes mellitus, retinal degeneration with blindness, cataracts, and small testes in males.

(9) Cohen syndrome is characterized by truncal obesity, hypotonia, muscle weakness, and mild mental retardation. Characteristic craniofacial features include a high nasal bridge, maxillary hypoplasia, downslanting palpebral fissures, high arched palate, short philtrum, strabismus, small jaw, open mouth, and prominent maxillary incisors. In addition, narrow hands and feet, short metacarpals and metatarsals, simian crease, hyperextensible joints, lumbar lordosis, and mild scoliosis are often present.

(10) Carpenter syndrome is characterized by brachycephaly with craniosynostosis, lateral displacement of inner canthi and apparent exophthalmos, flat nasal bridge, low-set ears, retrognathism, and high arched palate. The extremities may show brachydactyly, syndactyly, and polydactyly. Mental retardation is present.

(11) Albright hereditary osteodystrophy (i.e., pseudohypoparathyroidism type I) occurs as short stature, round face, short metacarpals and metatarsals, mental retardation, cataracts, coarse skin, brittle hair and nails, as well as hypocalcemia and hyperphosphatemia.

(12) Cushing syndrome is characterized by truncal obesity, with hypertension caused by high levels of cortisol arising from the adrenal cortex. Other features include "moon facies," plethora, hirsutism, buffalo hump, and striae. Prolonged exogenous administration of ACTH or corticosteroids can cause similar features referred to as

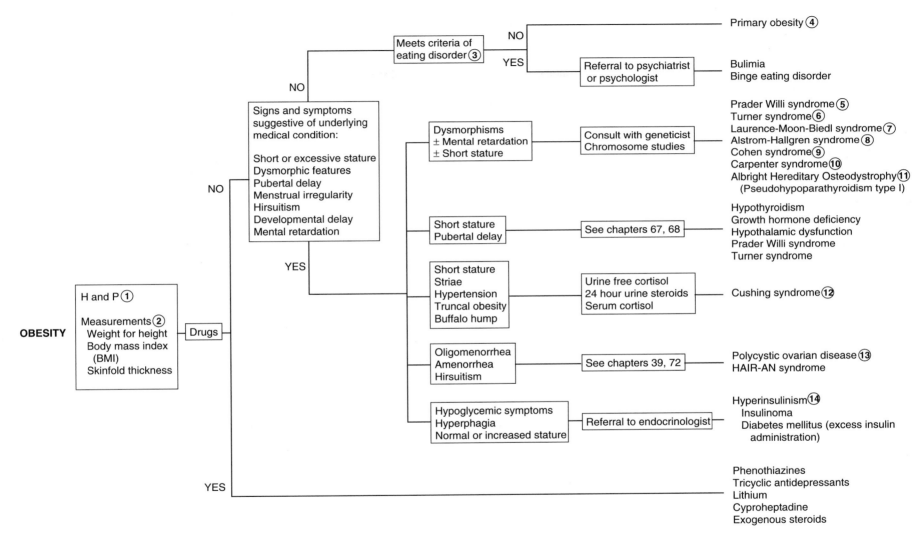

OBESITY

H and P ①

Measurements ②
  Weight for height
  Body mass index
    (BMI)
  Skinfold thickness

Drugs

NO

Signs and symptoms
suggestive of underlying
medical condition:

Short or excessive stature
Dysmorphic features
Pubertal delay
Menstrual irregularity
Hirsuitism
Developmental delay
Mental retardation

NO

Meets criteria of
eating disorder ③

NO → Primary obesity ④

YES → Referral to psychiatrist
or psychologist → Bulimia
Binge eating disorder

YES

Dysmorphisms
± Mental retardation
± Short stature → Consult with geneticist
Chromosome studies →
Prader Willi syndrome ⑤
Turner syndrome ⑥
Laurence-Moon-Biedl syndrome ⑦
Alstrom-Hallgren syndrome ⑧
Cohen syndrome ⑨
Carpenter syndrome ⑩
Albright Hereditary Osteodystrophy ⑪
  (Pseudohypoparathyroidism type I)

Short stature
Pubertal delay → See chapters 67, 68 →
Hypothyroidism
Growth hormone deficiency
Hypothalamic dysfunction
Prader Willi syndrome
Turner syndrome

Short stature
Striae
Hypertension
Truncal obesity
Buffalo hump → Urine free cortisol
24 hour urine steroids
Serum cortisol → Cushing syndrome ⑫

Oligomenorrhea
Amenorrhea
Hirsuitism → See chapters 39, 72 →
Polycystic ovarian disease ⑬
HAIR-AN syndrome

Hypoglycemic symptoms
Hyperphagia
Normal or increased stature → Referral to endocrinologist →
Hyperinsulinism ⑭
  Insulinoma
  Diabetes mellitus (excess insulin
    administration)

YES →
Phenothiazines
Tricyclic antidepressants
Lithium
Cyproheptadine
Exogenous steroids

HAIR-AN= Hyperandrogenism, insulin resistance and acanthosis nigricans   Nelson chapter 43

Obesity (continued)

cushingoid appearance. There may be signs of virilization, including hirsutism, acne, deepening of the voice, and clitoral enlargement in girls. Growth impairment occurs except when significant virilization is present, resulting in a period of normal or increased growth. Delayed puberty, amenorrhea, and oligomenorrhea in girls past menarche may occur. Laboratory findings include elevated evening cortisol levels (loss of normal diurnal rhythm with decreased evening cortisol levels) and increased urinary excretion of free cortisol and 17-hydroxycorticosteroids.

(13) The classic polycystic ovaries syndrome is characterized by obesity, hirsutism, and secondary amenorrhea, with bilaterally enlarged polycystic ovaries. Laboratory findings are variable, but there is often an increased ratio of luteinizing hormone to follicle-stimulating hormone. Dehydroepiandrosterone sulfate (DHAS) levels are normal or moderately elevated. Total testosterone level is usually normal, but serum free testosterone level may be elevated and sex hormone-binding globulin level decreased. Hyperandrogenism (HA) is often associated with insulin resistance (IR) and acanthosis nigricans (AN), otherwise known as the HAIR-AN syndrome. The mechanism of this syndrome is unknown; however, there is a defect in membrane insulin receptors. Testing for hyperinsulinism (i.e., fasting blood insulin and glucose) is therefore indicated in women with persistent anovulation, android obesity, or acanthosis nigricans.

(14) Hyperinsulinemia may be due to an insulin-secreting pancreatic tumor, hypersecretion of the pancreatic beta cells, or hypothalamic lesion. It may also be caused by excessive amounts of insulin in patients with diabetes mellitus.

BIBLIOGRAPHY

Dietz WH, Robinson TN: Assessment and treatment of childhood obesity. Pediatr Rev 14:337–344, 1993.

Klish WJ. Childhood obesity. Pediatr Rev 19:312–315, 1998.

Spitzer RL, Williams JBW, Kroenke K, et al: Utility of a new procedure for diagnosing mental disorders in primary care: The PRIME-MD 1000 study. JAMA 272:1749–1756, 1994.

Wolraich ML, Felice ME, Drotar D (eds): The classification of child and adolescent mental diagnoses in primary care. In: Diagnostic and Statistical Manual for Primary Care (DSM-PC), Child and Adolescent Version. Elk Grove Village, IL: American Academy of Pediatrics; 1996.

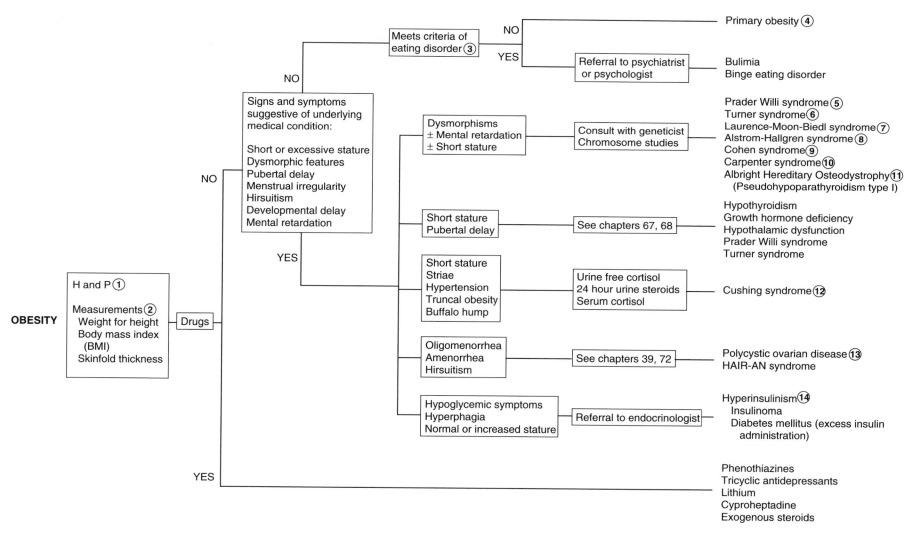

OBESITY

H and P ①

Measurements ②
Weight for height
Body mass index
(BMI)
Skinfold thickness

Drugs

NO

Signs and symptoms
suggestive of underlying
medical condition:

Short or excessive stature
Dysmorphic features
Pubertal delay
Menstrual irregularity
Hirsuitism
Developmental delay
Mental retardation

NO

Meets criteria of
eating disorder ③

NO → Primary obesity ④

YES → Referral to psychiatrist
or psychologist → Bulimia
Binge eating disorder

YES

Dysmorphisms
± Mental retardation
± Short stature → Consult with geneticist
Chromosome studies

Prader Willi syndrome ⑤
Turner syndrome ⑥
Laurence-Moon-Biedl syndrome ⑦
Alstrom-Hallgren syndrome ⑧
Cohen syndrome ⑨
Carpenter syndrome ⑩
Albright Hereditary Osteodystrophy ⑪
(Pseudohypoparathyroidism type I)

Short stature
Pubertal delay → See chapters 67, 68

Hypothyroidism
Growth hormone deficiency
Hypothalamic dysfunction
Prader Willi syndrome
Turner syndrome

Short stature
Striae
Hypertension
Truncal obesity
Buffalo hump → Urine free cortisol
24 hour urine steroids
Serum cortisol → Cushing syndrome ⑫

Oligomenorrhea
Amenorrhea
Hirsuitism → See chapters 39, 72 → Polycystic ovarian disease ⑬
HAIR-AN syndrome

Hypoglycemic symptoms
Hyperphagia
Normal or increased stature → Referral to endocrinologist

Hyperinsulinism ⑭
Insulinoma
Diabetes mellitus (excess insulin
administration)

YES → Phenothiazines
Tricyclic antidepressants
Lithium
Cyproheptadine
Exogenous steroids

HAIR-AN= Hyperandrogenism, insulin resistance and acanthosis nigricans   Nelson chapter 43

Chapter 75 Polyuria

Polyuria is an excessive urine volume, usually > 900 ml/m^2/day. It may be associated with increased thirst and drinking (polydipsia) and may be accompanied by nocturia or enuresis. Some conditions may appear as increased frequency of urination without increased volume (e.g., urinary tract infections, urge syndrome). They may be difficult to distinguish from true polyuria by history alone and are therefore included in the algorithm.

(1) History may include polyphagia, polydipsia, and weight loss, which may indicate diabetes mellitus. Children may be prone to infections with *Candida* or pyogenic skin infections. It is important to review fluid intake patterns. Children with psychogenic polydipsia often drink more during the day. Infants with polyuria due to diabetes insipidus (DI) often have failure to thrive and episodes of severe dehydration. There may be hyperthermia, vomiting, and constipation. Children with DI do not perspire and may have anorexia. DI secondary to a CNS lesion may occur as visual changes, sexual precocity, growth failure, and short stature. It is important to ask about a history of brain surgery or injury.

(2) Urinalysis revealing nitrite, leukocyte esterase, white blood cells (WBC), and often bacteria suggests infection. (See Ch. 30.) The presence of glucose with or without ketones suggests diabetes mellitus; the presence of protein or blood may indicate renal disease. (See Chs. 32 and 33.) A urine specific gravity > 1.015 makes DI unlikely. Urine and serum osmolality may be needed for complete evaluation.

(3) Diabetes mellitus is characterized by glucosuria and hyperglycemia, with a corresponding increase in serum and urine osmolality. The polyuria is due to an osmotic diuresis. Other substances that may produce osmotic diuresis are mannitol, glycerol, urea, and radiologic contrast materials. Type I or insulin-dependent diabetes mellitus is more common in children. In early stages there may be vomiting, dehydration, and polyuria. In the later stages there may be Kussmaul respirations, severe abdominal pain, and CNS changes, leading ultimately to coma. In addition to glucosuria and hyperglycemia, there is ketonuria, ketonemia, and a metabolic acidosis. Type II or non–insulin-dependent diabetes mellitus is more common in adults, but it may be seen in older children and adolescents, particularly with obesity or family history. Ketosis is infrequent. An oral glucose tolerance test may confirm the diagnosis of type II diabetes. Secondary diabetes may be seen with cystic fibrosis or ingestion of drugs or poisons (e.g., rat poison Vacor). Certain genetic syndromes may also be associated with diabetes mellitus including Prader-Willi syndrome. Autoimmune diseases (e.g., Hashimoto thyroiditis, multiple endocrine deficiency syndrome) may also be associated with type I diabetes.

(4) Renal glucosuria may be a congenital disorder or associated with Fanconi syndrome and other renal tubular disorders affecting renal absorption of glucose. A transient glucosuria may also occur with stressful events, with or without mild hyperglycemia. This finding may indicate a decreased capacity for insulin secretion, and patients may need closer follow-up and glucose tolerance testing for diabetes mellitus.

(5) The water deprivation test is useful in differentiating DI from psychogenic DI. Diabetes insipidus is characterized by low urine specific gravity (usually < 1.005), low urine osmolality, and normal serum osmolality when hydration is adequate. With water restriction or deprivation the serum sodium increases, as well as serum osmolality, whereas the patient remains unable to concentrate urine. The ratio of urine to plasma osmolality is < 1.0. This test should be conducted in a controlled setting and discontinued if the body weight decreases by more than 3%. In psychogenic DI, the serum sodium level is low normal but patients are able to concentrate urine. With water deprivation there is increased urine specific gravity and osmolality. The ratio of urine to serum osmolality is at least 2:1. There is no weight loss and the volume of urine decreases.

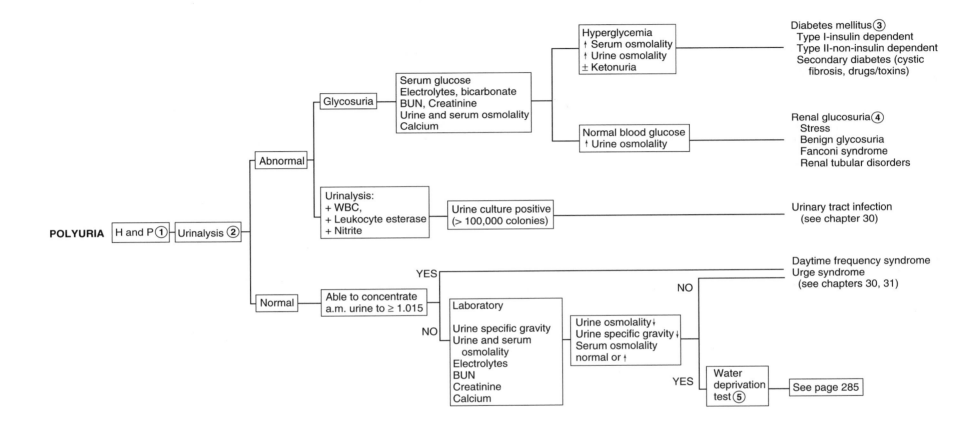

POLYURIA — H and P ① — Urinalysis ②

Abnormal

Glycosuria

Serum glucose
Electrolytes, bicarbonate
BUN, Creatinine
Urine and serum osmolality
Calcium

Hyperglycemia
↑ Serum osmolality
↑ Urine osmolality
± Ketonuria

Diabetes mellitus ③
Type I-insulin dependent
Type II-non-insulin dependent
Secondary diabetes (cystic
fibrosis, drugs/toxins)

Normal blood glucose
↑ Urine osmolality

Renal glucosuria ④
Stress
Benign glycosuria
Fanconi syndrome
Renal tubular disorders

Urinalysis:
+ WBC,
+ Leukocyte esterase
+ Nitrite

Urine culture positive
(> 100,000 colonies)

Urinary tract infection
(see chapter 30)

Normal

Able to concentrate
a.m. urine to ≥ 1.015

YES

Daytime frequency syndrome
Urge syndrome
(see chapters 30, 31)

NO

Laboratory

Urine specific gravity
Urine and serum
  osmolality
Electrolytes
BUN
Creatinine
Calcium

Urine osmolality↓
Urine specific gravity↓
Serum osmolality
normal or ↑

NO

YES

Water
deprivation
test ⑤

See page 285

Nelson chapters 568, 599

Polyuria *(continued)*

(6) In nephrogenic DI, the kidney does not respond to antidiuretic hormone. It may be a primary condition (X-linked recessive), which usually appears in male infants as polyuria, polydipsia, and hypernatremic dehydration. Secondary DI may be seen in conditions causing a loss of medullary concentrating gradient, such as renal failure, tubular defects, and obstructive uropathy. Diseases such as sickle cell disease may cause renal damage and often may be associated with isosthenuria (urine specific gravity = 1.010). Drugs (e.g., lithium) or metabolic diseases (e.g., hypokalemia, hypercalcemia) may decrease the effect of antidiuretic hormone on the tubule causing DI.

(7) Any lesion affecting the neurohypophyseal unit may cause central DI. These include suprasellar and chiasmatic tumors (e.g., craniopharyngiomas, optic gliomas, germinomas). Infections (encephalitis) as well as infiltrative processes (leukemia, sarcoidosis, tuberculosis, histiocytosis, actinomycosis) may also be causes. Wolfram syndrome is associated with insulin-dependent diabetes mellitus, diabetes insipidus, optic atrophy, deafness, and neurogenic bladder. Imaging (CT/MRI) may be considered to exclude brain tumors, injuries, or infiltrative processes. In patients with accompanying growth failure or short stature, pituitary tests and thyroid function tests may be considered. A radioimmunoassay for vasopressin is available. Low levels indicate central DI.

BIBLIOGRAPHY

Libber SM, Plotnick LP: Polyuria. In Hoekelman RA, Friedman SB, Nelson NM, Seidel HM (eds): Primary Pediatric Care, 2nd ed. St. Louis: CV Mosby, 1992.

POLYURIA (continued)

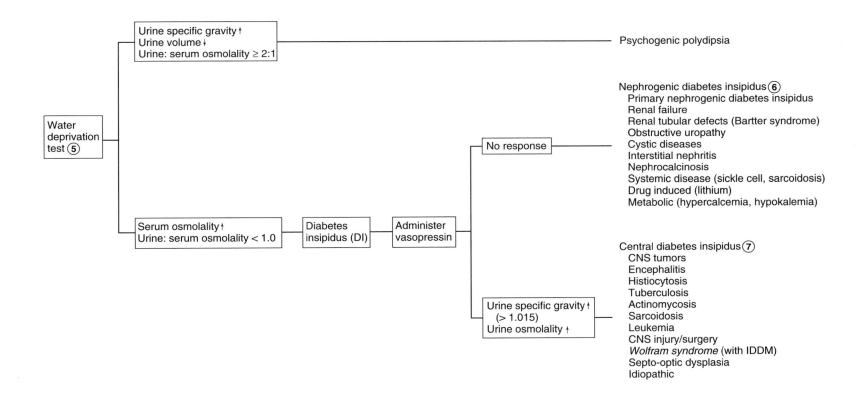

Water deprivation test ⑤

Urine specific gravity ↑
Urine volume ↓
Urine: serum osmolality ≥ 2:1
→ Psychogenic polydipsia

Serum osmolality ↑
Urine: serum osmolality < 1.0
→ Diabetes insipidus (DI) → Administer vasopressin

No response →
Nephrogenic diabetes insipidus ⑥
  Primary nephrogenic diabetes insipidus
  Renal failure
  Renal tubular defects (Bartter syndrome)
  Obstructive uropathy
  Cystic diseases
  Interstitial nephritis
  Nephrocalcinosis
  Systemic disease (sickle cell, sarcoidosis)
  Drug induced (lithium)
  Metabolic (hypercalcemia, hypokalemia)

Urine specific gravity ↑
(> 1.015)
Urine osmolality ↑
→
Central diabetes insipidus ⑦
  CNS tumors
  Encephalitis
  Histiocytosis
  Tuberculosis
  Actinomycosis
  Sarcoidosis
  Leukemia
  CNS injury/surgery
  Wolfram syndrome (with IDDM)
  Septo-optic dysplasia
  Idiopathic

IDDM= Insulin dependent diabetes mellitus

GENERAL

Chapter 76 *Fever Without a Source*

The most commonly used definition of fever is a rectal temperature ≥38°C (100.4°F). Fever without a source (FWS) is the acute onset of fever in a previously well child in whom no likely cause for the fever is evident after a thorough history and physical examination.

Guidelines for the management of the infant between birth and 36 months of age have been published with the purpose of identifying bacteremic infants and improving their outcomes. The validity and usefulness of these guidelines are debated. There is a greater consensus regarding infants younger than 3 months old, particularly younger than 28 days old. More debate occurs regarding the guidelines for the 3- to 36-month age group. Since *Streptococcus pneumoniae* is overwhelmingly the most common cause of bacteremia in the febrile young infant and in the one over 2 to 3 months, the widespread use of the new conjugated pneumococcal vaccine should significantly reduce the incidence of bacteremia. This may result in current guidelines, including our own, being less applicable.

Serious bacterial infections in the infant and child include meningitis, bacteremia (sepsis), osteomyelitis, septic arthritis, urinary tract infections, pneumonias, and bacterial enteritis.

If a child appears ill or toxic, regardless of culture results, he or she should be hospitalized for further evaluation and treatment.

(1) A rectal temperature is the best method of assessment of body core temperature. It is the recommended method when evaluating infants younger than 3 months of age. Tympanic thermometry may be acceptable for older children even with otitis media. Temperature-sensitive pacifiers and forehead strips are not considered reliable in young children. The role of bundling in the elevation of body temperature is controversial. One guideline suggests retaking the temperature of an infant 15 to 30 minutes after unbundling. If the fever diminishes and the infant appears healthy and has not received an antipyretic, the infant can be considered afebrile.

A medical history of sickle cell disease or immunodeficiency is very significant and will alter the approach to a febrile child. The algorithm is not recommended for these high-risk children.

The response to antipyretics does not help discern between a serious bacterial infection and a viral illness.

Infants with fever documented at home by a reliable caretaker should be treated the same as if the fever were documented by a health care worker.

There are no clear guidelines for infants with reports of tactile but unmeasured fever at home. Careful clinical judgment should be exercised. In the evaluation of a child with fever, the reliability of the caretakers to comply with recommended follow-up should be considered.

By definition, the physical examination of a child with FWS is nonlocalizing. The exception is otitis media in febrile children older than 3 months with a fever > 39°C (102.2°F). These children are considered at risk for bacteremia and should be approached as having FWS.

(2) Criteria identifying infants as "low risk" for serious bacterial infections may aid in the management of infants younger than 3 months of age. Clinical evaluation has been deemed unreliable to identify serious bacterial infections in these infants. The mean probability in infants younger than 12 weeks of age and nontoxic who meet the low-risk criteria is 0.2%.

(3) For children between 3 and 36 months of age, a WBC ≥15,000/μl is 75% sensitive but not very specific for bacteremia; 13% of children with a WBC above 15,000/μl are bacteremic, most commonly with *S. pneumoniae*, compared with 2.6% of those with a WBC below 15,000/μl.

Although the risk of bacteremia increases with higher absolute band counts, the relationship is not predictable. Polymorphonuclear neutrophil counts, toxic cell granulation, and neutrophil vacuolization have also been analyzed and do not offer any advantages over the total WBC in predicting bacteremia.

Urinalysis is helpful in identifying urinary tract infections. For children older than 1 year of age with symptoms of a urinary tract infection, the urine dipstick (specifically the leukocyte esterase and nitrite tests) and microscopic analysis for bacteria are nearly 100% sensitive. These results are not as reliable at younger ages. (see Ch. 30)

Stool analysis is important if diarrhea is present. Blood, mucus, or more than 5 WBCs per high-powered field (hpf) suggest bacterial enteritis. In these cases, a stool culture should be obtained and empirical antibiotic treatment should be initiated.

(4) Urine cultures should be obtained by suprapubic aspiration or catheterization from infants and from children when a clean-catch specimen cannot be obtained, if they are going to be treated with antibiotics. Stool cultures should be obtained if either bloody diarrhea or more than 5 WBCs/hpf on a stool specimen is present.

(5) The recommended empirical antibiotic therapy in young infants is ceftriaxone (50 mg/kg IM).

(6) In addition to meeting low-risk criteria, reliable parents and follow-up must be factors for a child to qualify to be treated as an outpatient with intramuscular injection of ceftriaxone.

(7) Current guidelines recommend inpatient evaluation for all infants younger than 28 days of age. In most institutions, these infants are treated empirically, although observation without antibiotics is an alternative management strategy.

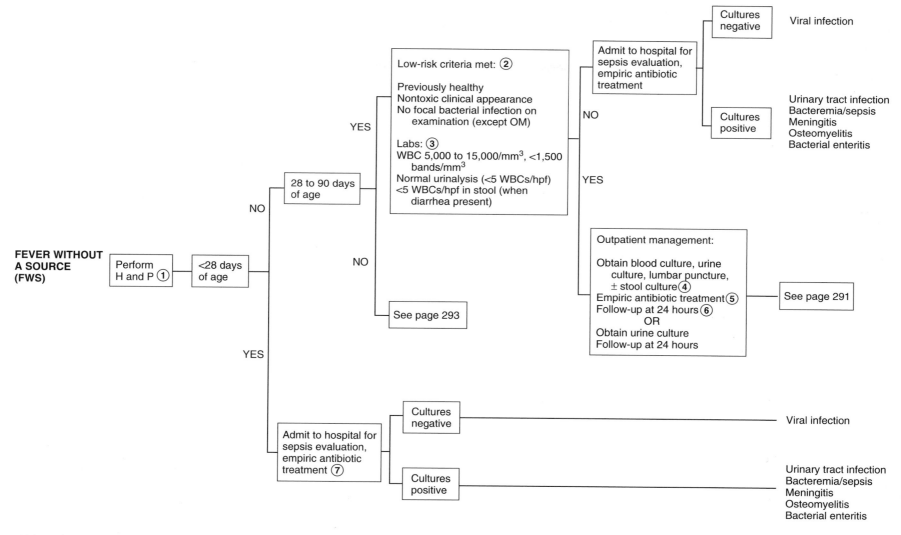

FEVER WITHOUT A SOURCE (FWS)

Perform H and P ①

<28 days of age

- NO → **28 to 90 days of age**
  - YES → **Low-risk criteria met: ②**

    Previously healthy
    Nontoxic clinical appearance
    No focal bacterial infection on examination (except OM)

    Labs: ③
    WBC 5,000 to 15,000/mm³, <1,500 bands/mm³
    Normal urinalysis (<5 WBCs/hpf)
    <5 WBCs/hpf in stool (when diarrhea present)

    - NO → **Admit to hospital for sepsis evaluation, empiric antibiotic treatment**
      - Cultures negative → Viral infection
      - Cultures positive → Urinary tract infection / Bacteremia/sepsis / Meningitis / Osteomyelitis / Bacterial enteritis
    - YES → **Outpatient management:**

      Obtain blood culture, urine culture, lumbar puncture, ± stool culture ④
      Empiric antibiotic treatment ⑤
      Follow-up at 24 hours ⑥
      OR
      Obtain urine culture
      Follow-up at 24 hours
      → See page 291
  - NO → See page 293

- YES → **Admit to hospital for sepsis evaluation, empiric antibiotic treatment ⑦**
  - Cultures negative → Viral infection
  - Cultures positive → Urinary tract infection / Bacteremia/sepsis / Meningitis / Osteomyelitis / Bacterial enteritis

Nelson chapter 172
Practical Strategies chapter 59

8 A second dose of ceftriaxone is recommended until 48-hour culture results are available.

9 Most recommend hospitalization of children with bacteremia due to pathogens other than pneumococcus.

10 Children with a suspected or proven urinary tract infection who appear severely ill or are vomiting should be hospitalized for intravenous antibiotic therapy. For children who are not severely ill, more conservative approaches may be acceptable.

FEVER WITHOUT SOURCE
(continued)

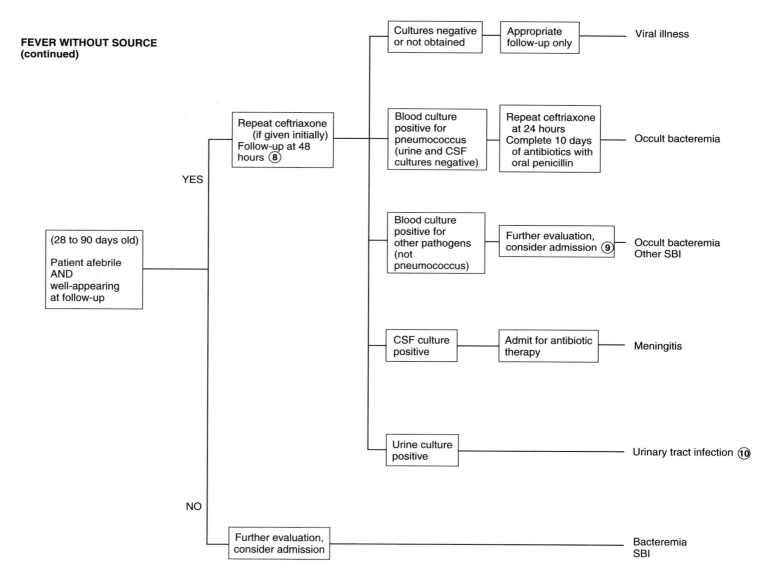

SBI= Serious bacterial infection

(11) It is reasonable in the well-appearing febrile 3- to 36-month-old child with mild symptoms and whose fever occurs early in the course of illness to observe closely, assuming the parents are reliable. Careful instructions should be given to parents to return if the fever persists more than 2 to 3 days.

Many children with FWS are in the prodromal phase of an infectious illness and develop more specific signs or symptoms within several hours to days of first being evaluated. In some diseases, such as Rocky Mountain spotted fever, leptospirosis, and measles, the fever may precede more specific signs by up to 3 days. In illnesses such as roseola, viral hepatitis, infectious mononucleosis, typhus, typhoid fever, and Kawasaki disease, a longer interval may occur between fever onset and more specific findings.

(12) Febrile drug reactions can occur secondary to atropine, salicylate, cocaine, amphetamine, neuroleptic agents, and LSD in addition to antibiotics.

(13) Vaccine reactions may be a source of fever. Diphtheria-tetanus-pertussis (DTP) may cause a fever acutely, although the febrile response to the currently used acellular version (DTaP) is less severe than it was to the previously widely used whole-cell DTP.

The measles-mumps-rubella (MMR) vaccine may cause a fever 7 to 10 days after administration, often accompanied by a rash.

(14) Chest X-rays are only recommended in children with respiratory signs or symptoms. Stool cultures should be performed only if the child has diarrhea.

(15) Based on data that questions the benefits of empirical antibiotic therapy in reducing the risk of a serious bacterial infection in a small number of children versus the cost and consequences of unnecessary therapy in the large number of children, an evaluation limited to a urinalysis and close follow-up is a reasonable approach to the well-appearing young febrile child. Certainly, parental reliability regarding observation of their child and compliance with recommended follow-up should factor into treatment decisions. Practice guidelines frequently used today do not reflect the change in epidemiology of occult bacteremia that has occurred since the widespread use of vaccines against *Haemophilus influenzae* type b. As previously mentioned, the use of the conjugate pneumococcal vaccine will likely result in a significant change in the approach to the febrile child between 3 and 36 months of age.

Increasing antibiotic resistance mandates that empirical therapy be used very selectively. In the absence of an elevated WBC, empirical therapy may be reasonable when the fever is very high (>40°C [104°F]). Current guidelines primarily recommend empirical treatment with intramuscular injection of ceftriaxone. Studies with oral antibiotics have shown that oral amoxicillin is effective in eradicating most cases of pneumococcal bacteremia. With the decreased incidence of *H. influenzae* type b disease, this is probably an acceptable regimen. The omission of a lumbar puncture before treating is considered safe in older children with FWS who are nontoxic, especially if they had been immunized against *H. influenzae* type b.

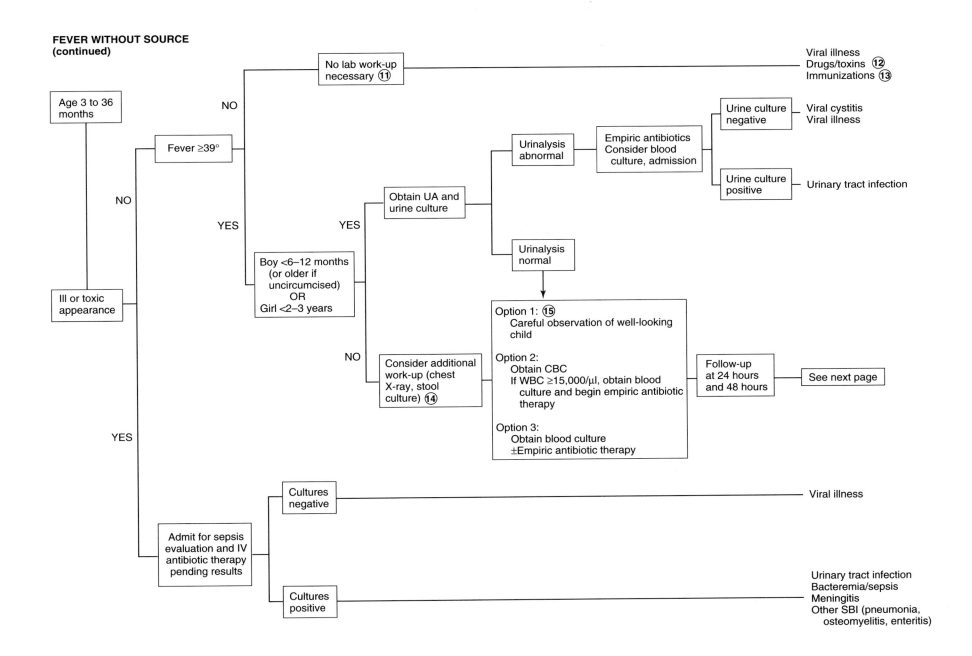

Age 3 to 36 months

NO

Fever ≥39°

NO

No lab work-up necessary ⑪

Viral illness
Drugs/toxins ⑫
Immunizations ⑬

YES

YES

Obtain UA and urine culture

Urinalysis abnormal

Empiric antibiotics
Consider blood culture, admission

Urine culture negative — Viral cystitis / Viral illness

Urine culture positive — Urinary tract infection

Boy <6–12 months (or older if uncircumcised) OR Girl <2–3 years

NO

Consider additional work-up (chest X-ray, stool culture) ⑭

Urinalysis normal

Option 1: ⑮
Careful observation of well-looking child

Option 2:
Obtain CBC
If WBC ≥15,000/µl, obtain blood culture and begin empiric antibiotic therapy

Option 3:
Obtain blood culture
±Empiric antibiotic therapy

Follow-up at 24 hours and 48 hours

See next page

Ill or toxic appearance

YES

Admit for sepsis evaluation and IV antibiotic therapy pending results

Cultures negative — Viral illness

Cultures positive — Urinary tract infection / Bacteremia/sepsis / Meningitis / Other SBI (pneumonia, osteomyelitis, enteritis)

(16) Occult bacteremia occurs in approximately 1.6% of nontoxic febrile children between 3 and 36 months of age (based on a prospective cohort study performed in the post–*H. influenzae* type b era). The most common cause is pneumococcus. Patients with pneumococcal bacteremia can continue to be treated as outpatients as long as they appear well. When bacteremia is caused by other pathogens, the patient should be admitted for a complete sepsis evaluation and treatment while results of sensitivity testing are pending.

(17) Like many aspects of occult bacteremia, the optimum management of the child who is well appearing but not afebrile at follow-up is unresolved. Certainly, children with more virulent pathogens (*H. influenzae* type b, *Neisseria meningitidis*) are more likely to be treated aggressively; less agreement exists regarding the child with pneumococcal bacteremia who is febrile but appears well at follow-up. One reasonable approach is to obtain a repeat blood culture in all patients and a lumbar puncture in those younger than 12 months of age. Strongly consider one in all others. Subsequent appropriate treatment options may be outpatient therapy with ceftriaxone or admission for intravenous therapy with antibiotics.

BIBLIOGRAPHY

Alpern ER, Henretig FM: Fever. In Fleisher G, Ludwig S: Textbook of Pediatric Emergency Medicine, 4th ed, p 257. Baltimore: Williams & Wilkins, 2000.

Bachur R, Harper MB: Reevaluation of outpatients with *Streptococcus pneumoniae* bacteremia. Pediatrics 105:502, 2000.

Baraff LJ, Bass JW, et al: Practice guidelines for the management of infants and children 0 to 36 months of age with fever without source. Pediatrics 92(1):1, 1993.

Hoberman A, Wald ER, et al: Oral versus initial intravenous therapy for urinary tract infections in young febrile children. Pediatrics 104:79, 1994.

Kramer MS, Shapiro ED: Management of the young febrile child: A commentary on recent practice guidelines. Pediatrics 100:123, 1997.

Lee GM, Harper MB: Risk of bacteremia for febrile young children in the post-*Haemophilus* influenzae type b era. Arch Pediatr Adolesc Med 152:624, 1998.

Lorin MI, Feigin RD: Fever without localizing signs and fever of unknown origin. In Feigin RD, Cherry JD (eds): Textbook of Pediatric Infectious Diseases, 4th ed, p 820. Philadelphia, WB Saunders Company, 1998.

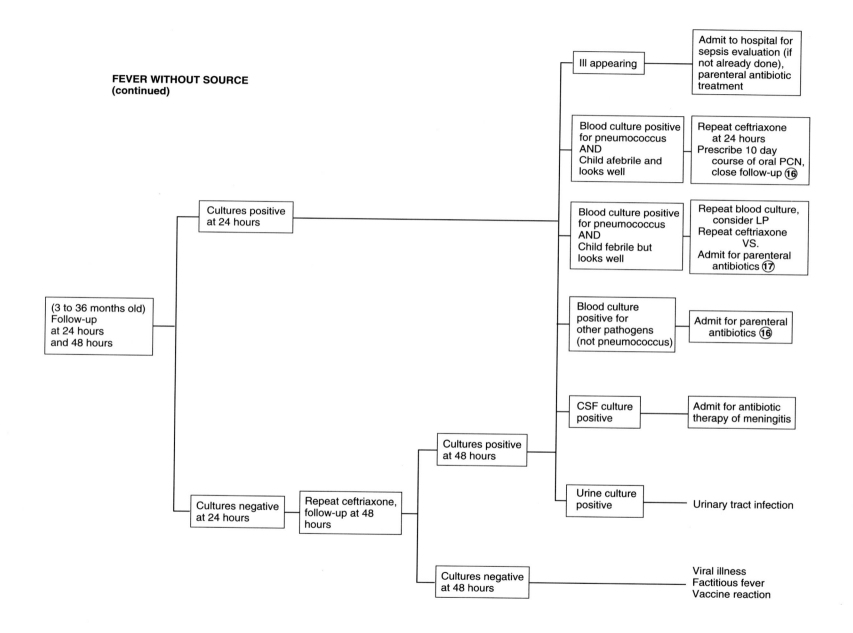

FEVER WITHOUT SOURCE
(continued)

One definition of fever of unknown origin (FUO) is an immunologically normal host with an oral or rectal temperature greater than 38°C (100.4°F) at least twice weekly for longer than 3 weeks, a noncontributory history and physical examination, a normal chest X-ray, and a normal urinalysis. A fever lasting longer than a week without an obvious source despite a complete history and physical examination, normal chest X-ray, and normal urinalysis also mandates careful evaluation. The longer the fever persists, the greater likelihood of a significant illness, and the more extensive the workup should be.

The evaluation of FUO is influenced by a number of factors that cannot be fully included in a single algorithm without making it unacceptably complex. Each evaluation should be affected by factors specific to each case; for example, the age of a patient and the patient's ability to report specific complaints, underlying medical conditions, and exposures all serve to guide the evaluation of FUO in a given child. The history is a critical factor in determining the cause of an FUO.

The most common causes of FUO in children are infections, autoimmune disease, and neoplasia. Approximately 25% of cases remain undiagnosed. Many are atypical manifestations of common childhood infectious diseases. Some disorders (e.g., juvenile rheumatoid arthritis) require an extended period of observation and repeated evaluation to diagnose. If the diagnosis does not become evident early in the evaluation of FUO, consultation with an infectious disease specialist is recommended.

1 A thorough history and physical examination will often focus the evaluation of FUO. The pattern of fever may be suggestive of a disorder, although it is usually not consistent enough to aid in diagnosis. Obtain a history for cardiac problems, gastrointestinal disease, and abdominal surgeries, which may put a patient at risk for abdominal abscesses. The past medical history should also review potential risk factors for human immunodeficiency virus (HIV) infection including transfu-

sions. A history of severe head trauma may be a clue for central fevers. Children younger than 6 years of age are more likely to have certain infections (e.g., respiratory, urinary tract, localized). In older children connective tissue disorders, tuberculosis, inflammatory bowel disease, and lymphoma are more likely.

The diet history should inquire about the possibility of infection related to the ingestion of contaminated water, unpasteurized whole milk, raw meat, game meat, or shellfish.

The social history should include a history of animal (domestic, farm, wild) exposure, insect or tick bites, and travel because many infectious diseases are endemic to certain areas (Lyme disease, Rocky Mountain spotted fever). Ask about sick contacts and contacts with people who have traveled; artifacts, rocks, or soil that have been brought from distant areas could serve as vectors.

On the physical examination, stool should always be checked for occult blood. Sexually active females should always have a pelvic examination. Rashes are especially important. Repeated skin examination can be helpful in revealing a diagnostic clue. Muscle tenderness may be a sign of connective tissue disorders or certain infections (e.g., trichinosis, enterovirus).

2 Nearly any medication can be associated with an allergic reaction, including fever. Some drugs (e.g., phenothiazines, anticholinergic drugs) impair sweating. Discontinuation of the drug followed by disappearance of the fever is suggestive of drug fever, although sometimes fever persists days to weeks as a result of slow excretion of the drug.

3 The extent of urgency of the evaluation depends on the degree of illness in the child. Hospitalization is not usually necessary to evaluate FUO. It does offer the advantage, however, of close observation and following up on every lead.

Blood cultures should be obtained aerobically unless anaerobic infection is suspected. Repeated cultures may be necessary to diagnose certain con-

ditions such as endocarditis, osteomyelitis, or deep-seated abscesses causing bacteremia. Specific media need to be requested if *Francisella tularemia* infection, leptospirosis, or *Yersinia* infection is suggested.

Chest X-rays are recommended because they will be abnormal in 10% to 15% of patients with FUO.

The purified protein derivative (PPD) test for tuberculosis with a *Candida* control (or other antigens) is usually recommended. Anergy specific for the PPD (and not the *Candida*) may occur in certain cases of tuberculosis. Further investigation (chest X-ray ± liver biopsy, skin biopsy, or bone marrow biopsy) may be indicated if clinical suspicion is high.

Both the CBC and erythrocyte sedimentation rate (ESR) are often abnormal but nonspecific. Serology tests are recommended when the ESR is extremely elevated (>100). The pathway for "normal results" should be followed in this setting; an extremely elevated ESR is more likely to occur in the setting of inflammatory disorders, localized infections, and malignancy than in other systemic infections.

4 Malaria may be transmitted by a mosquito vector from an infected person who has traveled in an endemic area to someone who has not traveled. In persons who took appropriate antimalarial drugs while traveling, the disease may not manifest until several months later.

5 The finding of hilar adenopathy on a chest X-ray should raise suspicion for sarcoidosis, tuberculosis, or malignancy.

6 Typhoid fever (from infection with *Salmonella typhi*) is transmitted via animals and food products. Symptoms are frequently nonspecific, and repeated blood and stool cultures or serology should lead to a diagnosis. Leptospirosis is transmitted by contact with animals or contaminated soil or water, and it is no longer primarily restricted to rural areas. Brucellosis is another common infectious cause of FUO in children;

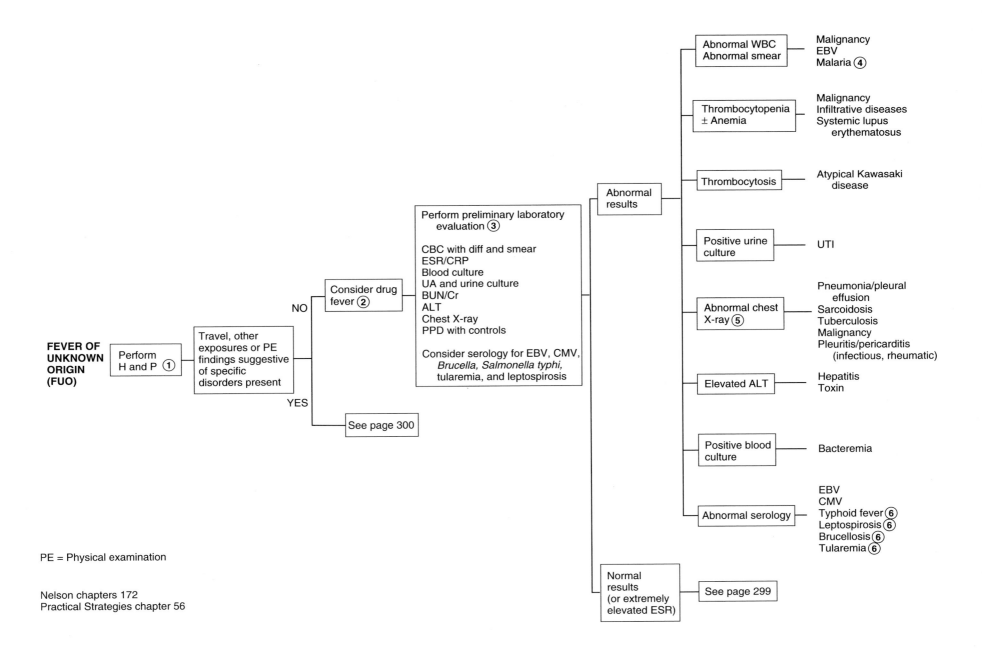

FEVER OF UNKNOWN ORIGIN (FUO) → Perform H and P ① → Travel, other exposures or PE findings suggestive of specific disorders present

NO → Consider drug fever ②

YES → See page 300

Perform preliminary laboratory evaluation ③

CBC with diff and smear
ESR/CRP
Blood culture
UA and urine culture
BUN/Cr
ALT
Chest X-ray
PPD with controls

Consider serology for EBV, CMV, *Brucella, Salmonella typhi,* tularemia, and leptospirosis

Abnormal results

Abnormal WBC Abnormal smear → Malignancy / EBV / Malaria ④

Thrombocytopenia ± Anemia → Malignancy / Infiltrative diseases / Systemic lupus erythematosus

Thrombocytosis → Atypical Kawasaki disease

Positive urine culture → UTI

Abnormal chest X-ray ⑤ → Pneumonia/pleural effusion / Sarcoidosis / Tuberculosis / Malignancy / Pleuritis/pericarditis (infectious, rheumatic)

Elevated ALT → Hepatitis / Toxin

Positive blood culture → Bacteremia

Abnormal serology → EBV / CMV / Typhoid fever ⑥ / Leptospirosis ⑥ / Brucellosis ⑥ / Tularemia ⑥

Normal results (or extremely elevated ESR) → See page 299

PE = Physical examination

Nelson chapters 172
Practical Strategies chapter 56

symptoms are nonspecific, and a history of exposure to animals or animal products should prompt specific investigations for it. Ingestion of squirrel or rabbit meat may be a risk factor for tularemia.

(7) Juvenile rheumatoid arthritis (JRA) is usually only diagnosed after an extended period of observation and evolution of more characteristic symptoms. The systemic form is most likely to present as an FUO; arthritis may not develop for months, and serology may remain negative for an extended period. A slit lamp examination performed by an ophthalmologist may reveal uveitis.

(8) Technetium-labeled WBC scans are very useful in identifying inflammatory bowel disease, most abscesses, and most osteomyelitis. These scans are not as sensitive for osteomyelitis of the spine. A bone scan may aid in detecting bone infections or malignancy not diagnosed by the technetium scan or CT.

(9) Fever is more common in children than adults with inflammatory bowel disease. Evaluation should be done in cases of prolonged FUO, even without specific gastrointestinal symptoms (especially if weight loss or impaired growth has occurred or if there is anemia, an elevated ESR, or occult blood in the stool).

(10) A factitious fever may be produced by intentional (i.e., Munchausen syndrome by proxy) or unintentional inappropriate heating of the thermometer or skin or mucosal surface before taking the temperature. Factitious fevers should be suspected when no recognizable circadian rhythm of the fevers can be identified. Be suspicious if vasoconstriction, sweating, tachypnea, and tachycardia are not associated with the fever.

(11) The outcome of children with undiagnosed FUO is variable. In those without a diagnosis after a preliminary laboratory evaluation, some will eventually be diagnosed after observation and evolution of other symptoms (e.g., familial Mediterranean fever). In others (~25%), fevers will continue to recur without a diagnosis. In many the fever will eventually resolve. In general, the outcome for children with FUO is better than for adults with FUO.

FEVER OF UNKNOWN ORIGIN
(continued)

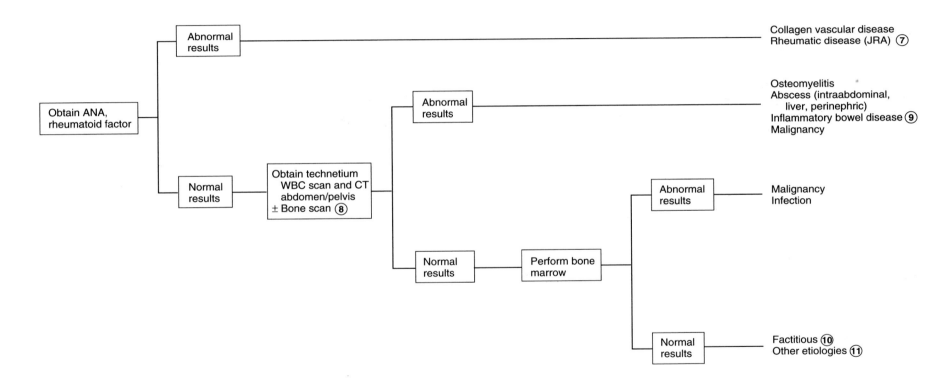

JRA = Juvenile rheumatoid arthritis

(12) The algorithm lists diagnoses suggested by particular elements of the history and physical examination. Repeating the history is important because parents and patients frequently remember historical elements that may be contributory. Physical findings often evolve.

(13) Acute bacterial endocarditis is usually fulminant in onset, but the subacute form is more insidious and usually found in someone with a preexisting cardiac lesion. Repeated blood cultures may be negative. Echocardiography may initially be negative.

(14) In children, FUO is more likely to occur due to nonpulmonary tuberculosis than pulmonary tuberculosis. A high index of suspicion based on a history of possible contacts should initiate further investigation of liver and bone marrow if chest X-ray and skin testing are negative or inconclusive.

(15) A CBC, chest X-ray, and sinus CT or X-ray should be obtained when patients have complaints of prolonged upper respiratory symptoms, regardless of the severity of the complaints.

(16) Toxoplasmosis is most often acquired by ingestion of oocytes excreted by cats.

(17) Liver abscesses are occasionally found in the normal host. They are more common in the immunocompromised patient. Blood cultures and liver function tests are often normal. Imaging may be necessary for diagnosis.

(18) Osteomyelitis is often, but not always, clinically evident especially in young infants. Sometimes infection of the pelvic bone will occur as FUO. Whole-body bone or gallium scans may aid in this diagnosis.

(19) Fever repeatedly occurring in warm environments and absence of sweating while febrile may suggest ectodermal dysplasia or factitious fever. Dental defects and sparse hair occur in the ectodermal dysplasias.

(20) Severe brain damage may result in dysfunction of thermoregulation. Rarely, neurologically intact children have fevers due to central dysfunction.

(21) Recurrent episodes of fever and joint and abdominal complaints characterize familial Mediterranean fever.

(22) Both hypothermia and extreme fevers occur in familial dysautonomia. Excessive sweating, insensitivity to pain, ataxia, and progressive scoliosis are also characteristic.

(23) Infantile cortical hyperostosis (i.e., Caffey disease) is suggested by swelling of soft tissues over the face and jaws, cortical thickening of long bones and flat bones, and tenderness over affected bony areas.

BIBLIOGRAPHY

Lorin MI, Feigin RD: Fever without localizing signs and fever of unknown origin. In Feigin RD, Cherry JD (eds): Textbook of Pediatric Infectious Diseases, 4th ed, p 820. Philadelphia: WB Saunders Company, 1998.

FEVER OF UNKNOWN ORIGIN

Travel, other exposures or PE findings suggestive of specific disorders present ⑫

(Boxes list suggestive findings in no particular order)

Exposure to wild or domesticated animals

Zoonoses ⑥
    Tularemia
    Typhoid fever
    Brucellosis
    Leptospirosis
    Q fever
    Rat bite fever
    Psittacosis

Rash or petechiae

Lyme disease
Juvenile rheumatoid arthritis ⑦
Acute rheumatic fever
Endocarditis ⑬
Dermatomyositis
Systemic lupus erythematosus
Kawasaki disease
Rocky Mountain spotted fever
Histiocytosis
Serum sickness
Tularemia
EBV

Travel OR exposure to persons recently traveled

Coccidiomycosis
Histoplasmosis
Malaria ④
Blastomycosis
Lyme disease
Rocky Mountain spotted fever
Tuberculosis (TB) ⑭
Ehrlichiosis
Babesiosis
Typhoid fever
Other endemic diseases

Mild upper respiratory symptoms ⑮

Sinusitis
Pulmonary disease
    (pneumonia, TB, abscess, sarcoid)
Wegener's granulomatosis
Malignancy

Ingestion of contaminated food or milk
OR pica

Visceral larva migrans
Toxoplasmosis ⑯
Typhoid fever
Brucellosis
Rat bite fever

Weight loss or impaired linear growth, vague abdominal complaints

Inflammatory bowel disease ⑨
Intra-abdominal abscesses ⑰
Malignancy

Bone, joint or muscle pain or tenderness

Osteomyelitis ⑱
Malignancy
Trichinosis
Dermatomyositis
Polyarteritis
Arboviral infections

Abnormal cardiac exam

Carditis (rheumatic fever)
Endocarditis ⑬
Juvenile rheumatoid arthritis ⑦
Systemic lupus erythematosus
Viral pericarditis
Myocarditis

Other physical abnormalities (neurologic, cutaneous, dental)

Ectodermal dysplasia ⑲
CNS/hypothalamic disorders ⑳
Familial Mediterranean fever ㉑
Familial dysautonomia ㉒
Infantile cortical hyperostosis ㉓

Chapter 78 *Recurrent Infections*

Recurrent infections are a frequent complaint, but only rarely are they caused by primary disorders of the immune system. More likely explanations for recurrent infections are upper respiratory tract infections, respiratory allergies, or a single prolonged infection, which may wax and wane, in otherwise normal children. Immunodeficiencies can occur secondary to infection, drugs, malnutrition, or protein loss.

Data gathered from the history and physical examination should help categorize a patient as probably well, probably allergic, chronically ill, or probably immunodeficient.

1 Obtain a detailed history of the frequency and nature of the recurrent infections. High fevers and purulent secretions suggest bacterial infections and may warrant an evaluation for an immune deficiency. Recurrent infections of a single site suggest allergy or local mechanical problems (e.g., anatomic obstruction, foreign bodies).

For young infants, an in-depth birth history should be obtained, including exposure to maternal infections (herpes simplex, rubella, cytomegalovirus) and risk factors for human immunodeficiency virus (HIV). If the infant was premature, inquire about associated complications (e.g., bronchopulmonary dysplasia, blood transfusions). A history of delayed umbilical cord separation with marked leukocytosis suggests a leukocyte adhesion abnormality. Inquire about any chronic medical problems, conditions requiring indwelling equipment (e.g., catheters, shunts, prosthetic devices), and conditions disrupting the integrity of mucocutaneous barriers (e.g., dermal sinus tracks, burns, surgical wounds).

The family history should inquire specifically about immunodeficiency disorders as well as allergic disease, unexplained infant deaths, and risk factors for HIV in family members. The social history should inquire about risk factors for HIV in the patient plus exposure to environmental irritants (smoke, other fumes), animals, chemicals, and school or daycare attendance. Inquire about travel and any changes in the child's routine that may expose the child to new allergens or infectious contacts.

Findings suggestive of allergic disease on physical examination include a transverse nasal crease, allergic ''shiners,'' posterior pharyngeal cobblestoning, and swollen pale nasal mucosa. Children experiencing chronic respiratory infections may demonstrate scarred tympanic membranes, postnasal drip, and cervical adenopathy. Lymphadenopathy suggests chronic disease; absent lymph tissue (i.e., tonsils, lymph nodes, absent thymus on chest X-ray) suggest a congenital lymphocyte (immune) defect.

2 Approximately half of the children with a complaint of recurrent infections are normal healthy children who are experiencing frequent upper respiratory tract infections. Children who have a large family or attend daycare will experience 6 to 10 viral infections, mostly upper respiratory tract and gastrointestinal infections, a year until age 3 to 5. A minimal workup is usually all that is necessary.

3 Rarely, the CBC may reveal an unsuspected malignancy or neutropenia. Further workup would be based on specific results.

4 Approximately 30% of children with recurrent respiratory symptoms have allergies. A chest X-ray is indicated to rule out foreign bodies or anatomic abnormalities if the child is experiencing coughing or wheezing. It may not be necessary otherwise. An allergic disorder is suggested by a serum IgE level of greater than 50 IU/ml in a child younger than 1 year old or greater than 100 IU/ml in an older child.

5 Approximately 10% of children presenting with recurrent infections have an underlying chronic nonimmunologic problem. Malnutrition, chronic illnesses, and protein-losing enteropathies alter immune function. Structural or anatomic defects (e.g., cleft palate, congenital heart disease, pulmonary sequestration) are risk factors for recurrent local infections. Growth may be normal or below average. Suggestive findings on physical examination include abnormal lung examination, digital clubbing, abdominal distention, hepatosplenomegaly, muscle wasting, and pallor.

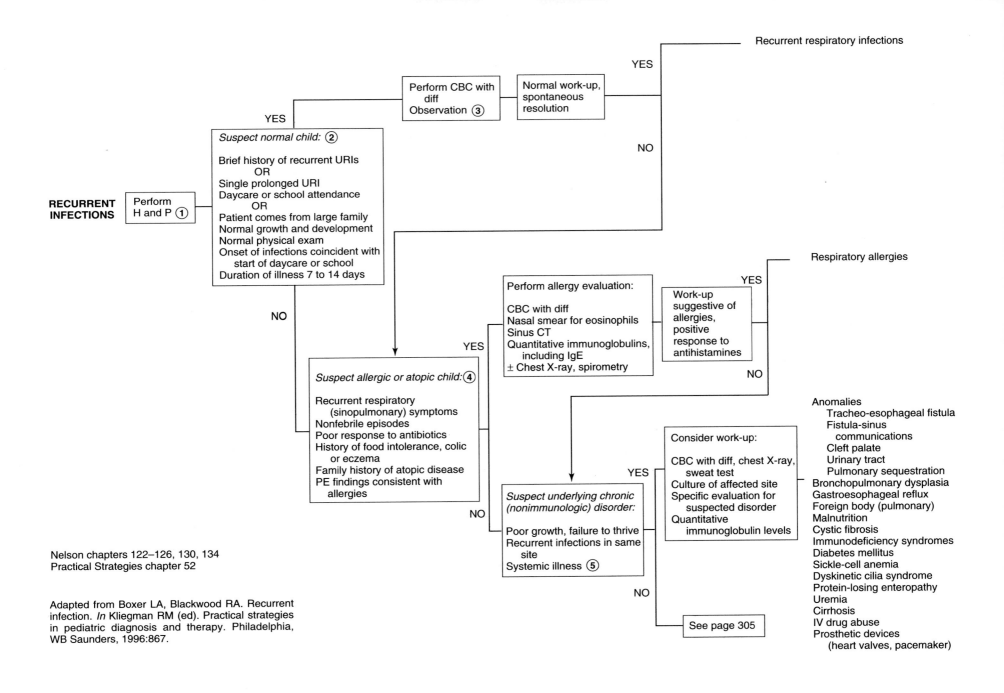

RECURRENT INFECTIONS → Perform H and P ①

Suspect normal child: ②

Brief history of recurrent URIs
OR
Single prolonged URI
Daycare or school attendance
OR
Patient comes from large family
Normal growth and development
Normal physical exam
Onset of infections coincident with start of daycare or school
Duration of illness 7 to 14 days

YES → Perform CBC with diff Observation ③ → Normal work-up, spontaneous resolution

YES → Recurrent respiratory infections

NO

Suspect allergic or atopic child: ④

Recurrent respiratory (sinopulmonary) symptoms
Nonfebrile episodes
Poor response to antibiotics
History of food intolerance, colic or eczema
Family history of atopic disease
PE findings consistent with allergies

YES → Perform allergy evaluation:

CBC with diff
Nasal smear for eosinophils
Sinus CT
Quantitative immunoglobulins, including IgE
± Chest X-ray, spirometry

→ Work-up suggestive of allergies, positive response to antihistamines

YES → Respiratory allergies

NO

NO

Suspect underlying chronic (nonimmunologic) disorder:

Poor growth, failure to thrive
Recurrent infections in same site
Systemic illness ⑤

YES → Consider work-up:

CBC with diff, chest X-ray, sweat test
Culture of affected site
Specific evaluation for suspected disorder
Quantitative immunoglobulin levels

NO → See page 305

Anomalies
   Tracheo-esophageal fistula
   Fistula-sinus communications
   Cleft palate
   Urinary tract
   Pulmonary sequestration
Bronchopulmonary dysplasia
Gastroesophageal reflux
Foreign body (pulmonary)
Malnutrition
Cystic fibrosis
Immunodeficiency syndromes
Diabetes mellitus
Sickle-cell anemia
Dyskinetic cilia syndrome
Protein-losing enteropathy
Uremia
Cirrhosis
IV drug abuse
Prosthetic devices (heart valves, pacemaker)

Nelson chapters 122–126, 130, 134
Practical Strategies chapter 52

Adapted from Boxer LA, Blackwood RA. Recurrent infection. *In* Kliegman RM (ed). Practical strategies in pediatric diagnosis and therapy. Philadelphia, WB Saunders, 1996:867.

(6) Only about 10% of children presenting with recurrent infections will have an underlying immunodeficiency. Recurrent pneumonias are the most common complaint, although children with immunodeficiencies usually experience infections of different sites and severity.

In addition to criteria listed on the algorithm, immunodeficiency would also be suspected in children with unexpected complications, infections in unusual sites (brain, liver), and three or more serious respiratory or bacterial infections per year. In general, children with disorders of antibodies, complements, or phagocytic cells have recurrent infections with encapsulated bacteria but may grow and develop normally. Children with T-cell disorders are more likely to develop failure to thrive and opportunistic infections (e.g., *Candida*, toxoplasmosis, cytomegalovirus, tuberculosis, *Pneumocystis carinii* pneumonia) early in life.

(7) Note that testing for HIV antibody is not routinely recommended unless obvious risk factors are present.

(8) Wiskott-Aldrich syndrome is an X-linked recessive disorder characterized by abnormal lymphocytes, platelets, and phagocytes. Patients experience recurrent infections with encapsulated bacteria and opportunistic pathogens, hemorrhage, and atopic dermatitis. Immunoglobulin levels vary. IgG is usually normal, IgA and IgE elevated, and IgM decreased. Patients respond to some antigens normally but cannot respond to polysaccharide antigens at all (pneumococcal vaccine, *Haemophilus influenzae* type b vaccine). T-cell levels and the helper:suppressor ratio is normal, but their function is abnormal.

(9) Chédiak-Higashi syndrome is characterized by partial albinism, neutropenia, and abnormal giant cytoplasmic granules in the leukocytes. Recurrent infections of the skin, respiratory tract, and mucous membranes typically occur. Bleeding time is usually prolonged. The presence of large melanosomes in melanocytes can confirm the diagnosis. Neuropathies, ataxia, and nystagmus may also occur. Chemotactic function is abnormal when assayed in control serum.

(10) Congenital asplenia may occur as part of a syndrome in association with congenital heart disease; functional asplenia occurs in children with sickle cell disease. Asplenic children are at especially high risk for infection by pneumococci and *H. influenzae* as well as *Salmonella*, *Staphylococcus aureus*, gram-negative enteric bacilli, and meningococci. Howell-Jolly bodies and pitted or pocked erythrocytes on the peripheral blood smear suggest asplenia. Children who have undergone surgical splenectomy are also at increased risk of serious bacterial infections, although their risk may be slightly lower because of the previous development of opsonizing antibodies.

RECURRENT INFECTIONS
(continued)

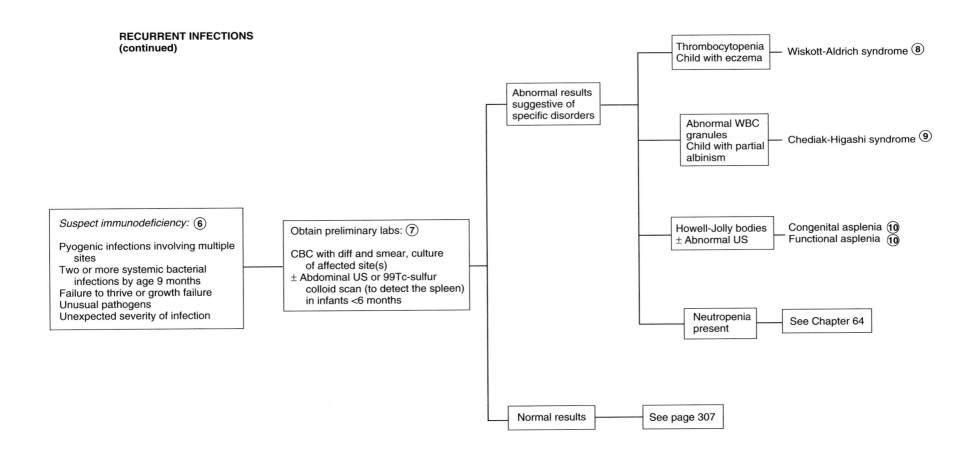

Suspect immunodeficiency: ⑥

Pyogenic infections involving multiple
  sites
Two or more systemic bacterial
  infections by age 9 months
Failure to thrive or growth failure
Unusual pathogens
Unexpected severity of infection

Obtain preliminary labs: ⑦

CBC with diff and smear, culture
  of affected site(s)
± Abdominal US or 99Tc-sulfur
  colloid scan (to detect the spleen)
  in infants <6 months

Abnormal results
suggestive of
specific disorders

Thrombocytopenia
Child with eczema — Wiskott-Aldrich syndrome ⑧

Abnormal WBC
granules
Child with partial
albinism — Chediak-Higashi syndrome ⑨

Howell-Jolly bodies
± Abnormal US — Congenital asplenia ⑩
Functional asplenia ⑩

Neutropenia
present — See Chapter 64

Normal results — See page 307

Recurrent Infections (continued)

(11) It is normal for infants to experience a variable physiologic hypogammaglobulinemia between 4 and 9 months of life. When prolonged or severe, recurrent viral and pyogenic infections may occur. The number of B cells and T cells is normal, and the infants respond appropriately to immunizations even though their immunoglobulin levels remain low until age 12 to 36 months.

(12) IgA deficiency is the most common primary immunodeficiency. Affected children may be asymptomatic or have recurrent respiratory, gastrointestinal, and urogenital tract infections; autoimmune disease (e.g., celiac disease, systemic lupus erythematosus) may also be associated.

Four types of IgG subclass deficiencies are recognized as possible causes of recurrent infections. The total IgG level is usually normal. A group of rare disorders characterized by decreased synthesis of IgG and IgA but increased levels of IgM has been described. T-cell function may be normal or abnormal; recurrent pyogenic infections begin in the first few years of life.

(13) Severe combined immunodeficiency syndromes are a group of disorders of severe abnormalities in B- and T-cell function. Onset of symptoms is in the first few months of life with recurrent pneumonias, failure to thrive, chronic diarrhea, and severe candidal infections. Subtypes include X-linked recessive, reticular dysgenesis, Swiss-type, bare lymphocyte syndrome, adenosine deaminase deficiency, purine nucleoside phosphorylase deficiency, and interleukin-2 deficiency.

(14) DiGeorge syndrome occurs due to abnormal development of the branchial pouches. The thymus, parathyroid glands, face, ears, aortic arch, and heart are all affected. Diagnosis is usually early in life based on the congenital heart defects. The immunodeficiency is related to inadequate thymic function. The total lymphocyte count may range from very low to normal, but T-cell levels are usually depressed. Immunoglobulin levels may be normal, but antibody response to antigens is abnormal.

(15) Cartilage-hair hypoplasia (short-limbed dwarfism) is an autosomal recessive immunodeficiency with skeletal abnormalities and sparse, unpigmented hair. Both B and T cell functions are affected; the immunodeficiency worsens with time.

(16) X-linked agammaglobulinemia (i.e., Bruton agammaglobulinemia) is an X-linked recessive disorder of severe hypogammaglobulinemia or agammaglobulinemia. Affected infants usually present with recurrent bacterial infections (e.g., otitis media, sinusitis, pneumonia, meningitis) at age 6 to 9 months after maternal antibody levels have waned. Occasionally, a child may remain asymptomatic for a longer period (up to 2 years). These children have marked hypoplasia of lymphoid tissue on physical examination.

(17) Common variable immunodeficiency is a group of disorders characterized by severe hypogammaglobulinemia. It is often associated with a spruelike syndrome with diarrhea, protein-losing enteropathies, and failure to thrive. Chronic respiratory infections are the most common manifestation; *Giardia* infection is also common. These children have low circulating levels of IgG, IgM, and IgA but normal or increased numbers of B cells.

(18) Secondary defects of the immune system, including the complement system, may occur owing to problems such as HIV infection, splenic dysfunction, malignancy, immunosuppression (e.g., chemotherapy, transplantation), and various causes of neutropenia.

(19) Ataxia-telangiectasia is an autosomal recessive disorder characterized by immunodeficiency, neurologic dysfunction, endocrine abnormalities, oculocutaneous telangiectasia, and a high rate of malignancy. The presenting symptom is usually ataxia. Varying degrees of both B- and T-cell dysfunction occur.

(20) The complement system acts synergistically with the other components of the immune system to enhance the immune response to infectious agents. Congenital deficiencies of all the components of the complement cascade have been described. Disorders that can result in a secondary deficiency or defective function of complement factors include severe combined immunodeficiency, systemic lupus erythematosus, malnutrition, sickle cell disease, acute postinfectious nephritis, burns, and disorders involving immune complex formation.

The clinical presentation of complement disorders depends on the components affected. Complement disorders should be suspected in children with collagen vascular diseases, chronic nephritis, recurrent pyogenic infections, meningococcal or gonococcal infections, angioedema, partial lipodystrophy, or a second episode of septicemia at any age. The total hemolytic complement activity (CH_{50}) test is the most useful screening test for complement disorders. Measurement of serum C3 and C4 levels is also readily available.

(21) Disorders of the phagocytic cells occur with cutaneous abscesses, mucous membrane lesions, lymphadenitis, pulmonary infections, lung and liver abscesses, and gastrointestinal problems due to granulomatous obstruction. Specific testing can identify disorders of motility and chemotaxis, adhesion (leukocyte adherence defects), specific granule defects (Chédiak-Higashi syndrome), and disorders of microbicidal activity (chronic granulomatous disease, myeloperoxidase deficiency). (See Ch. 64.)

(22) Chronic granulomatous disease is a rare disorder of the microbicidal function of neutrophils. Catalase-positive microorganisms (*S. aureus, S. marcescens*) are ingested but not killed, owing to a defect in oxidative function. Recurrent pneumonitis, dermatitis, and lymphadenitis are the most common manifestations. Onset may occur early in infancy or as late as young adulthood.

BIBLIOGRAPHY

Sorenson RU, Moore C: Immunology in the pediatrician's office. Pediatr Clin North Am 41:691–714, 1994.

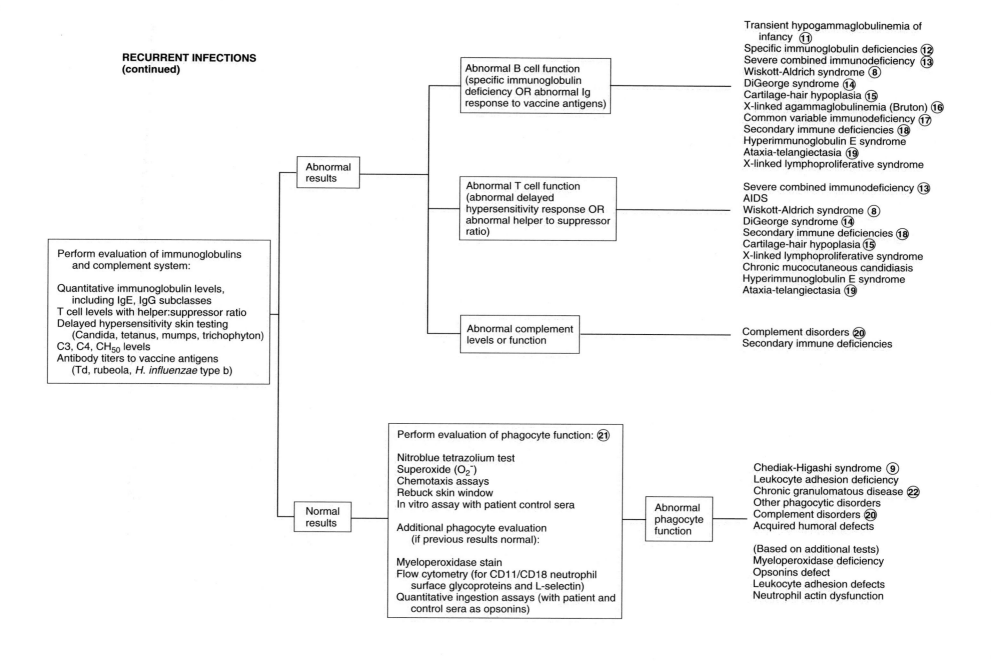

RECURRENT INFECTIONS
(continued)

Perform evaluation of immunoglobulins
  and complement system:

Quantitative immunoglobulin levels,
  including IgE, IgG subclasses
T cell levels with helper:suppressor ratio
Delayed hypersensitivity skin testing
  (Candida, tetanus, mumps, trichophyton)
C3, C4, CH_{50} levels
Antibody titers to vaccine antigens
  (Td, rubeola, *H. influenzae* type b)

Abnormal
results

Abnormal B cell function
(specific immunoglobulin
deficiency OR abnormal Ig
response to vaccine antigens)

Transient hypogammaglobulinemia of
  infancy ⑪
Specific immunoglobulin deficiencies ⑫
Severe combined immunodeficiency ⑬
Wiskott-Aldrich syndrome ⑧
DiGeorge syndrome ⑭
Cartilage-hair hypoplasia ⑮
X-linked agammaglobulinemia (Bruton) ⑯
Common variable immunodeficiency ⑰
Secondary immune deficiencies ⑱
Hyperimmunoglobulin E syndrome
Ataxia-telangiectasia ⑲
X-linked lymphoproliferative syndrome

Abnormal T cell function
(abnormal delayed
hypersensitivity response OR
abnormal helper to suppressor
ratio)

Severe combined immunodeficiency ⑬
AIDS
Wiskott-Aldrich syndrome ⑧
DiGeorge syndrome ⑭
Secondary immune deficiencies ⑱
Cartilage-hair hypoplasia ⑮
X-linked lymphoproliferative syndrome
Chronic mucocutaneous candidiasis
Hyperimmunoglobulin E syndrome
Ataxia-telangiectasia ⑲

Abnormal complement
levels or function

Complement disorders ⑳
Secondary immune deficiencies

Normal
results

Perform evaluation of phagocyte function: ㉑

Nitroblue tetrazolium test
Superoxide (O_2^-)
Chemotaxis assays
Rebuck skin window
In vitro assay with patient control sera

Additional phagocyte evaluation
  (if previous results normal):

Myeloperoxidase stain
Flow cytometry (for CD11/CD18 neutrophil
  surface glycoproteins and L-selectin)
Quantitative ingestion assays (with patient and
  control sera as opsonins)

Abnormal
phagocyte
function

Chediak-Higashi syndrome ⑨
Leukocyte adhesion deficiency
Chronic granulomatous disease ㉒
Other phagocytic disorders
Complement disorders ⑳
Acquired humoral defects

(Based on additional tests)
Myeloperoxidase deficiency
Opsonins defect
Leukocyte adhesion defects
Neutrophil actin dysfunction

A reasonable definition of an irritable infant is one younger than 1 year of age who is deemed by their caretaker to be crying excessively or to be "fussy" without an apparent reason. Although many children presenting with this history will be normal, up to 61% of afebrile children presenting to an emergency department with prolonged excessive crying will have an underlying serious cause. The challenge to the practitioner is to identify those infants who are affected by a serious organic or life-threatening disorder. Although there are numerous causes of infant irritability, only those not obvious by history and physical examination and those that may be inadvertently overlooked are included here.

1 A thorough history and physical examination will yield a diagnosis in a majority of crying infants who present for evaluation. Febrile infants or those presenting with respiratory distress or other clinical instability will be evaluated and managed according to their clinical presentation. In irritable infants presenting without an obvious etiology, the history will reveal the diagnosis in approximately 20%, the physical examination in 41%, and preliminary laboratory or imaging studies in another 20%.

The feeding history may suggest problems associated with overfeeding or underfeeding or problems related to breast-feeding. A social history may indicate recent events that could disrupt the infant's normal patterns. A history of sick contacts may also be helpful. A thorough unclothed physical examination is essential. Corneal staining with fluorescein to look for corneal abrasions should be standard, as should retinoscopy. Eversion of the eyelids may aid in identifying a foreign body. Rectal examination can aid in the diagnosis of constipation.

2 Judgment must be used in determining whether certain subtle or minor physical findings (e.g., abrasions, insect bites, stomatitis) can be diagnostic. In cases of severe or persistent irritability, additional evaluation remains necessary.

3 Tourniquet syndrome refers to a thin filamentous material (hair, thread) that has wrapped around an appendage and is causing vascular compromise. Finger, toes, penis, and even the uvula have been reported as affected sites. Edema and duskiness that accompany the condition make diagnosis difficult by obscuring the strangulating item. A site of well-demarcated discoloration or swelling on a distal appendage should raise suspicion for this cause. Rapid diagnosis is necessary to minimize morbidity. Surgical intervention is frequently needed, especially for cases of penile strangulation.

4 Hand-foot syndrome (i.e., acute sickle dactylitis) is often the first clinical manifestation of sickle cell disease. Infants present with irritability and painful, usually symmetric, swelling of the hands and feet. Irritability related to other causes of hemolytic anemia is most likely to occur in severe cases with associated cardiovascular decompensation.

5 If the initial history and physical examination do not suggest a diagnosis, consider the ability to console the infant during the evaluation. An infant who can be consoled during the initial period of observation and has normal results on physical examination is not likely to have a serious illness. On the contrary, persistent crying during the evaluation is highly suggestive of a serious illness. The decision of how long to observe a child before initiating a workup should be individualized based on the degree of irritability and the age of the child.

6 A head CT should be strongly considered before performing a lumbar puncture (LP), especially if signs or symptoms suggesting infection are absent.

7 Because many persistently inconsolable infants do have a serious illness, in-hospital observation should be strongly considered until a diagnosis can be established.

8 Because only 50% of infants with meningitis initially present with fever, this diagnosis is very important to rule out in the irritable infant. And because the differential of the irritable afebrile infant includes nonmeningeal intracranial causes, a head CT should be obtained before performing an LP in these infants to rule out increased intracranial pressure.

9 Acidosis, hypernatremia, hypocalcemia, and hypoglycemia are serious causes of irritability in infants. Inborn errors of metabolism should be considered when there is associated vomiting, neurologic symptoms, failure to thrive, or a positive family history, including unexplained neonatal deaths.

10 Limited information is available regarding maternal drug use and irritability in the breast-fed infant. Maternal use of decongestants and illicit drugs (e.g., cocaine, opiates, marijuana) is probably associated with infant irritability. Irritability may also be a sign of neonatal drug withdrawal; withdrawal usually occurs in the first week of life but may be delayed up to 2 to 3 weeks if the mother was using methadone. Consider postnatal exposure to cocaine (active or passive) as another cause of infant irritability.

11 Evidence of erupting teeth, increased salivation, and relief with chewing on a cold or blunt object suggests teething. Unless clinically obvious, the diagnosis should remain one of exclusion.

12 A common definition of colic is recurrent episodes of excessive crying or fussiness at predictable times of the day, usually the evening, lasting more than 3 hours, and occurring on more than 3 days per week in otherwise normal infants. Onset is usually around 3 weeks of age, and the condition typically resolves by 3 to 4 months of age. Parental education and reassurance are necessary and important.

13 Normal crying may be reported as excessive by inexperienced or stressed parents. Nor-

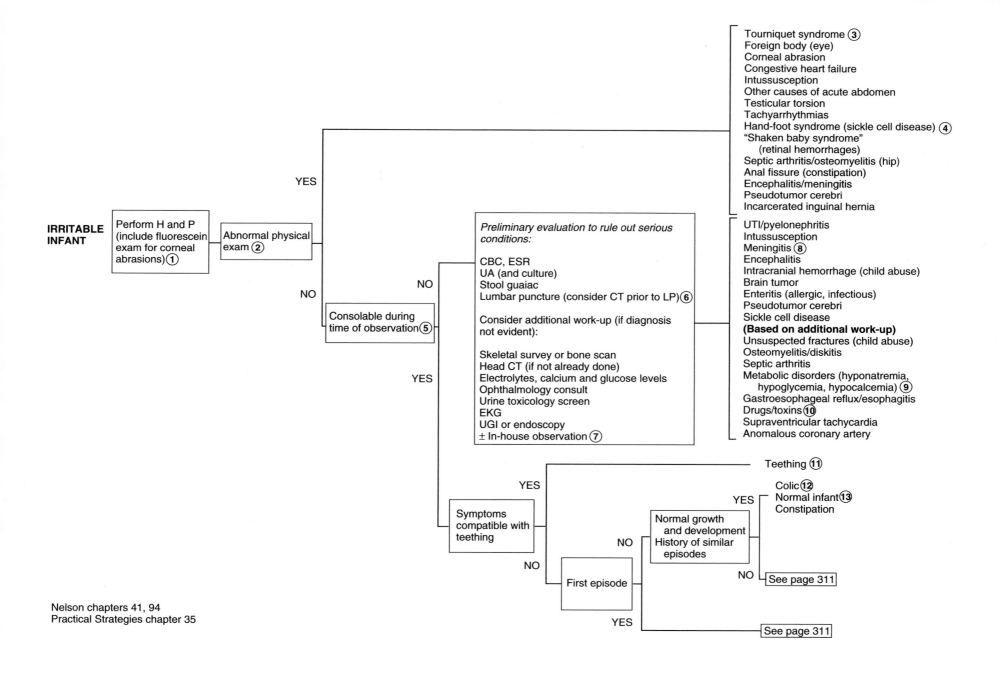

IRRITABLE INFANT

Perform H and P (include fluorescein exam for corneal abrasions) ①

Abnormal physical exam ②

YES

- Tourniquet syndrome ③
- Foreign body (eye)
- Corneal abrasion
- Congestive heart failure
- Intussusception
- Other causes of acute abdomen
- Testicular torsion
- Tachyarrhythmias
- Hand-foot syndrome (sickle cell disease) ④
- "Shaken baby syndrome"
  (retinal hemorrhages)
- Septic arthritis/osteomyelitis (hip)
- Anal fissure (constipation)
- Encephalitis/meningitis
- Pseudotumor cerebri
- Incarcerated inguinal hernia

NO

Consolable during time of observation ⑤

NO

Preliminary evaluation to rule out serious conditions:

CBC, ESR
UA (and culture)
Stool guaiac
Lumbar puncture (consider CT prior to LP) ⑥

Consider additional work-up (if diagnosis not evident):

Skeletal survey or bone scan
Head CT (if not already done)
Electrolytes, calcium and glucose levels
Ophthalmology consult
Urine toxicology screen
EKG
UGI or endoscopy
± In-house observation ⑦

- UTI/pyelonephritis
- Intussusception
- Meningitis ⑧
- Encephalitis
- Intracranial hemorrhage (child abuse)
- Brain tumor
- Enteritis (allergic, infectious)
- Pseudotumor cerebri
- Sickle cell disease
- **(Based on additional work-up)**
- Unsuspected fractures (child abuse)
- Osteomyelitis/diskitis
- Septic arthritis
- Metabolic disorders (hyponatremia, hypoglycemia, hypocalcemia) ⑨
- Gastroesophageal reflux/esophagitis
- Drugs/toxins ⑩
- Supraventricular tachycardia
- Anomalous coronary artery

YES

Symptoms compatible with teething

YES

Teething ⑪

NO

First episode

NO

Normal growth and development
History of similar episodes

YES

Colic ⑫
Normal infant ⑬
Constipation

NO

See page 311

YES

See page 311

Nelson chapters 41, 94
Practical Strategies chapter 35

mally, crying increases from birth until 6 to 8 weeks of age, with an average maximum of 2.5 to 3 hours per day.

(14) If the stool tests positive for blood, a diagnostic and often therapeutic "air enema" should be strongly considered to rule out intussusception. Intussusception typically occurs as the sudden onset of frequent severe episodes of pain. Infants are initially normal between episodes and gradually become weaker and more lethargic. Vomiting and grossly bloody and mucousy ("currant jelly") stools may also occur. (See Ch. 25.) Positive stool guaiac tests may also occur with constipation, suggested by a history of hard stools or fissures on examination. Fissures result in bright red streaks coating the stool; they can occur even in the absence of constipation.

(15) Follow-up should be recommended within 24 hours for any irritable infant, even if the infant can be consoled. In addition, parents should be counseled carefully about worrisome signs and symptoms and reasons to follow-up sooner. In infants who can be consoled but experience repeated episodes of excessive crying not consistent with colic, careful follow-up is essential. Laboratory or imaging evaluation should be considered to rule out some of the more subtle causes of persistent crying.

(16) Irritability associated with immunizations may be due to the injection or the vaccine. Because the whole-cell diphtheria-tetanus-pertussis (DTP) vaccine has been replaced with the acellular version, fewer irritable reactions have been reported. Crying related to vaccines is usually brief but will occasionally last up to 3 hours. The children may warrant some investigation or at least prolonged observation or close follow-up.

(17) Mild cases of cow's milk protein hypersensitivity may occur as very nonspecific gastrointestinal symptoms (e.g., spitting, slightly loose stools, irritability). Consider a trial of a casein hydrolysate formula in the infant with fussiness and some minimal gastrointestinal symptoms.

BIBLIOGRAPHY

Pawel BB, Henretig FM: Crying and colic in early infancy. In Fleisher G, Ludwig S (eds): Textbook of Pediatric Emergency Medicine, 4th ed, p 193. Baltimore: Williams & Wilkins, 2000.

Poole R: The infant with acute, unexplained, excessive crying. Pediatrics 88:450, 1991.

IRRITABLE INFANT (continued)

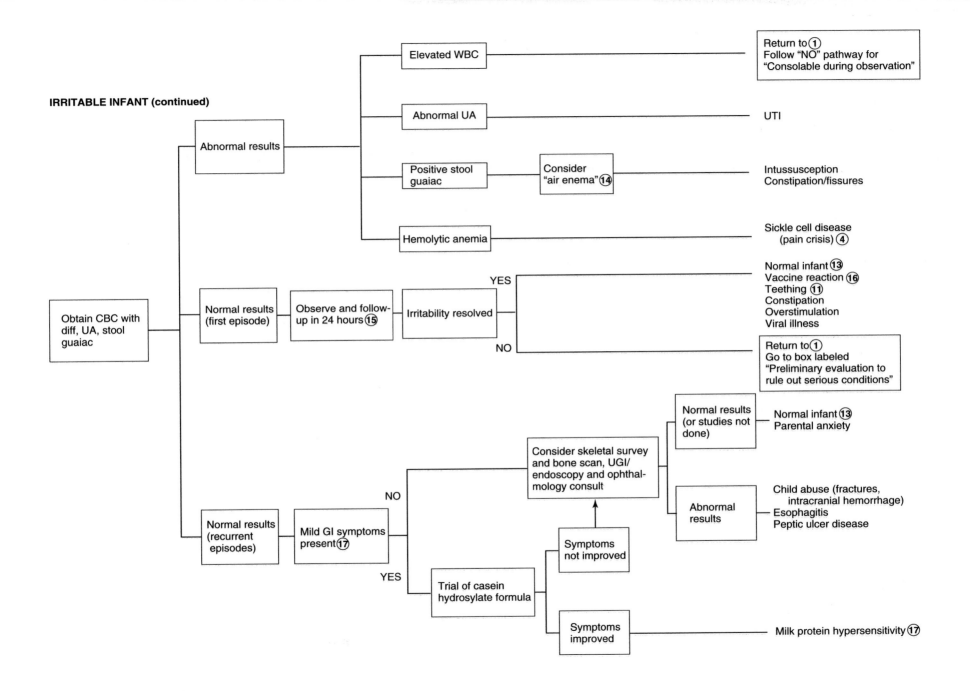

Chapter 80 *Failure to Thrive*

Failure to thrive (FTT) refers to implied growth failure (i.e., poor weight gain ± affected linear growth) in infants and young children. One commonly used definition is a weight persistently below the third or fifth percentile for the child's age in the absence of constitutional delay. Another definition is a deceleration of growth velocity with subsequent crossing of at least two major percentile lines on the growth chart.

Traditionally, FTT has been categorized as either organic or nonorganic (psychosocial). Nonorganic causes outnumber organic ones; in many cases an organic cause is exacerbated by nonorganic factors. Of the organic causes of FTT, CNS developmental abnormalities are the most common.

(1) Careful, nonjudgmental observation of the parent-child interaction is important. Sensitive questions about how difficult the child is to take care of, the parents' impression of the problem, and the relationship and shared responsibilities between the parents should be asked. Ask parents how they felt about the infant after birth. Postpartum depression can affect bonding and have a negative impact on the feeding interactions and increase the risk of neglect. FTT due to inadequate intake may be related to financial limitations of the parents.

A thorough history and physical examination, including a good review of systems, is essential in the evaluation of the child with FTT. Inquire specifically about risk factors for human immunodeficiency virus (HIV) infection and travel to or from a developing country. A family history of growth patterns (e.g., short stature, constitutional growth delay) may also be helpful. Accurate measurements and plotting a growth curve are essential. Weight generally drops off before length or head circumference in acute malnutrition. Most measurement errors occur in regard to length.

The severity of wasting can be categorized by determining the ratio of actual weight and the median expected weight for length. Growth is considered normal if the ratio is > 90% of the median weight for height, moderate if the value is 70% to 80% of the value, and severe if < 70%. Be aware of the potential paradox of normalization of the weight-for-height ratio in prolonged cases of malnutrition (after linear growth is affected).

Growth charts for premature infants are available and may be used up to 1 to 2 years of age. Once a child has reached 40 weeks of gestational age, conventional charts may be used.

(2) Most causes of developmental delay can result in FTT. A small head that predates the FTT suggests a neurologic cause, such as a hypoxic-ischemic encephalopathy or a congenital viral infection including HIV. Dysmorphic features suggest chromosomal abnormalities. Prenatal exposure to anticonvulsants or alcohol are also risk factors for developmental delay and FTT. Other examples include neuromuscular disorders, including cerebral palsy, congenital syndromes, and metabolic disorders.

(3) Oral-motor dysfunction is common in children with developmental delay. The condition may be subtle and tends to manifest when a child begins taking more textured solid foods. Evaluation by a speech pathologist, including an oropharyngeal motility study, may be necessary.

(4) Although organic causes of failure to thrive are more the exception than the rule, a careful history and physical examination will usually suggest the underlying medical problem. Any disease, depending on its severity and chronicity, may produce FTT.

(5) Obtaining a good diet history is often difficult; asking parents to provide a 24-hour dietary recall or a food diary for 2 to 3 days is often helpful. Quantifying water and milk and juice intake may be helpful. Ask about formula preparation and substitution and the process of feeding and mealtimes in the household. For example, inquire about whether everyone in the family eats their meals together and whether any distractions are present during meals. Even in cases in which a psychosocial cause is obvious, a CBC and possibly lead level in children older than 6 months should be obtained because iron deficiency and lead toxicity can cause an impaired appetite, exacerbating a nutritional FTT.

(6) Other psychosocial factors include a poor parent-child relationship, a distractible child or poor environment, or poor interactions such as coercive feeding.

(7) A serum protein and albumin level may aid in determining the severity of the problem. Additional tests should be considered according to the suspected disorder.

(8) If a cause is not apparent after a thorough history, physical examination, and preliminary laboratory evaluation, hospitalization or a series of home nurse visits may help identify inadequate calorie intake or psychosocial problems.

(9) When the preliminary evaluation and a period of observation does not suggest the cause, further consideration should be given to organic disorders, especially those that may occur as subtle symptoms. Gastroesophageal reflux may occur without obvious spitting or vomiting, and malabsorption disorders without obvious diarrhea.

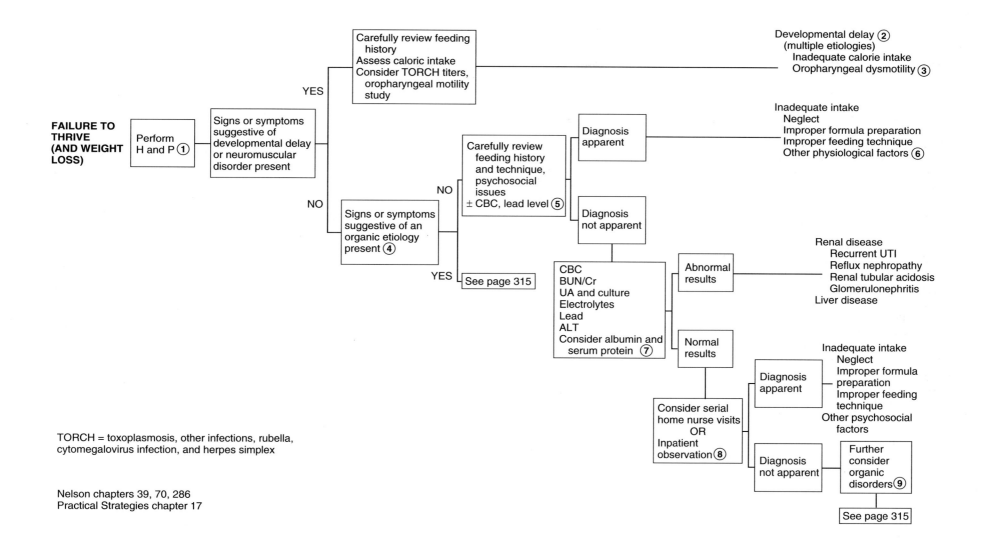

FAILURE TO THRIVE (AND WEIGHT LOSS)

Perform H and P ①

Signs or symptoms suggestive of developmental delay or neuromuscular disorder present

YES → Carefully review feeding history
Assess caloric intake
Consider TORCH titers, oropharyngeal motility study

→ Developmental delay ② (multiple etiologies)
Inadequate calorie intake
Oropharyngeal dysmotility ③

NO → Signs or symptoms suggestive of an organic etiology present ④

→ **NO** → Carefully review feeding history and technique, psychosocial issues ± CBC, lead level ⑤

→ Diagnosis apparent → Inadequate intake
Neglect
Improper formula preparation
Improper feeding technique
Other physiological factors ⑥

→ Diagnosis not apparent

→ **YES** → See page 315

CBC
BUN/Cr
UA and culture
Electrolytes
Lead
ALT
Consider albumin and serum protein ⑦

→ Abnormal results → Renal disease
Recurrent UTI
Reflux nephropathy
Renal tubular acidosis
Glomerulonephritis
Liver disease

→ Normal results → Consider serial home nurse visits OR Inpatient observation ⑧

→ Diagnosis apparent → Inadequate intake
Neglect
Improper formula preparation
Improper feeding technique
Other psychosocial factors

→ Diagnosis not apparent → Further consider organic disorders ⑨ → See page 315

TORCH = toxoplasmosis, other infections, rubella, cytomegalovirus infection, and herpes simplex

Nelson chapters 39, 70, 286
Practical Strategies chapter 17

10 If gastrointestinal causes are not identified in a child with a history of vomiting, neuroimaging should also be considered since increased intracranial pressure may be the cause.

11 Children with Hirschsprung disease may have a history of delayed passage of meconium, Down syndrome, or positive family history. Most cases will be diagnosed in the first days of life with abdominal distention, vomiting, and constipation. Occasionally, older children will present with FTT, abdominal distention, and constipation. A few will demonstrate intermittent diarrhea. Absent stool on rectal examination and immediate passage of stool after the rectal examination are also suggestive. A rectal suction biopsy demonstrating absent ganglion cells is necessary for diagnosis.

12 Inborn errors of metabolism in the neonate are typically severe and life threatening. The infants are usually normal at birth and rapidly deteriorate over the hours to days after their birth. Signs and symptoms are nonspecific and include vomiting, lethargy, poor feeding, convulsions, and coma. These infants are often presumed to have sepsis. The physical examination may be normal or may reveal signs related to the CNS, hepatomegaly, or, occasionally, a characteristic odor that may aid in diagnosis.

A high index of suspicion is necessary and should be increased by a history of consanguinity and/or a family history of neonatal deaths. For a metabolic workup, blood and urine should be obtained during episodes of suggestive symptoms. Blood tests should include CBC, electrolytes, pH, glucose, ammonia, lactate, carnitine, and serum amino acids. Urine should be analyzed for ketones, reducing substances, organic acids, amino acids, and carnitine. Urine δ-aminolevulinic acid and porphobilinogen should also be obtained if porphyria is being considered. Porphyria generally occurs as other symptoms (e.g., abdominal pain, photosensitivity, rashes, tingling) in addition to vomiting. Amylase or lipase should be considered, particularly in younger children or in older children who also complain of abdominal pain.

Mild variants of most inborn errors do occur and have an insidious presentation. Be suspicious when there is a history of unexplained mental retardation, seizures, or unusual odor (especially if manifest during an acute illness), or a family history of metabolic disorders or unexplained infant deaths. Some children will experience intermittent episodes of severe illness, including unexplained vomiting, acidosis, and mental deterioration or coma.

13 Celiac disease commonly presents as intestinal symptoms in the first 2 years of life after the introduction of wheat products into the diet.

14 Milk or formula protein intolerance is usually accompanied by frequent loose and sometimes bloody stools. Vomiting is not always significant.

15 Cystic fibrosis may appear at birth with meconium ileus or later with steatorrhea, FTT, and cough. Not all cases develop pancreatic insufficiency; of those that do, the malabsorption may not be evident until after the neonatal period. Shwachman-Diamond syndrome is characterized by pancreatic insufficiency in addition to chronic neutropenia, which may result in recurrent respiratory infections. (See Ch. 64.)

16 Even the most exhaustive efforts and thorough evaluation may occasionally fail to determine the cause of a case of FTT. Maintaining involvement and recurrent evaluation over time may be the key to diagnosis.

17 Extremely premature infants (<1000 g) may remain short (small) throughout their lives but should maintain a normal growth rate and weight-for-height ratio.

18 Constitutional growth delay is a variant pattern of normal growth. Children present with short stature in early to middle childhood and eventually experience delayed puberty. There is frequently a history of delayed puberty, a late adolescent growth spurt, and a cessation of growth at a late age in family members. Physical examination is normal, laboratory tests are normal, and bone age is delayed.

19 Eating disorders should always be carefully considered in adolescents, regardless of associated complaints.

20 In children without other obvious associated disorders, iatrogenic causes of anorexia (e.g., drug therapy, unpalatable therapeutic diets) and depression should be considered.

21 It is important to inquire about risk factors for HIV because it may occur only as FTT with lymphadenopathy and developmental delay. Associated infections are not always present.

22 Nearly any chronic disease can lead to FTT secondary either to altered intake, increased needs, or excessive irritability.

BIBLIOGRAPHY

Bithoney WG, Dubowitz H, Egan H: Failure to thrive/growth deficiency. Pediatr Rev 13:453, 1992.

Frank DA, Silva M, Needleman R: Failure to thrive: Mystery, myth, and method. Contemp Pediatr 10:114, 1993.

Tolia V: Failure to thrive. In Wyllie R, Hyams J (eds): Pediatric Gastrointestinal Disease: Pathophysiology, Diagnosis, Management, 2nd ed, p 51. Philadelphia: WB Saunders Company, 1999.

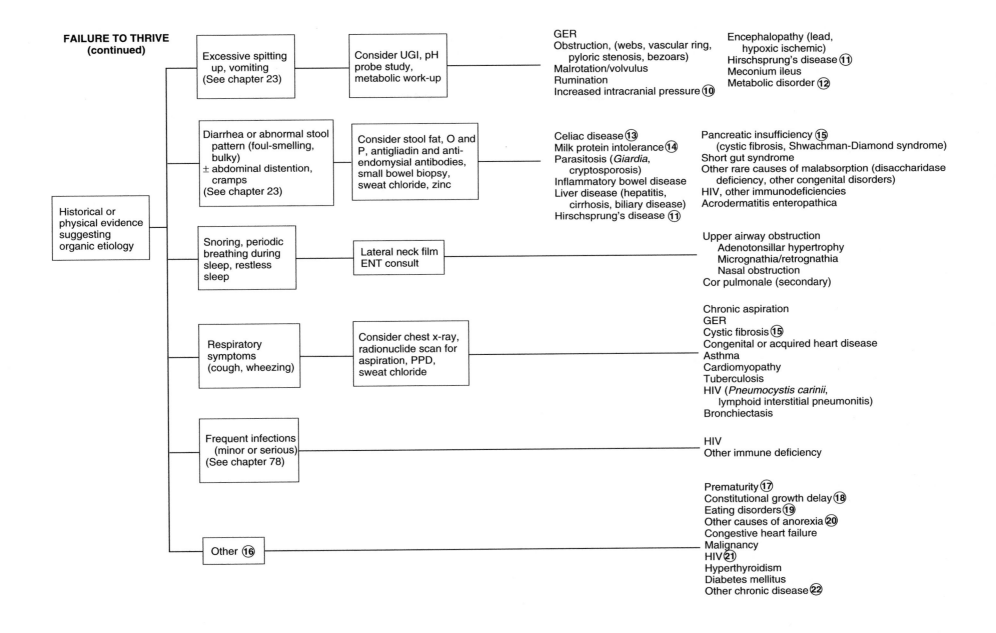

FAILURE TO THRIVE
(continued)

Historical or physical evidence suggesting organic etiology

Excessive spitting up, vomiting (See chapter 23)

Consider UGI, pH probe study, metabolic work-up

GER
Obstruction, (webs, vascular ring, pyloric stenosis, bezoars)
Malrotation/volvulus
Rumination
Increased intracranial pressure ⑩

Encephalopathy (lead, hypoxic ischemic)
Hirschsprung's disease ⑪
Meconium ileus
Metabolic disorder ⑫

Diarrhea or abnormal stool pattern (foul-smelling, bulky) ± abdominal distention, cramps (See chapter 23)

Consider stool fat, O and P, antigliadin and anti-endomysial antibodies, small bowel biopsy, sweat chloride, zinc

Celiac disease ⑬
Milk protein intolerance ⑭
Parasitosis (*Giardia*, cryptosporosis)
Inflammatory bowel disease
Liver disease (hepatitis, cirrhosis, biliary disease)
Hirschsprung's disease ⑪

Pancreatic insufficiency ⑮ (cystic fibrosis, Shwachman-Diamond syndrome)
Short gut syndrome
Other rare causes of malabsorption (disaccharidase deficiency, other congenital disorders)
HIV, other immunodeficiencies
Acrodermatitis enteropathica

Snoring, periodic breathing during sleep, restless sleep

Lateral neck film ENT consult

Upper airway obstruction
Adenotonsillar hypertrophy
Micrognathia/retrognathia
Nasal obstruction
Cor pulmonale (secondary)

Respiratory symptoms (cough, wheezing)

Consider chest x-ray, radionuclide scan for aspiration, PPD, sweat chloride

Chronic aspiration
GER
Cystic fibrosis ⑮
Congenital or acquired heart disease
Asthma
Cardiomyopathy
Tuberculosis
HIV (*Pneumocystis carinii*, lymphoid interstitial pneumonitis)
Bronchiectasis

Frequent infections (minor or serious) (See chapter 78)

HIV
Other immune deficiency

Other ⑯

Prematurity ⑰
Constitutional growth delay ⑱
Eating disorders ⑲
Other causes of anorexia ⑳
Congestive heart failure
Malignancy
HIV ㉑
Hyperthyroidism
Diabetes mellitus
Other chronic disease ㉒

Sleep problems or disturbances are a common concern of parents. They may be classified as dyssomnias (disturbance in amount or timing of sleep), parasomnias (abnormal sleep behaviors such as nightmares and night terrors), and disruptions due to other physical or mental conditions. It is important to understand the normal maturation of the sleep cycle of newborns, infants, and children. In the first year, infants often wake many times during the night, but they may not always cry. The average newborn sleeps about 16.5 hours a day, with relatively undifferentiated sleep cycles. Sleep wake cycles become more clearly established by 3 to 4 months of age, with an increasing proportion of nighttime sleep. However, there is a great deal of individual variation. In evaluating sleep disorders, it is important to identify inappropriate parental expectations, excessive parental anxiety or stress, as well as parental behaviors that may reinforce the sleep problems.

① History and physical examination should first of all identify any underlying organic etiology for the sleep disturbance. This may be easier to identify in cases of an acute change in sleep due to illness or injury. A drug and medication history should include caffeine-containing beverages and over-the-counter medications such as cold preparations. Maternal behaviors and attachment as well as psychosocial stress have an important role in sleep problems. Perinatal factors such as birth asphyxia and prematurity contribute to increased wakefulness.

② There are many organic causes of sleep problems. These include acute illness, such as otitis media, upper respiratory tract infection, and urinary tract infection. Other possible causes include teething, food allergy, atopic disease, gastroesophageal reflux, and diaper dermatitis. Injuries such as corneal abrasion, occult fracture, and secondary to child abuse should be identified. It is important not to miss anatomic causes such as obstructive airway disease.

③ If possible, parents should be asked to keep a sleep log. This should include the following information: the time the child awoke in the morning, the time and duration of daytime naps, the time the child is put to bed at night, the time the child fell asleep, the time(s) awakened at night and what the parent did, and the time the parent fell asleep and woke up. It is also important to review sleep practices and influences. The term sleep hygiene is used to describe habits acquired for readying for, falling, and staying asleep. Bedtime settling practices create sleep associations and include rituals and routines used such as bedtime stories or songs, rocking, or comforting. The child's temperament and ability to self-soothe (e.g., thumb sucking, transitional objects) are important in the ability to fall asleep and maintain sleep. Feeding practices play an important role. Breast-fed infants may be more likely to wake up for feeding. Co-sleeping is controversial. In countries where co-sleeping is common it does not seem to be associated with sleep problems; studies in the United States suggest an association. It is important to be sensitive to parental attitudes and beliefs regarding co-sleeping. One must also determine whether the co-sleeping arrangement is due to the parent's beliefs or a response to a sleep problem.

④ Sleep onset association disorder describes a child who requires certain activities to fall asleep, such as rocking, singing, playing, or feeding. Some associations may be helpful in preparing the child for bed (reading), others may create problems (rocking) if the child tends to wake up and require the same behavior repeated to fall asleep.

⑤ Trained night feeders are babies who have a prolonged need for nighttime feeding. Beyond 6 months of age most night feeding may be considered a learned behavior. It is present in approximately 5% of children aged 6 months to 3 years. It may be considered a form of sleep onset association disorder because the child requires food or drink to return to sleep.

⑥ Parasomnias or disorders of arousal include night terrors and nightmares as well as sleep walking and talking. Night terrors occur early in the night during partial arousal from deep non–rapid eye movement (REM) sleep. The child may cry or scream and show signs of agitation; the child may appear disoriented or confused and seems unaware of the parent's presence. He or she may be difficult to arouse and on awakening usually has no memory of the event. This occurs most commonly in children aged 2 to 6 years. Nightmares usually occur later during the night during REM sleep. The child usually remembers the dream vividly, seems upset on waking, but can be comforted by the parent. The peak age at onset of nightmares is 3 to 5 years, but they can occur at any age, presumably even in preverbal children. Sleep walking (somnambulism) occurs, like sleep terrors, during non-REM sleep. The most common age at onset is between 4 to 8 years of age. Safety of the child is the primary concern with this disorder. Sleep talking (somniloquy) is not specific to any stage of sleep and has no clinical significance except that it may occur during nightmares or night terrors.

⑦ Obstructive sleep apnea is due to recurring episodes of upper airway obstruction and is associated with hypoxemia and hypercapnia. There may be a history of snoring and mouth breathing with episodes of apnea. It is often associated with airway obstruction due to hypertrophy of the tonsils and adenoids. Sleep apnea is associated with micrognathia, Pierre-Robin syndrome, Arnold-Chiari syndrome, and the Pickwickian syndrome. It often results in daytime hypersomnia.

⑧ The child's temperament plays an important role, with struggles for autonomy and attention-seeking behaviors further complicating the situation. Bedtime struggles are common in the first 4 years. They usually begin after 6 to 9 months of age with the acquisition of developmental skills-such as object permanence with consequent sepa-

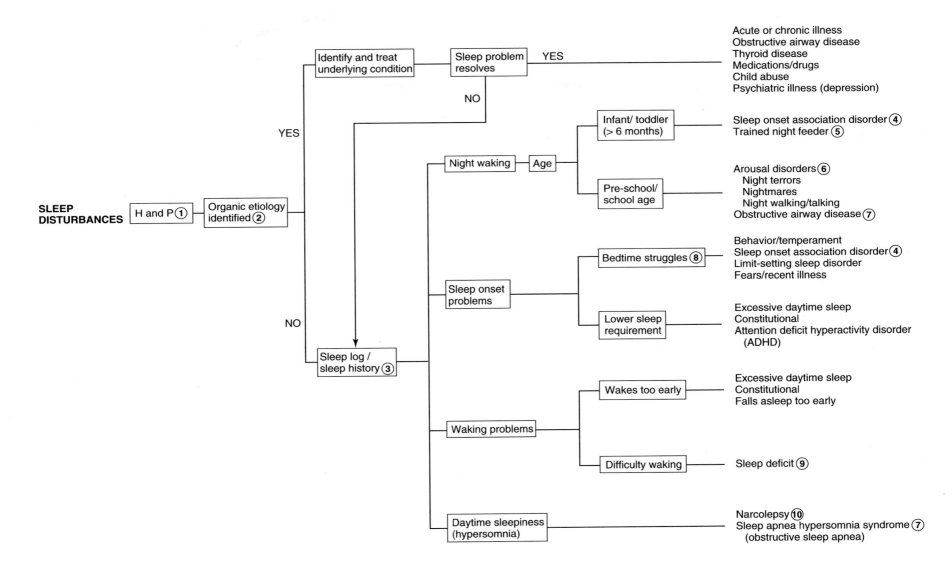

SLEEP DISTURBANCES — H and P ① — Organic etiology identified ②

YES → Identify and treat underlying condition → Sleep problem resolves → **YES**

- Acute or chronic illness
- Obstructive airway disease
- Thyroid disease
- Medications/drugs
- Child abuse
- Psychiatric illness (depression)

NO → Sleep log / sleep history ③

NO → Sleep log / sleep history ③

Night waking → Age

- Infant/ toddler (> 6 months) →
  - Sleep onset association disorder ④
  - Trained night feeder ⑤
- Pre-school/ school age →
  - Arousal disorders ⑥
    - Night terrors
    - Nightmares
    - Night walking/talking
  - Obstructive airway disease ⑦

Sleep onset problems

- Bedtime struggles ⑧ →
  - Behavior/temperament
  - Sleep onset association disorder ④
  - Limit-setting sleep disorder
  - Fears/recent illness
- Lower sleep requirement →
  - Excessive daytime sleep
  - Constitutional
  - Attention deficit hyperactivity disorder (ADHD)

Waking problems

- Wakes too early →
  - Excessive daytime sleep
  - Constitutional
  - Falls asleep too early
- Difficulty waking →
  - Sleep deficit ⑨

Daytime sleepiness (hypersomnia) →
- Narcolepsy ⑩
- Sleep apnea hypersomnia syndrome ⑦ (obstructive sleep apnea)

Nelson chapter 20.5

ration anxiety and the ability to pull to stand, which the child may use to avoid going to bed. Another problem may be the parent's inability to set limits (i.e., limit-setting sleep disorder). Difficulty settling to sleep may occur during an acute illness and may persist after recovery.

(9) A child who has difficulty waking up in the morning often has a sleep deficit. This is most common in adolescents because of increased activities and demands on their time. There is often an increased physiologic need for sleep at this time as well.

(10) Narcolepsy is a rare disorder with a characteristic irresistible daytime sleepiness. It may be associated with cataplexy (i.e., sudden loss of muscle tone) and rarely with hallucinations and sleep paralysis. It is rare in children; however, 25% of adults with narcolepsy report initial presentation during adolescence. Confirmation of the diagnosis requires referral to a sleep laboratory for polysomnography.

BIBLIOGRAPHY

Adair RH, Bauchner H: Sleep problems in childhood. Curr Probl Pediatr 23:147–170, 1993.

Anders TF, Carskadon MA, Dement WC: Sleep and sleepiness in children and adolescents. Pediatr Clin North Am 27:29–43, 1980.

Blum NJ, Carey WB: Sleep problems among infants and young children. Pediatr Rev 17:87–93, 1996.

Lozoff B, Zuckerman B: Sleep problems in children. Pediatr Rev 10:17–24, 1988.

Schmitt BD: When baby just won't sleep. Contemp Pediatr, May 1985, pp 38–52.

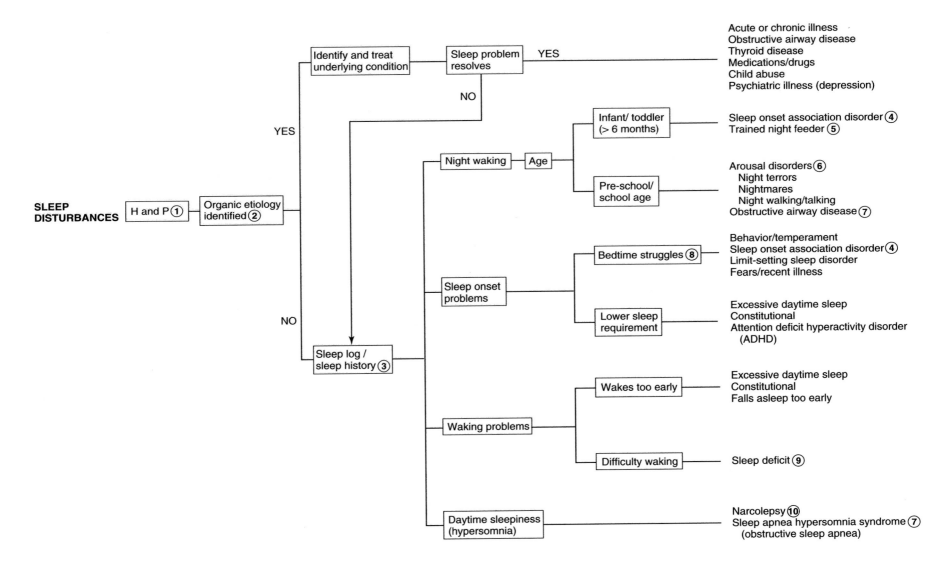

Nelson chapter 20.5

FLUIDS AND ELECTROLYTES

Acidemia is a blood pH less than 7.35. Excessive acidity of body fluids (acidosis) may be acute or chronic, primarily metabolic (decreased plasma bicarbonate), or primarily respiratory (increased partial pressure of CO_2). It may occur as part of a mixed acid-base disorder.

1 In acute acidosis, inquire about diarrhea or other gastrointestinal losses, medications, and possibility of ingestions. In young infants a history of poor feeding, failure to thrive, vomiting, lethargy, or seizures may indicate an inborn error of metabolism. Poor growth may be a clue to renal tubular acidosis in older children. Nonspecific symptoms of acidosis may include hyperventilation and Kussmaul breathing (i.e., deep, rapid respirations). Unusual breath odors may suggest diabetic ketoacidosis or ingestions.

2 The diagnosis is made by laboratory values. The pH reflecting extracellular free hydrogen ion $[H^+]$ concentration, partial pressure of CO_2 (PCO_2), and plasma bicarbonate level (HCO_3^-) are considered in clinical acid-base disorders. Their relationship is described by this modified version of the Henderson-Hasselbach equation:

$$[H^+] = 24 \times PCO_2 / HCO_3^-$$

When the HCO_3^- level is decreased, an increased respiratory rate occurs as a compensatory mechanism to try to maintain a normal pH. Renal compensation (i.e., secretion of excess H^+ and reabsorption of bicarbonate) is necessary to ultimately correct the acidosis because the lungs cannot create an absolute loss or gain of H^+ ions.

In mixed acid-base disorders, a combination of simple disorders occurs, such as in the child with chronic lung disease who experiences a combined metabolic alkalosis and respiratory acidosis. Guidelines exist for expected renal and respiratory compensation of acidemia. Mixed disorders should be suspected when the compensatory response differs from the predicted response. Compensation never overcorrects the pH and rarely corrects the pH to normal values.

Urine pH and urine electrolytes should be included in the preliminary analysis if renal tubular acidosis is suspected. A serum osmolality value will aid in narrowing the diagnosis of a metabolic acidosis with an increased anion gap.

3 Neuromuscular disorders that can result in a respiratory acidosis include brainstem or spinal cord disorders, including tumors, Guillain-Barré syndrome, polio, myasthenia gravis, muscular dystrophy, botulism, encephalopathy, and drugs (e.g., depressants, sedatives).

4 The anion gap (AG) reflects unmeasured anions, which, in combination with bicarbonate (HCO_3^-) and chloride (Cl^-), counterbalance the positive charge of the sodium (Na^+) ions.

$$AG = Na^+ - (Cl^- + HCO_3^-)$$

The normal anion gap is 12 mEq/l (range: 8 to 16 mEq/l). Elevation occurs secondary to an excess accumulation of acids (endogenous or ingested) or inadequate excretion of acids. Hyperchloremia occurs in a metabolic acidosis with a normal anion gap. An anion gap lower than expected may occur in the presence of hyperkalemia, hypercalcemia, hypoalbuminemia, hypermagnesemia, bromide intoxication, or laboratory error.

5 Ingestions should be suspected in young children or depressed adolescents at risk for suicide with an acute onset of symptoms (usually multisystemic), a history of previous accidental ingestions, or an altered level of consciousness.

6 A difference of greater than 10 to 15 mOsm/l between the measured serum osmolality and calculated serum osmolality suggests unmeasured osmotic particles (e.g., methanol, ethylene glycol).

$$\text{Calculated serum osmolality} = 2 [\text{serum } Na^+ + K^+] + BUN/2.8 + glucose/18$$

7 Ethylene glycol (radiator antifreeze) ingestion causes neurologic symptoms, respiratory failure, cardiovascular collapse, and renal failure. The increased anion gap is due to the accumulation of the metabolite formic acid. Lactic acidosis also frequently occurs.

8 Methanol (wood alcohol) ingestion causes gastrointestinal and neurologic symptoms. A severe blinding retinitis can also occur. The anion gap is due to the metabolites glyoxylic acid, formic acid, and oxalic acid. Lactic acidosis also occurs.

9 Salicylate ingestion in children is characterized by neurologic symptoms (e.g., coma, altered mental status, seizures) and hyperventilation. Fever may be prominent in infants. Younger children are more susceptible to metabolic acidosis. Respiratory alkalosis is the predominant acid-base abnormality in older patients.

10 Starvation, glycogen storage disease (type 1), and inborn errors of amino acid or organic acid metabolism are less common causes of ketoacidosis.

11 Lactic acidosis with blood lactate levels ≥ 5 mEq/l most commonly occurs due to hypotension, hypovolemia, or sepsis. Exercise, ethanol ingestion, and inborn errors of carbohydrate and energy metabolism are other causes.

12 An increased anion gap in renal failure occurs because impaired H^+ excretion prevents appropriate regeneration of HCO_3^-. Anions such as sulfate and phosphate also accumulate.

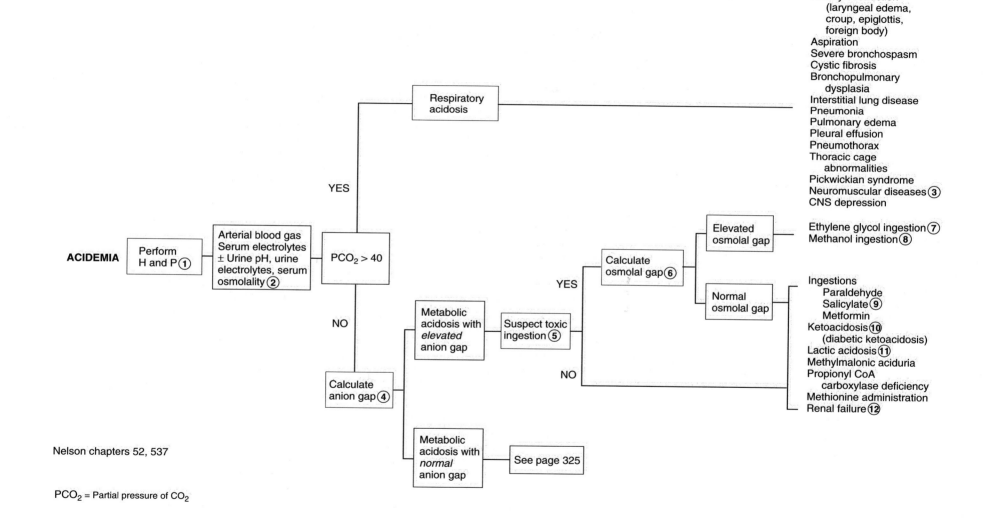

Airway obstruction
  (laryngeal edema,
  croup, epiglottis,
  foreign body)
Aspiration
Severe bronchospasm
Cystic fibrosis
Bronchopulmonary
  dysplasia
Interstitial lung disease
Pneumonia
Pulmonary edema
Pleural effusion
Pneumothorax
Thoracic cage
  abnormalities
Pickwickian syndrome
Neuromuscular diseases ③
CNS depression

Respiratory
acidosis

Elevated
osmolal gap

Ethylene glycol ingestion ⑦
Methanol ingestion ⑧

ACIDEMIA

Perform
H and P ①

Arterial blood gas
Serum electrolytes
± Urine pH, urine
electrolytes, serum
osmolality ②

PCO₂ > 40

YES

NO

YES

NO

Calculate
osmolal gap ⑥

Normal
osmolal gap

Ingestions
  Paraldehyde
  Salicylate ⑨
  Metformin
Ketoacidosis ⑩
  (diabetic ketoacidosis)
Lactic acidosis ⑪
Methylmalonic aciduria
Propionyl CoA
  carboxylase deficiency
Methionine administration
Renal failure ⑫

Metabolic
acidosis with
elevated
anion gap

Suspect toxic
ingestion ⑤

Calculate
anion gap ④

Metabolic
acidosis with
normal
anion gap

See page 325

Nelson chapters 52, 537

PCO₂ = Partial pressure of CO₂

Acidemia (continued)

13 Hyperkalemia develops without the effect of aldosterone. It may occur due to primary aldosterone deficiency or result from acquired kidney disease resulting in low renin levels.

14 Type IV renal tubular acidosis (RTA) is characterized by a deficiency of or impaired distal tubular response to aldosterone.

15 In pseudohypoaldosteronism both renin and aldosterone levels are elevated, but the response of the distal tubule to the aldosterone is impaired.

16 Certain medications (e.g., potassium-sparing diuretics, nonsteroidal antiinflammatory drugs, β-blocking agents, angiotensin-converting enzyme inhibitors, cyclosporine) can cause a functional hypoaldosteronism.

17 Urine pH should be measured on a fresh urine specimen. Serum electrolytes should be collected at the same time for the HCO_3^- level. The urine specimen can be taken at any time but should be obtained while the patient is still acidotic.

The urine pH reflects only free H^+ (less than 1% of the total H^+ excreted). It is often helpful to consider it in conjunction with a measure of net acid excretion, primarily urine ammonium concentration. Synthesis of ammonia (NH_3) and its subsequent excretion as ammonium (NH_4^+) are increased in most cases of systemic acidosis. The urinary anion gap is used to estimate the production of ammonium ion:

$$\text{Urine AG} = (\text{Urine Na}^+ + \text{Urine K}^+) - \text{Urine Cl}^-$$

The lower or more negative the gap, the greater the acid secretion in the form of NH_4^+.

18 RTA is characterized by an inability to adequately acidify the urine in the presence of a normal anion gap (hyperchloremic) acidosis. It may occur primarily or in association with multiple inherited disorders or acquired systemic disorders. In the distal and proximal subtypes, volume contraction results in an aldosterone-mediated hypokalemia.

In distal (type I or classic) RTA, a permanent deficiency of H^+ secretion by the distal tubules results in wasting of a portion of the filtered load of HCO_3^-. The HCO_3^- wasting persists even in the presence of severe systemic acidosis; urine pH is never more acidic than 5.8. The urine anion gap is a small or low negative value.

In proximal RTA (type II or HCO_3^- wasting) a defect in the proximal tubular reabsorption of HCO_3^- results in a higher load of HCO_3^- being presented to the distal tubule. In mild acidosis, this excess HCO_3^- is lost in the urine because its amount exceeds the capacity of the distal tubule for reabsorption in the normal distal tubule. In more severe acidosis a lower amount of HCO_3^- is filtered and is able to be reabsorbed in the normal distal tubule. Because distal acidification mechanisms are intact in proximal RTA, urine pH will become more acidic (pH < 5.5) under these circumstances. The urine anion gap is a high negative value, regardless of the severity or duration of the acidosis. Accompanying hypokalemia can be severe.

19 Rapid volume expansion with non–HCO_3^--containing solutions can cause transient small HCO_3^- losses in the urine.

20 Premature infants and neonates with renal function that is normal for maturation may demonstrate a mild metabolic acidosis due to a transient reduced threshold for HCO_3^- reabsorption. This normally corrects by 4 to 6 weeks in the premature infant and by 3 weeks in the term infant.

21 Increased HCO_3^- losses in diarrhea can contribute to a metabolic acidosis.

BIBLIOGRAPHY

Brewer ED: Disorders of acid-base balance. Pediatr Clin North Am 37:429–447, 1990.

Hanna JD, Scheinman JI, Chan JC: The kidney in acid-base balance. Pediatr Clin North Am 42:1365–1395, 1995.

ACIDEMIA (continued)

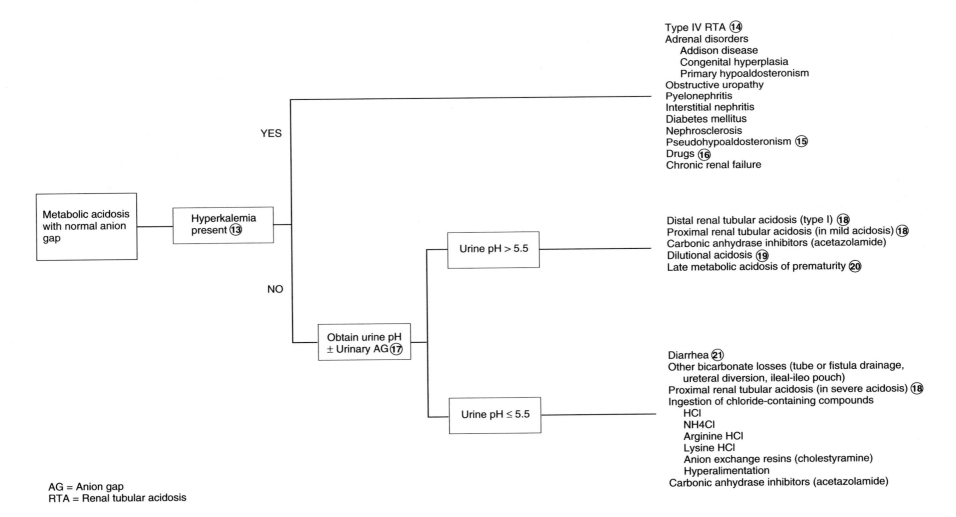

Type IV RTA ⑭
Adrenal disorders
    Addison disease
    Congenital hyperplasia
    Primary hypoaldosteronism
Obstructive uropathy
Pyelonephritis
Interstitial nephritis
Diabetes mellitus
Nephrosclerosis
Pseudohypoaldosteronism ⑮
Drugs ⑯
Chronic renal failure

Metabolic acidosis with normal anion gap

Hyperkalemia present ⑬

YES

NO

Obtain urine pH ± Urinary AG ⑰

Urine pH > 5.5

Distal renal tubular acidosis (type I) ⑱
Proximal renal tubular acidosis (in mild acidosis) ⑱
Carbonic anhydrase inhibitors (acetazolamide)
Dilutional acidosis ⑲
Late metabolic acidosis of prematurity ⑳

Urine pH ≤ 5.5

Diarrhea ㉑
Other bicarbonate losses (tube or fistula drainage,
    ureteral diversion, ileal-ileo pouch)
Proximal renal tubular acidosis (in severe acidosis) ⑱
Ingestion of chloride-containing compounds
    HCl
    NH4Cl
    Arginine HCl
    Lysine HCl
    Anion exchange resins (cholestyramine)
    Hyperalimentation
Carbonic anhydrase inhibitors (acetazolamide)

AG = Anion gap
RTA = Renal tubular acidosis

Alkalemia is a serum pH above 7.45. The term alkalosis refers to the process resulting in excess total body bicarbonate (HCO_3^-) or deficit of total body hydrogen. The disorder may be acute or chronic, primarily metabolic, or primarily respiratory or occur as a part of a mixed acid-base disorder.

(1) The history should inquire about underlying medical problems and medication use, as well as potential losses of gastrointestinal fluid (e.g., vomiting, diarrhea, nasogastric drainage). The diet history should inquire about the possibility of ingestion of natural licorice, but most licorice in the United States is artificially flavored. A prenatal history of polyhydramnios and history of prematurity may suggest a primary renal hypokalemic syndrome (e.g., Bartter syndrome). Older children should be asked about use of chewing tobacco because some brands may contain an acid with a mineralocorticoid effect.

(2) The pH (reflecting extracellular free hydrogen ion [H^+] concentration), partial pressure of CO_2 (PCO_2), and plasma HCO_3^- level are considered in clinical acid-base disorders. Their relationship is described by this modified version of the Henderson-Hasselbalch equation:

$$[H^+] = 24 \times PCO_2 / HCO_3^-$$

In response to an increased pH, the body normally attempts to decrease total serum HCO_3^- (renal compensation) and increase PCO_2 (respiratory compensation). In mixed acid-base disorders, a combination of simple disorders occurs, such as in the child with vomiting and diarrhea who may experience a metabolic alkalosis and metabolic acidosis. Guidelines exist for expected renal and respiratory compensation of alkalemia. Mixed disorders should be suspected when the compensatory response is different from the predicted response. If metabolic alkalosis is suggested, a spot urinary chloride level should be obtained.

(3) Respiratory alkalosis occurs when a primary decrease in PCO_2 causes an increase in the pH to greater than 7.45. Hyperventilation of various causes is the most common etiology. Tachypnea is often obvious initially. In chronic respiratory alkalosis, the respiratory rate may approach normal, with the patient taking deeper breaths.

(4) A metabolic alkalosis occurs when a primary increase in extracellular HCO_3^- causes a rise in the pH above 7.45. The etiology may be loss of H^+, gain of HCO_3^-, or loss of extracellular fluid with chloride losses exceeding HCO_3^- losses. Factors that prevent renal excretion of HCO_3^- (e.g., renal failure, volume depletion, profound hypokalemia) must be present to maintain a metabolic alkalosis. Volume depletion results in aldosterone-mediated sodium retention in exchange for potassium and H^+ secretion, which maintains an alkalosis (i.e., contraction alkalosis) with a paradoxical aciduria. Hypokalemia is a stimulus for additional renal H^+ secretion.

(5) If the etiology of a metabolic alkalosis is not clear from the history and physical examination, a spot urine chloride test will aid in the diagnosis.

(6) The loss of hydrochloric acid (HCl) due to vomiting or nasogastric fluid drainage leads to increased gastric HCl production, which is accompanied by systemic HCO_3^- production. The alkalosis is further maintained by volume depletion that results in aldosterone-mediated renal absorption of sodium in exchange for H^+ and potassium secretion.

(7) High urinary chloride losses (e.g., sodium chloride) occur shortly after beginning diuretic therapy. Urinary chloride losses are minimized with prolonged therapy because of chloride depletion and subsequent volume contraction. The volume contraction results in aldosterone-mediated sodium and closely linked chloride reabsorption and H^+ secretion.

(8) In congenital chloride-wasting diarrhea, a rare inherited disorder, a defect of the normal chloride-for-HCO_3^- exchange in the ileum and colon leads to increased gastrointestinal losses of chloride and subsequent metabolic alkalosis.

(9) Infants with cystic fibrosis require more sodium chloride than is contained in usual formulas or breast milk. High losses of sodium chloride in sweat that are not countered by dietary intake can cause volume contraction and mild metabolic alkalosis.

(10) Rapid recovery from compensated chronic respiratory acidosis can cause posthypercapnia metabolic alkalosis. This scenario is most likely to occur in infants with bronchopulmonary dysplasia who have experienced sodium chloride losses and volume depletion from diuretic use. After correction of the hypercapnia and despite normalization of the pH, renal HCO_3^- reabsorption is favored until volume and chloride depletion is corrected.

(11) Ingestion of exogenous sources of alkali (e.g., citrate, acetate, lactate, HCO_3^-) is occasionally sufficient to generate a metabolic alkalosis. Excessive transfusions with citrated blood or Plasmanate containing acetate are other possible causes.

(12) High levels of urinary chloride indicate some impairment of urinary reabsorption of chloride. The presence or absence of hypertension can help clarify the diagnosis.

(13) Mineralocorticoid excess typically results in volume expansion and hypertension. Congenital adrenal hyperplasia with deficiencies of the 11-hydroxylase or 17-hydroxylase enzymes results in levels of desoxycorticosterone (an aldosterone precursor) high enough to exert a significant mineralocorticoid effect. Natural licorice and some chewing tobaccos have glycyrrhizic acid that creates a mineralocorticoid effect.

(14) Bartter syndrome is a rare renal tubular disorder characterized by hypokalemic metabolic alkalosis, urinary chloride wasting, increased

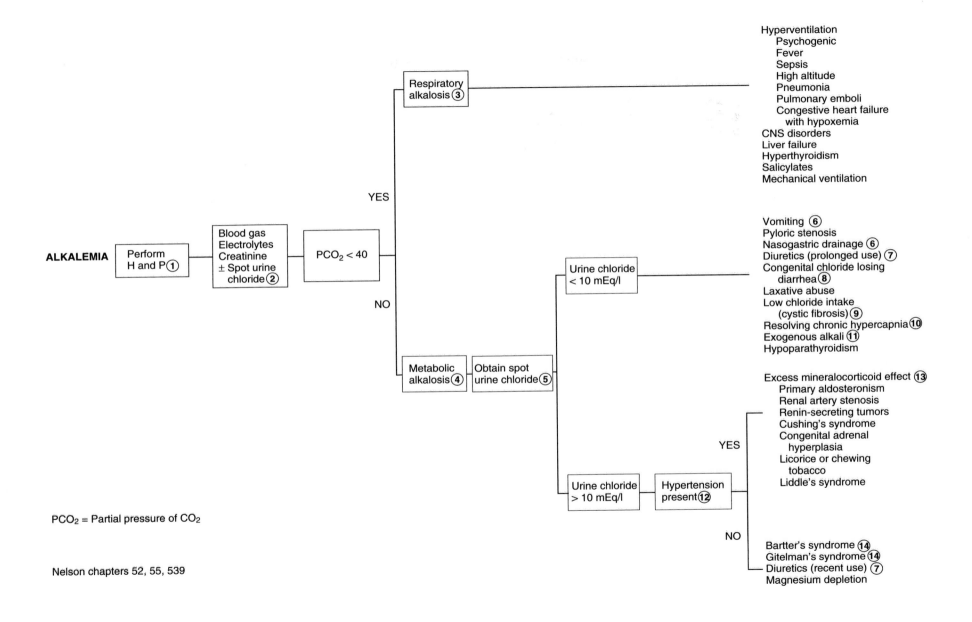

ALKALEMIA

Perform H and P ①

Blood gas
Electrolytes
Creatinine
± Spot urine chloride ②

$PCO_2 < 40$

YES → Respiratory alkalosis ③

Hyperventilation
  Psychogenic
  Fever
  Sepsis
  High altitude
  Pneumonia
  Pulmonary emboli
  Congestive heart failure
    with hypoxemia
CNS disorders
Liver failure
Hyperthyroidism
Salicylates
Mechanical ventilation

NO → Metabolic alkalosis ④ → Obtain spot urine chloride ⑤

Urine chloride < 10 mEq/l

Vomiting ⑥
Pyloric stenosis
Nasogastric drainage ⑥
Diuretics (prolonged use) ⑦
Congenital chloride losing
  diarrhea ⑧
Laxative abuse
Low chloride intake
  (cystic fibrosis) ⑨
Resolving chronic hypercapnia ⑩
Exogenous alkali ⑪
Hypoparathyroidism

Urine chloride > 10 mEq/l → Hypertension present ⑫

YES

Excess mineralocorticoid effect ⑬
  Primary aldosteronism
  Renal artery stenosis
  Renin-secreting tumors
  Cushing's syndrome
  Congenital adrenal
    hyperplasia
  Licorice or chewing
    tobacco
  Liddle's syndrome

NO

Bartter's syndrome ⑭
Gitelman's syndrome ⑭
Diuretics (recent use) ⑦
Magnesium depletion

PCO_2 = Partial pressure of CO_2

Nelson chapters 52, 55, 539

plasma renin and aldosterone levels, and normal to low blood pressure. Children exhibit failure to thrive, short stature, polyuria, polydipsia, and tendency to get dehydrated. Gitelman syndrome is a similar but more benign tubular disorder characterized by hypokalemia and urinary magnesium wasting. Children with this syndrome exhibit short stature after age 6 years and are prone to febrile seizures and hypomagnesemic-tetanic episodes. The two disorders can be distinguished by urinary calcium levels, which are high in Bartter syndrome and low in Gitelman syndrome.

BIBLIOGRAPHY

Avner E: Clinical disorders of water metabolism. Pediatr Ann 24:23, 1995.

Brewer ED: Disorders of acid-base balance. Pediatr Clin North Am 37:429–447, 1990.

Hanna JD, Scheinman JI, Chan JC: The kidney in acid-base balance. Pediatr Clin North Am 42:1365–1395, 1995.

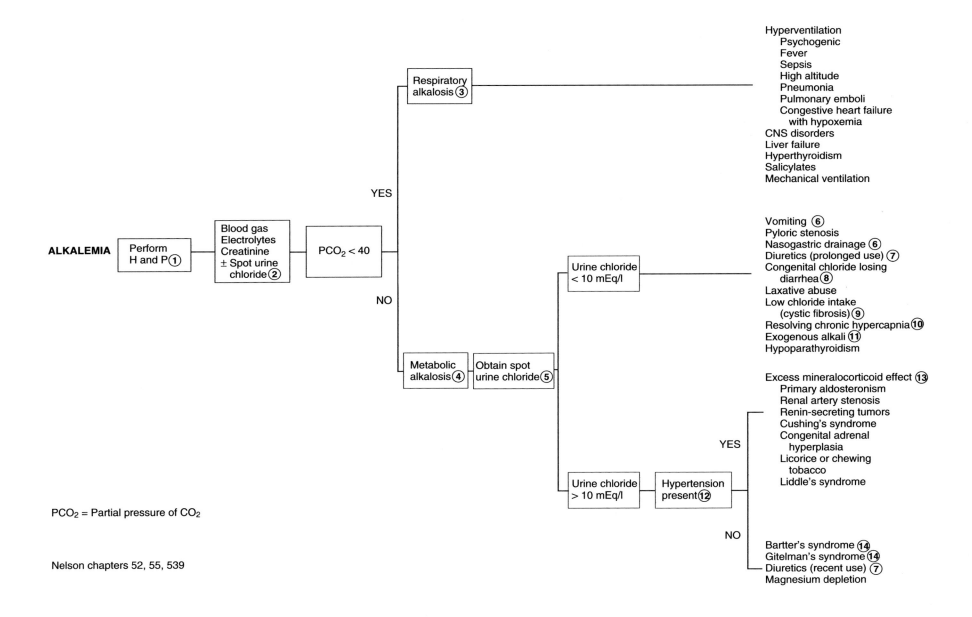

ALKALEMIA

Perform H and P ①

Blood gas
Electrolytes
Creatinine
± Spot urine chloride ②

$PCO_2 < 40$

YES → Respiratory alkalosis ③

Hyperventilation
    Psychogenic
    Fever
    Sepsis
    High altitude
    Pneumonia
    Pulmonary emboli
    Congestive heart failure
       with hypoxemia
CNS disorders
Liver failure
Hyperthyroidism
Salicylates
Mechanical ventilation

NO → Metabolic alkalosis ④ → Obtain spot urine chloride ⑤

Urine chloride < 10 mEq/l

Vomiting ⑥
Pyloric stenosis
Nasogastric drainage ⑥
Diuretics (prolonged use) ⑦
Congenital chloride losing diarrhea ⑧
Laxative abuse
Low chloride intake (cystic fibrosis) ⑨
Resolving chronic hypercapnia ⑩
Exogenous alkali ⑪
Hypoparathyroidism

Urine chloride > 10 mEq/l → Hypertension present ⑫

YES →
Excess mineralocorticoid effect ⑬
    Primary aldosteronism
    Renal artery stenosis
    Renin-secreting tumors
    Cushing's syndrome
    Congenital adrenal hyperplasia
    Licorice or chewing tobacco
    Liddle's syndrome

NO →
Bartter's syndrome ⑭
Gitelman's syndrome ⑭
Diuretics (recent use) ⑦
Magnesium depletion

PCO_2 = Partial pressure of CO_2

Nelson chapters 52, 55, 539

Sodium (Na⁺) is the primary cation of the extracellular fluid (ECF) compartment and is the major osmotically active solute in the ECF. Osmolality is the measurement of the number of solute particles in a unit of volume. It can be measured or estimated by the formula:

$$\text{Calculated serum osmolality} = 2[\text{serum Na}^+ + \text{K}^+] + \text{BUN}/2.8 + \text{glucose}/18$$

The body responds to changes in osmolality by increasing or suppressing thirst and antidiuretic hormone (ADH) release.

(1) Signs and symptoms of hypernatremia are nonspecific. Thirst will be increased as long as the brain's thirst centers are intact. Excessive thirst to the point it disrupts sleep or play and enuresis may be a clue to diabetes. Neurologic symptoms (e.g., irritability, lethargy, confusion, seizures) may be present in severe cases.

Inquire about volume losses (diarrhea, vomiting), oral intake, and urine output. Specifically ask about formula preparation and the possibility of excessive salt intake (e.g., of table salt or sea water). Polyuria and polydipsia may suggest diabetes mellitus or insipidus. Infants with fever, very low birth weight infants, and children with cystic fibrosis or heat stroke are at risk for hypernatremia because of excessive (hypotonic) sweat losses. Infants who cry excessively and are satisfied with water rather than milk should be evaluated for diabetes insipidus (DI). The medical history should also inquire about renal disease and CNS disease or hemorrhage, which may be a risk factor for central DI.

(2) The approach to hypernatremia is best initiated with an assessment of the patient's volume status. Hypovolemia manifests as lethargy, dry mucous membranes, and decreased skin turgor. Infants will exhibit decreased tearing and a sunken fontanel. Tachycardia, orthostatic hypotension, and oliguria are also common. Fever may occur as both a cause and an effect of hypernatremic dehydration. The signs of ECF volume losses are less pronounced in hypernatremic dehydration than in hyponatremic dehydration.

Patients appear to have a normal volume status (euvolemia) when total body water is decreased in the presence of normal or near-normal sodium content. This situation occurs secondary to inadequate water intake or solute-free water losses. These water losses may be extrarenal or renal (DI). Extrarenal losses will produce hypertonic urine. Urine sodium may be variable. Renal losses result in hypotonic urine.

Hypervolemia occurs when total body water is essentially normal in the presence of increased total body sodium. Manifestations of excess ECF volume include edema and congestive heart failure.

(3) Diarrhea is most likely to lead to hyponatremic or isonatremic dehydration; hypernatremic dehydration is likely if fluid intake is low (vomiting, anorexia), fever is present (increased free water insensible losses), or hypertonic fluids are being given. Lactulose for constipation or hepatic failure may cause diarrhea, resulting in hypernatremic dehydration.

(4) Insensible water losses from the respiratory tract occur due to hyperventilation or respiratory distress. Dermal losses are common in infants placed on a radiant warmer and in settings of increased ambient temperature.

(5) Although adipsia is rare, it can occur as a primary entity or secondary to hypothalamic lesions, hydrocephalus, or head trauma.

(6) Hypotonic urine and polyuria in the presence of hypernatremia suggest DI. DI is an inability to effectively conserve urinary water. Hypernatremia in DI most often occurs when access to water is restricted. Because young children do not usually have control over their fluid intake, most pediatric cases of DI occur as hypovolemia. DI may also occur secondary to lack of ADH production (central DI) or renal resistance to ADH (nephrogenic DI).

(7) A water deprivation test should be carefully monitored in the hospital and should be done during daytime hours rather than overnight. During water deprivation, the body weight should not be allowed to decline by more than 3%.

(8) The response to intramuscular aqueous vasopressin (0.1 to 0.2 units/kg) will help to confirm the diagnosis of DI and distinguish between central and renal causes.

(9) Central DI is probably the diagnosis if, after administration of vasopressin, the urine:serum ratio becomes greater than 1, although psychogenic polydipsia needs to be ruled out. Patients with psychogenic polydipsia (i.e., water intoxication) will usually concentrate urine when fluids are withheld. Diagnosis is occasionally difficult because the maximal urinary concentration achievable after dehydration is lowered in prolonged cases of psychogenic polydipsia. If the administration of vasopressin produces a higher urinary concentration than dehydration does, DI is the diagnosis regardless of the level of urinary concentration.

Central DI may be primary (familial or nonfamilial) or occur secondary to head trauma or several disease states (suprasellar or intrasellar tumors, granulomatous disease, histiocytosis, CNS infection or hemorrhage). ADH release can also be inhibited by stress (e.g., pain from surgery or trauma) and certain drugs and medications (e.g., α-adrenergic agonists, alcohol, opiate antagonists, phenytoin, clonidine) and carbon monoxide poisoning. The disorder has also been associated with cleft lip and palate.

(10) Nephrogenic DI may be congenital or secondary to multiple types of renal disease. Males with primary nephrogenic DI are likely to have a significant history of polyuria, polydipsia, and previous episodes of hypernatremic dehydration. Females with a primary defect have milder symptoms and tend to be diagnosed later in life.

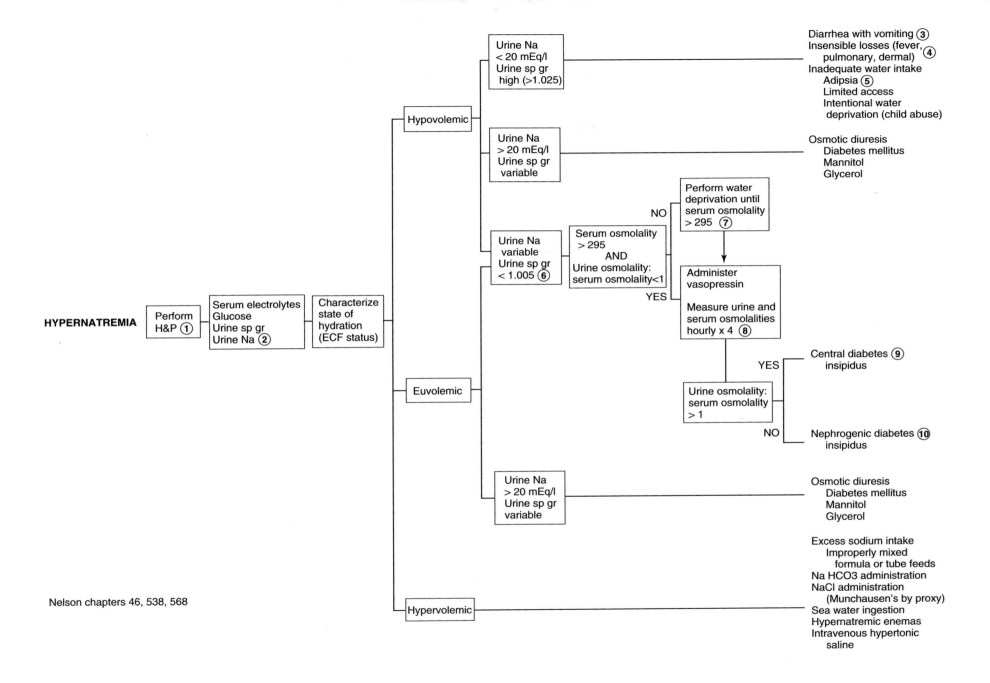

HYPERNATREMIA

Perform H&P (1)

Serum electrolytes
Glucose
Urine sp gr
Urine Na (2)

Characterize state of hydration (ECF status)

Hypovolemic

Urine Na < 20 mEq/l
Urine sp gr high (>1.025)

Diarrhea with vomiting (3)
Insensible losses (fever, pulmonary, dermal) (4)
Inadequate water intake
  Adipsia (5)
  Limited access
  Intentional water deprivation (child abuse)

Urine Na > 20 mEq/l
Urine sp gr variable

Osmotic diuresis
  Diabetes mellitus
  Mannitol
  Glycerol

Euvolemic

Urine Na variable
Urine sp gr < 1.005 (6)

Serum osmolality > 295
AND
Urine osmolality: serum osmolality<1

NO → Perform water deprivation until serum osmolality > 295 (7)

YES → Administer vasopressin

Measure urine and serum osmolalities hourly x 4 (8)

Urine osmolality: serum osmolality > 1

YES → Central diabetes insipidus (9)

NO → Nephrogenic diabetes insipidus (10)

Urine Na > 20 mEq/l
Urine sp gr variable

Osmotic diuresis
  Diabetes mellitus
  Mannitol
  Glycerol

Hypervolemic

Excess sodium intake
  Improperly mixed formula or tube feeds
Na HCO3 administration
NaCl administration
  (Munchausen's by proxy)
Sea water ingestion
Hypernatremic enemas
Intravenous hypertonic saline

Nelson chapters 46, 538, 568

It can also be caused by drugs or medications (e.g., lithium, demeclocycline, methoxyflurane, amphotericin B, cyclophosphamide, propoxyphene, cisplatin, angiographic dyes, osmotic diuretics), hypokalemia, and hypercalcemia.

BIBLIOGRAPHY

Avner E: Clinical disorders of water metabolism. Pediatr Ann 24:23, 1995.
Conley SB: Hypernatremia. Pediatr Clin North Am 37:365–372, 1990.

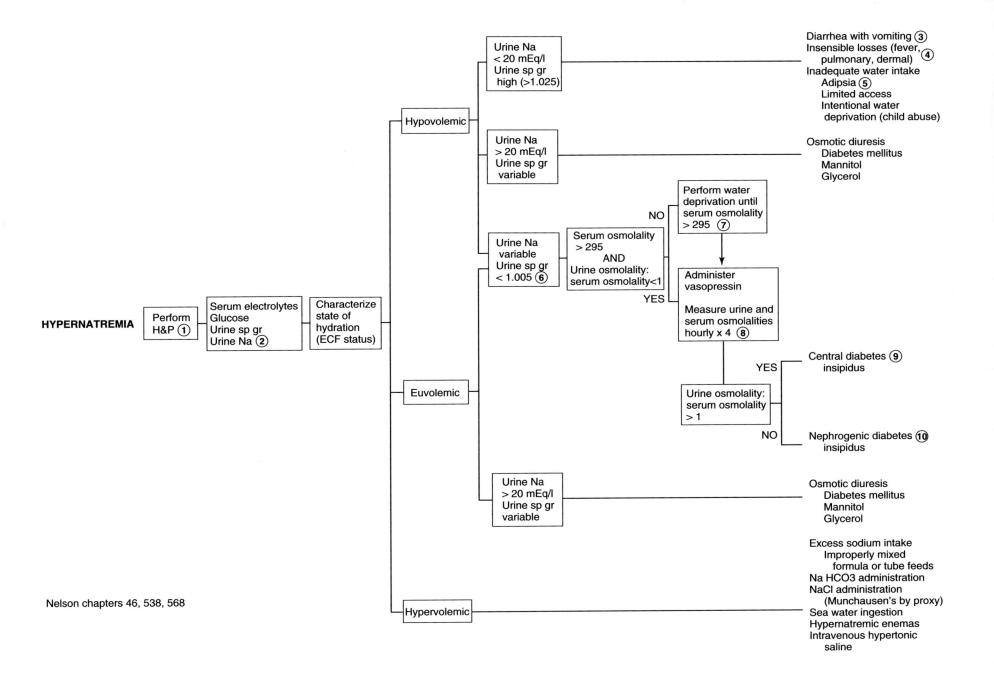

HYPERNATREMIA

Perform H&P ①

Serum electrolytes
Glucose
Urine sp gr
Urine Na ②

Characterize state of hydration (ECF status)

Hypovolemic

Urine Na < 20 mEq/l
Urine sp gr high (>1.025)

Diarrhea with vomiting ③
Insensible losses (fever, pulmonary, dermal) ④
Inadequate water intake
  Adipsia ⑤
  Limited access
  Intentional water deprivation (child abuse)

Urine Na > 20 mEq/l
Urine sp gr variable

Osmotic diuresis
  Diabetes mellitus
  Mannitol
  Glycerol

Euvolemic

Urine Na variable
Urine sp gr < 1.005 ⑥

Serum osmolality > 295
AND
Urine osmolality: serum osmolality<1

NO → Perform water deprivation until serum osmolality > 295 ⑦

YES → Administer vasopressin

Measure urine and serum osmolalities hourly x 4 ⑧

Urine osmolality: serum osmolality > 1

YES → Central diabetes insipidus ⑨

NO → Nephrogenic diabetes insipidus ⑩

Urine Na > 20 mEq/l
Urine sp gr variable

Osmotic diuresis
  Diabetes mellitus
  Mannitol
  Glycerol

Hypervolemic

Excess sodium intake
  Improperly mixed formula or tube feeds
Na HCO3 administration
NaCl administration (Munchausen's by proxy)
Sea water ingestion
Hypernatremic enemas
Intravenous hypertonic saline

Nelson chapters 46, 538, 568

Chapter 85 *Hyponatremia*

Sodium (Na^+) is the primary cation of the extracellular fluid (ECF) compartment and is the major osmotically active solute in the ECF. Osmolality is the measurement of the number of solute particles in a unit of volume. It can be measured or estimated by the formula:

$$\text{Calculated serum osmolality} = 2 \text{ [serum } Na^+ + K^+\text{]} + BUN/2.8 + \text{glucose}/18$$

The body responds to changes in osmolality by increasing or suppressing thirst and antidiuretic hormone (ADH) release.

(1) The history should inquire about gastrointestinal losses (e.g., vomiting, diarrhea). Ask about fluid intake, urine output, medications, and possibility of a toxic ingestion. For infants, inquire specifically about formula preparation and amount of free water ingested. Ingestions should be suspected in young children aged 1 to 5 years old with an acute onset of symptoms, a history of previous accidental ingestions, neurologic symptoms, or an unusual breath odor. Signs of hyponatremia usually manifest when the sodium level falls rapidly below 120 mEq/l. Signs and symptoms may include apathy, anorexia, nausea, vomiting, altered mental status, and seizures. Musculoskeletal symptoms include cramps and weakness.

(2) If the preliminary laboratory evaluation reveals a significantly elevated blood urea nitrogen and creatinine value *not* believed to be caused by dehydration, a pediatric nephrologist should be consulted for further evaluation of presumed renal failure.

(3) Hyponatremia most commonly occurs in conjunction with a hypotonic state. The presence of lipemic serum or clinical clues suggestive of diabetes mellitus (e.g., polyuria, polydipsia, weight loss, hyperglycemia) or a possible ingestion should prompt consideration of nonhypotonic states.

(4) Older methods of electrolyte measurement determined sodium in mEq/l of plasma as opposed to plasma water, which could yield an artificially low sodium value (pseudohyponatremia) in the presence of hyperlipidemia (nephrotic syndrome) or hyperproteinemia, which is rare in children. Newer methods use ion-selective electrodes to measure serum sodium activity directly in plasma water and do not produce this artifact.

(5) Hyponatremia occurs in a hypertonic setting when an osmotically active solute has been added to the ECF. A difference of greater than 10 to 15 mOsm/l between the measured serum osmolality and the calculated serum osmolality is suggestive of a nonglucose solute in the ECF and may be the first clue to certain ingestions (e.g., of methanol, ethanol).

(6) Assessment of the patient's overall volume status is essential in the evaluation of hyponatremia.

Hypovolemia (dehydration) manifests as lethargy, dry mucous membranes, and decreased skin turgor. Infants will exhibit decreased tearing and a sunken fontanel. Tachycardia, orthostatic hypotension, and oliguria are also common.

Patients appear to have a normal volume status (euvolemia) when total body sodium is normal or near normal in the presence of a slight excess of body water. Most patients presenting with euvolemic hyponatremia have a syndrome of inappropriate antidiuretic hormone secretion (SIADH). Although characterized as euvolemic, many of these patients will have a slightly increased but clinically unimportant ECF volume.

Hypervolemia occurs when total body water is increased to a greater degree than total body sodium in either edema-forming states or renal failure.

HYPONATREMIA

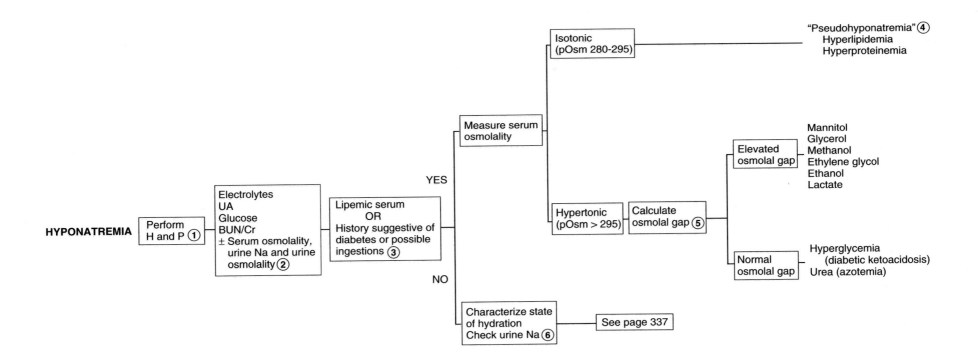

Perform H and P ①

Electrolytes
UA
Glucose
BUN/Cr
± Serum osmolality,
  urine Na and urine
  osmolality ②

Lipemic serum
OR
History suggestive of
diabetes or possible
ingestions ③

YES

Measure serum osmolality

Isotonic
(pOsm 280–295)

"Pseudohyponatremia" ④
Hyperlipidemia
Hyperproteinemia

Hypertonic
(pOsm > 295)

Calculate osmolal gap ⑤

Elevated osmolal gap

Mannitol
Glycerol
Methanol
Ethylene glycol
Ethanol
Lactate

Normal osmolal gap

Hyperglycemia
  (diabetic ketoacidosis)
Urea (azotemia)

NO

Characterize state
of hydration
Check urine Na ⑥

See page 337

Nelson chapters 46, 569

(7) Renal disorders causing sodium wasting include nephritis, medullary cystic disease, polycystic kidney disease, and obstructive uropathies. Premature infants may have limited reabsorption of sodium leading to salt wasting.

In proximal renal tubular acidosis (RTA), reduced proximal tubular reabsorption of bicarbonate results in an obligatory loss of sodium. Type IV RTA is caused by either a lack of aldosterone or an insensitivity to it (i.e., pseudohypoaldosteronism), resulting in increased renal losses of sodium.

(8) Conditions in which isotonic fluid translocates to a "third space" include burns, pancreatitis, muscle trauma, peritonitis, ascites, and other effusions.

(9) Water intoxication as a cause of hyponatremia occurs in children receiving intravenous fluids in the presence of some level of impaired water excretion. For instance, infants are less efficient at excreting water and, therefore, are at higher risk for water intoxication. Infants younger than 6 months of age fed excessive amounts of water may also develop hyponatremia and seizures. Rare causes include tap water enemas and swallowed swimming pool water. Psychogenic polydipsia is most likely to occur in mentally disturbed patients.

(10) The syndrome of SIADH is characterized by a sustained or intermittent secretion of ADH that is inappropriate based on the volume status and serum osmolality. The urine osmolality is generally higher than the serum osmolality and higher than expected for the degree of hyponatremia. The urine sodium is usually higher than expected for the degree of hyponatremia in SIADH. The diagnosis is one of exclusion and should only be made in the presence of normal renal, adrenal, pituitary, and thyroid function, and in the absence of hypovolemia, dehydration, and edema. The condition can occur due to numerous causes, including CNS disorders, pulmonary disorders, tumors, and medications. Postoperative pain and stress are also causes.

(11) In glucocorticoid deficiency, ADH release is not maximally suppressed. The condition resembles SIADH, except that it will respond to exogenous glucocorticoid.

(12) A reset osmostat is a variant of SIADH affecting chronically ill children. The plasma osmolality level at which ADH release occurs is reset downward, so that these patients have chronic hyponatremia. Water loading decreases ADH secretion, and sodium loading increases ADH secretion and concentrates the urine.

(13) Hypervolemia occurs when total-body water is increased to a greater degree than total-body sodium. Patients usually have an impaired ability to excrete water and may have decreased intravascular volume. A manifestation of excess ECF volume is peripheral edema, as noted in cirrhosis and heart failure. All cases are further complicated by an increased secretion of ADH, which leads to further water retention.

BIBLIOGRAPHY

Avner E: Clinical disorders of water metabolism. Pediatr Ann 24:23, 1995.
Berry PL, Belsha CW: Hyponatremia. Pediatr Clin North Am 37:351–363, 1990.
Trachtman H: Sodium and water homeostasis. Pediatr Clin North Am 42:1343–1363, 1995.

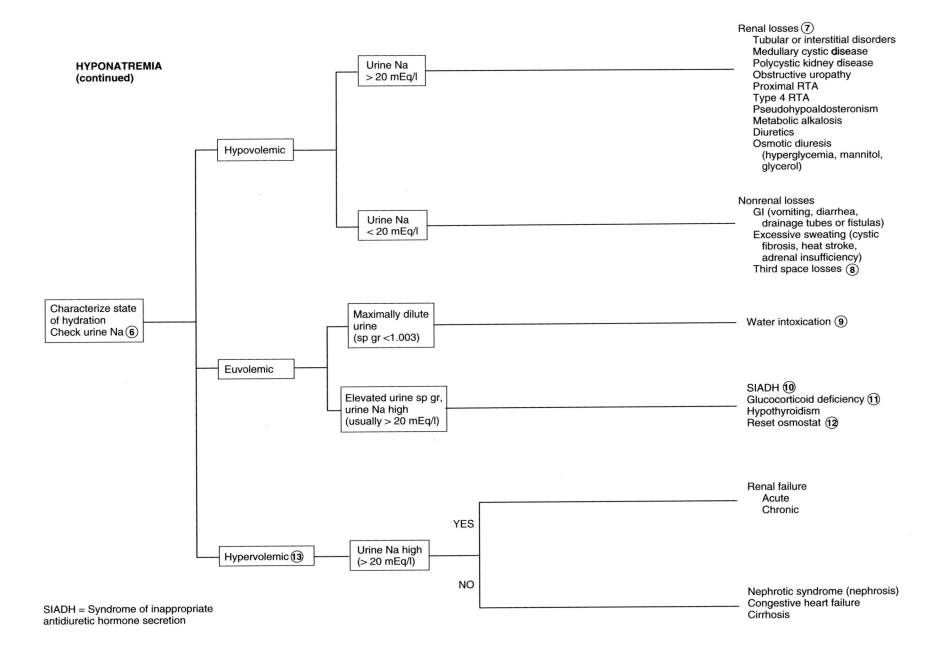

HYPONATREMIA
(continued)

Characterize state
of hydration
Check urine Na ⑥

Hypovolemic

Urine Na
> 20 mEq/l

Renal losses ⑦
   Tubular or interstitial disorders
   Medullary cystic disease
   Polycystic kidney disease
   Obstructive uropathy
   Proximal RTA
   Type 4 RTA
   Pseudohypoaldosteronism
   Metabolic alkalosis
   Diuretics
   Osmotic diuresis
      (hyperglycemia, mannitol,
      glycerol)

Urine Na
< 20 mEq/l

Nonrenal losses
   GI (vomiting, diarrhea,
      drainage tubes or fistulas)
   Excessive sweating (cystic
      fibrosis, heat stroke,
      adrenal insufficiency)
   Third space losses ⑧

Euvolemic

Maximally dilute
urine
(sp gr <1.003)

Water intoxication ⑨

Elevated urine sp gr,
urine Na high
(usually > 20 mEq/l)

SIADH ⑩
Glucocorticoid deficiency ⑪
Hypothyroidism
Reset osmostat ⑫

Hypervolemic ⑬

Urine Na high
(> 20 mEq/l)

YES

Renal failure
   Acute
   Chronic

NO

Nephrotic syndrome (nephrosis)
Congestive heart failure
Cirrhosis

SIADH = Syndrome of inappropriate
antidiuretic hormone secretion

Chapter 86 *Hypokalemia*

Potassium is the main cation of the intracellular fluid (ICF) compartment. The extracellular fluid (ECF) concentration is carefully regulated to maintain a value around 4 mEq/l. Potassium (K^+) plays a critical role in the excitability of nerve and muscle cells and contractility of muscles (smooth, skeletal, cardiac). Aldosterone normally regulates renal excretion of potassium. Aldosterone also causes sodium reabsorption and H^+ secretion in the distal tubule. Aldosterone similarly affects potassium excretion in the stool. Hypokalemia is defined as a serum potassium concentration < 3.5 mEq/l.

(1) The history should inquire about medications, underlying medical problems, and diet including the use of salt substitutes and pica. Muscle weakness, hyporeflexia, and intestinal ileus are manifestations of hypokalemia. Cardiac arrhythmias are the most serious complications. Flattened T waves, a short PR interval, and a prolonged QT interval are characteristic EKG abnormalities. A U wave may develop after the QRS complex. Patients may also be lethargic or confused and may have muscle cramping, rhabdomyolysis, and myoglobinuria in cases of severe potassium depletion.

(2) Acid-base disorders and disturbances in chloride or magnesium levels may contribute to potassium imbalance and will need to be corrected before correcting the potassium problem.

(3) Gastrointestinal losses of potassium are exacerbated by accompanying volume depletion and subsequent increased aldosterone effects.

(4) If the etiology of hypokalemia is unclear from the history, a urine potassium level may aid in distinguishing between renal and nonrenal losses.

(5) Transcellular shifts of potassium occur in an effort to maintain electrical neutrality in varying conditions. In metabolic acidosis, potassium shifts out of the cell in exchange for intracellular buffering of H^+. The opposite exchange occurs to a lesser degree in metabolic alkalosis. These shifts also occur in acid-base disturbances that are primarily respiratory, although to a lesser degree.

(6) Insulin, catecholamines, and β-agonists (albuterol) shift potassium intracellularly acutely.

(7) Potassium uptake by rapidly forming new red blood cells and platelets in the treatment of megaloblastic anemia can result in hypokalemia. Similarly, transfusion of frozen, washed red blood cells (not stored in acid-citrate-dextran) may lower potassium levels because of increased cellular uptake.

(8) Rarely, episodic weakness or paralysis can occur due to transient changes in potassium levels. In the hypokalemic version, triggers such as exercise, stress, or β₂-agonists, or eating a heavy meal cause a sudden intracellular shift of potassium. Barium poisoning from foods, not radiologic barium, can cause a similar paralysis. In the hyperkalemic version, symptoms follow rest after exercise or ingestion of potassium. Both are autosomal dominant disorders.

(9) Chronic clay ingestion contributes to hypokalemia by binding dietary potassium. Nutritional potassium deficiency is otherwise uncommon in patients with normal diets.

(10) Gentamicin, amphotericin B, and chemotherapeutic agents can damage renal tubules, resulting in potassium wasting. Hypercalcemic states also induce renal damage.

(11) Glycyrrhizic acid is a component of natural licorice, rarely used today, which can exert a mineralocorticoid effect. Many infants with Cushing syndrome may have tumors of the adrenal cortex, which result in overproduction of aldosterone as well as cortisol and other corticosteroids.

(12) Increased excretion of cations (K^+, H^+) accompanies excretion of nonreabsorbable anions as a means of maintaining electrical neutrality.

(13) Bartter syndrome is characterized by hypokalemia secondary to renal losses, normal blood pressure, and vascular insensitivity to pressor agents. Renin and aldosterone levels are elevated. Clinical manifestations include growth failure, weakness, constipation, polyuria, and dehydration. Gitelman and Liddle syndromes are other rare primary hypokalemic tubulopathies.

BIBLIOGRAPHY

Brem AS: Disorders of potassium homeostasis. Pediatr Clin North Am 37:419–427, 1990.

Watkins SL: Disorders of potassium balance. Pediatr Ann 24:31, 1995.

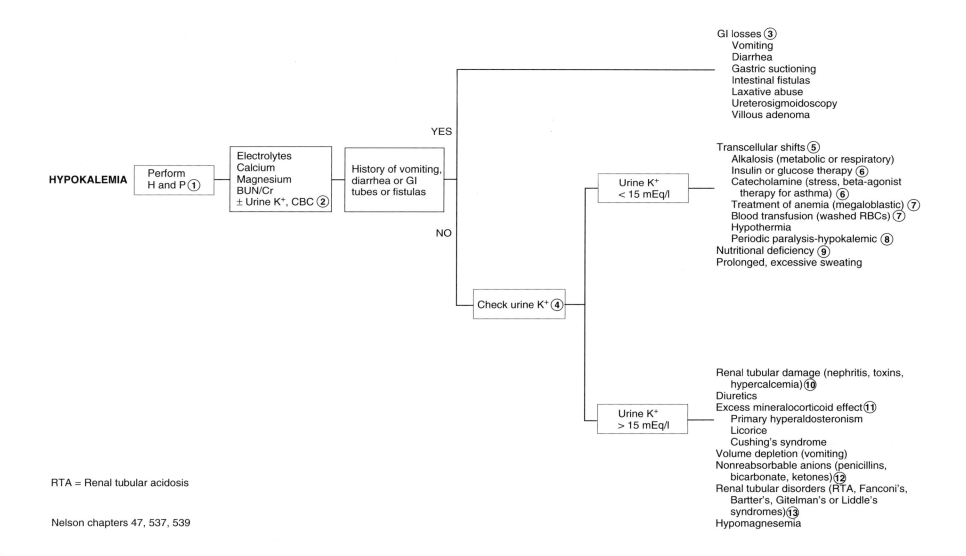

HYPOKALEMIA → Perform H and P ① → Electrolytes / Calcium / Magnesium / BUN/Cr / ± Urine K⁺, CBC ② → History of vomiting, diarrhea or GI tubes or fistulas

YES

GI losses ③
- Vomiting
- Diarrhea
- Gastric suctioning
- Intestinal fistulas
- Laxative abuse
- Ureterosigmoidoscopy
- Villous adenoma

NO → Check urine K⁺ ④

Urine K⁺ < 15 mEq/l

Transcellular shifts ⑤
- Alkalosis (metabolic or respiratory)
- Insulin or glucose therapy ⑥
- Catecholamine (stress, beta-agonist therapy for asthma) ⑥
- Treatment of anemia (megaloblastic) ⑦
- Blood transfusion (washed RBCs) ⑦
- Hypothermia
- Periodic paralysis-hypokalemic ⑧
Nutritional deficiency ⑨
Prolonged, excessive sweating

Urine K⁺ > 15 mEq/l

Renal tubular damage (nephritis, toxins, hypercalcemia) ⑩
Diuretics
Excess mineralocorticoid effect ⑪
- Primary hyperaldosteronism
- Licorice
- Cushing's syndrome
Volume depletion (vomiting)
Nonreabsorbable anions (penicillins, bicarbonate, ketones) ⑫
Renal tubular disorders (RTA, Fanconi's, Bartter's, Gitelman's or Liddle's syndromes) ⑬
Hypomagnesemia

RTA = Renal tubular acidosis

Nelson chapters 47, 537, 539

Chapter 87 *Hyperkalemia*

Potassium is the main cation of the intracellular fluid (ICF) compartment. The extracellular fluid (ECF) concentration is carefully regulated to maintain a value around 4 mEq/l. Potassium (K^+) plays a critical role in the excitability of nerve and muscle cells and contractility of muscles (smooth, skeletal, cardiac). Aldosterone normally regulates renal excretion of potassium. Aldosterone also causes sodium reabsorption and H^+ secretion in the distal tubule. Aldosterone similarly affects potassium excretion in the stool. Hyperkalemia is defined as a serum potassium concentration > 5.5 mEq/l.

(1) The history should inquire about medications, underlying medical problems, and diets, including the use of salt substitutes and pica. Hyperkalemia may manifest with muscle weakness, as well as tingling, paresthesias, and paralysis. EKG changes include narrow peaked T waves and shortened QT interval initially. At higher serum potassium levels, delayed depolarization results in a widened QRS and P wave that may precede more serious arrhythmias (e.g., ventricular fibrillation, asystole).

(2) Increased intake of potassium is a rare cause of hyperkalemia in children with normal renal function. Salt substitutes may be a cause.

(3) Acute or chronic renal disorders may be responsible for impaired excretion of potassium.

(4) Type IV renal tubular acidosis (RTA) is characterized by a deficiency of aldosterone. Pseudohypoaldosteronism is a subtype of type IV RTA that is characterized by high levels of aldosterone but an impaired distal tubular response to it.

(5) Trauma, use of cytotoxic agents, massive hemolysis, rhabdomyolysis, and, to a lesser extent, intense exercise can release potassium due to tissue breakdown.

(6) Transcellular shifts of potassium occur in an effort to maintain electrical neutrality in varying conditions. In metabolic acidosis, potassium shifts out of the cell in exchange for intracellular buffering of H^+. The opposite exchange occurs to a lesser degree in metabolic alkalosis. These shifts also occur in acid-base disturbances that are primarily respiratory, although to a lesser degree.

(7) Potassium accompanies the osmotic shift of water from ICF to ECF in hypertonic states.

(8) Rarely, episodic weakness or paralysis can occur due to transient changes in potassium levels. In the hyperkalemic version, symptoms follow rest after exercise or ingestion of potassium. In the hypokalemic version, triggers such as exercise, stress, β_2-agonists, or a heavy meal cause a sudden intracellular shift of potassium. Barium poisoning from foods, not radiologic barium, can cause a similar paralysis. Both are autosomal dominant disorders.

BIBLIOGRAPHY

Brem AS: Disorders of potassium homeostasis. Pediatr Clin North Am 37:419–427, 1990.
Watkins SL: Disorders of potassium balance. Pediatr Ann 24:31, 1995.

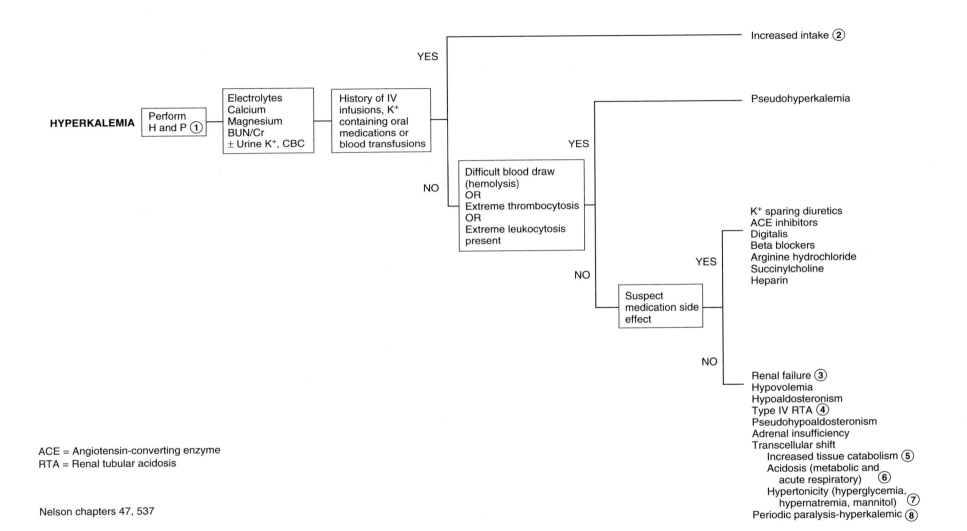

HYPERKALEMIA

Perform H and P ①

Electrolytes
Calcium
Magnesium
BUN/Cr
± Urine K^+, CBC

History of IV infusions, K^+ containing oral medications or blood transfusions

YES — Increased intake ②

NO

Difficult blood draw (hemolysis)
OR
Extreme thrombocytosis
OR
Extreme leukocytosis present

YES — Pseudohyperkalemia

NO

Suspect medication side effect

YES
K^+ sparing diuretics
ACE inhibitors
Digitalis
Beta blockers
Arginine hydrochloride
Succinylcholine
Heparin

NO
Renal failure ③
Hypovolemia
Hypoaldosteronism
Type IV RTA ④
Pseudohypoaldosteronism
Adrenal insufficiency
Transcellular shift
    Increased tissue catabolism ⑤
    Acidosis (metabolic and acute respiratory) ⑥
    Hypertonicity (hyperglycemia, hypernatremia, mannitol) ⑦
    Periodic paralysis-hyperkalemic ⑧

ACE = Angiotensin-converting enzyme
RTA = Renal tubular acidosis

Nelson chapters 47, 537

Serum calcium concentration in the extracellular fluid (ECF) is maintained by parathyroid hormone (PTH), which acts on the kidneys and bones, and by 1,25-dihydroxyvitamin D, which acts on the intestines and bones. About 50% of the calcium is in the biologically important ionized form, 40% is protein bound (i.e., mainly albumin), and 10% is complexed to anions (e.g., bicarbonate, citrate, sulfate, phosphate, and lactate). Mild hypocalcemia is usually asymptomatic. Symptoms and signs of more severe hypocalcemia include paresthesias of the extremities, Chvostek sign, Trousseau sign, muscle cramps or spasm, laryngospasm, tetany, and seizures. Cardiac manifestations include a prolonged QT interval, which may progress to heart block.

(1) Calcium levels are affected by serum albumin levels and by pH. A low serum albumin will lower the total serum calcium, and acidic pH will decrease protein binding and increase ionized calcium levels. It is important to obtain an ionized calcium level. If this test is not available, in order to correct for hypoalbuminemia, 0.2 mmol/l (0.8 mg/dl) of calcium must be added to the total calcium level for each 1 g/dl decrease in serum albumin from the normal 4.0 g/dl. Similarly, for each 0.1 decrease in pH ionized calcium rises by 0.05 mmol/L. However, these corrections are a poor substitute for ionized calcium level.

(2) Hypoalbuminemic states result in a lower serum calcium level. The ionized calcium that is the biologically important level is usually normal, but it should be confirmed. Causes include liver disease, protein-losing enteropathy, and nephrotic syndrome.

(3) Endotoxic shock is associated with hypocalcemia, although the mechanism is unknown. Hypocalcemia may also occur with rapid correction or overcorrection of acidosis.

(4) Aplasia or hypoplasia of the parathyroid glands is often associated with DiGeorge/velocardiofacial syndrome. Many of the children have transient neonatal hypocalcemia; however, the hypocalcemia may recur later in life. Associated anomalies include conotruncal heart defects, velopharyngeal insufficiency, cleft palate, renal anomalies, and partial to complete aplasia of the thymus with varying severities of immunodeficiency.

(5) Surgical hypoparathyroidism is a complication of thyroidectomy. This may occur even when the glands were identified and left undisturbed.

(6) Autoimmune hypoparathyroidism is usually associated with other autoimmune disorders such as Addison disease and chronic mucocutaneous candidiasis. Other associations, including vitiligo, alopecia areata, pernicious anemia, and malabsorption may not appear until adulthood. Parathyroid antibodies are present.

(7) Maternal hyperparathyroidism during pregnancy may cause a transient neonatal hypocalcemia. It may persist for weeks or months. Symptoms such as tetany may be delayed, especially in breast-fed infants.

(8) Vitamin D deficiency occurs in dark-skinned breast-fed infants who live in areas with less sunlight. It may also occur in infants fed with unfortified cow's milk. Inadequate exposure to ultraviolet light particularly in dark-skinned children may also cause vitamin D deficiency. Inadequate absorption of vitamin D or calcium may be seen in diseases such as celiac disease, liver disease including biliary cirrhosis, and cystic fibrosis. Phenobarbital and phenytoin interfere with metabolism of vitamin D. Renal failure also decreases vitamin D synthesis. Clinical manifestations of vitamin D deficiency include rickets, which occurs as a result of the body's attempt to maintain serum calcium levels.

(9) Vitamin D–dependent rickets (vitamin D–resistant rickets) type I usually presents between the ages of 3 to 6 months in children receiving adequate quantities of vitamin D. This is believed to be caused by decreased activity of the enzyme 25-hydroxy-1α-hydroxylase, resulting in decreased serum levels of 1,25-dihydroxyvitamin D. Alkaline phosphatase and PTH are increased, and serum phosphorus is low.

(10) In pseudohypoparathyroidism (i.e., Albright hereditary osteodystrophy), the parathyroid glands are normal or even hyperplastic. PTH levels are normal or elevated; however, there is a peripheral resistance to PTH. This syndrome is associated with tetany and a distinctive phenotype with brachydactyly, skeletal abnormalities, short stature, and mild mental retardation.

(11) Hyperphosphatemia may be associated with renal failure. It can occur secondary to rapid cell destruction due to chemotherapy (i.e., tumor-lysis syndrome). Trauma leading to rhabdomyolysis causes release of cellular phosphorus. Hyperphosphatemia may also result from exogenous phosphate in the form of laxatives and enemas.

(12) Pancreatitis causes release of pancreatic lipase, resulting in degradation of omental fat and binding of calcium in the peritoneum.

(13) "Hungry bone" syndrome may occur during initial therapy to correct chronic hyperparathyroidism, leading to a sudden fall in phosphorus and calcium levels. Calcium and phosphorus are rapidly absorbed into severely demineralized bones.

(14) Vitamin D–dependent rickets (type II) is a hereditary disorder due a receptor defect, resulting in hypocalcemia despite elevated levels of 1,25-dihydroxyvitamin D.

(15) Hypocalcemia may also occur with alkalosis or rapid correction or overcorrection of acidosis.

(16) Hypomagnesemia often coexists with hypocalcemia and may be due to decreased absorption (e.g., in malabsorption syndromes) or intake. Familial hypomagnesemia with secondary hypocalcemia usually appears between the second and sixth weeks of life. Aminoglycoside therapy may cause increased urinary losses of magnesium. PTH may be normal or decreased.

BIBLIOGRAPHY

Bushinsky DA, Monk RD: Calcium. Lancet 352:306–311, 1998.
Fouser L: Disorders of calcium, phosphorus, and magnesium. Pediatr Ann 24:38–46, 1995.

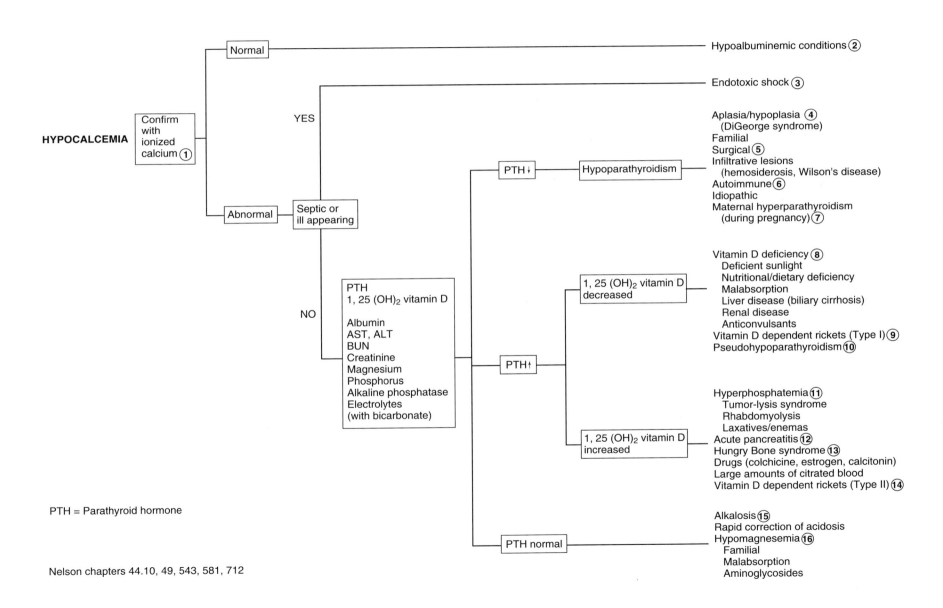

PTH = Parathyroid hormone

Nelson chapters 44.10, 49, 543, 581, 712

Chapter 89 Hypercalcemia

Serum calcium concentration in the extracellular fluid (ECF) is maintained by parathyroid hormone (PTH) and by 1,25-dihydroxyvitamin D. PTH acts on the kidneys and bones and stimulates the production of 1,25-dihydroxyvitamin D, which acts on the intestines and bones. About 50% of the calcium is in the biologically important ionized form, 40% is protein bound (mainly albumin), and 10% is complexed to anions (bicarbonate, citrate, sulfate, phosphate, and lactate). Calcium levels are affected by serum albumin levels and by pH. An elevated serum albumin concentration will appear to raise the total serum calcium concentration; an alkaline pH will increase protein binding and decrease ionized calcium levels. It is important to obtain an ionized calcium level.

Mild hypercalcemia is usually asymptomatic. With more severe hypercalcemia there may be neurologic features, ranging from drowsiness to depression, stupor, and coma. Gastrointestinal manifestations such as constipation, nausea, vomiting, anorexia, and ulcers may occur. Hypercalciuria leads to nephrogenic diabetes insipidus, resulting in polyuria. Other renal effects of hypercalcemia include nephrolithiasis and nephrocalcinosis.

(1) Primary hyperparathyroidism is caused by excessive production of PTH, owing to adenoma or hyperplasia. Incidence may be sporadic or may occur as part of the multiple endocrine neoplasia (MEN) syndromes, with involvement of the pancreas and the anterior pituitary. Hyperparathyroidism–jaw tumor syndrome is characterized by parathyroid adenomas and fibroosseous jaw tumors. Patients may also have polycystic kidney disease, renal hamartomas, and Wilms tumor.

(2) Secondary hyperparathyroidism is increased production of PTH in response to hypocalcemia, as in chronic renal failure. If this persists for a prolonged period, the glands begin to autonomously produce PTH even after the underlying reason for the hypocalcemia has been corrected, as after renal transplant. This is known as tertiary hyperparathyroidism and results in hypercalcemia.

(3) Hypercalcemia may occur in association with malignancies (e.g., neuroblastoma, leukemia, renal tumors). This may be due to ectopic production of PTH; however, ectopic production of PTH-related peptide (PTHrP) is more common.

(4) Ten percent of children with Williams syndrome have hypercalcemia. The cause is unknown. Features of the syndrome include feeding difficulties, elfin facies, growth delay, gregarious personality, supravalvular aortic stenosis, renovascular disease, and developmental delay.

(5) In familial hypocalciuric hypercalcemia (familial benign hypercalcemia), the patients are usually asymptomatic and the PTH levels are inappropriately normal. The calcium to creatinine clearance ratio is decreased in spite of the hypercalcemia.

(6) Idiopathic hypercalcemia of infancy manifests during the first year of life with failure to thrive and hypercalcemia. There is increased absorption of calcium. Levels of 1,25-dihydroxyvitamin D may be normal or elevated. PTH and phosphorus levels are normal.

(7) Ectopic production of vitamin D may occur with granulomatous disease, such as sarcoidosis (30%–50%) and tuberculosis. It may rarely occur with tumors. The excessive 1,25-dihydroxyvitamin D suppresses the production of PTH.

(8) Hypervitaminosis A results in excessive bone resorption. Thiazide diuretics cause increased renal calcium reabsorption. Milk-alkali syndrome is caused by the consumption of large amounts of calcium containing nonabsorbable antacids, leading to hypercalcemia, alkalemia, nephrocalcinosis, and renal insufficiency.

(9) Malignancy may cause hypercalcemia secondary to bone destruction. In thyrotoxicosis the PTH is suppressed. Hypercalcemia is due to excessive bone resorption caused by the thyroid hormone. Patients undergoing dialysis may develop hypercalcemia, especially if they receive calcium supplements or are dialyzed against a high calcium bath.

(10) Jansen-type metaphyseal chondrodysplasia is a rare genetic disorder with features of short-limbed dwarfism. Circulating levels of PTH and PTHrP are undetectable. The hypercalcemia is severe but asymptomatic.

BIBLIOGRAPHY

Bushinsky DA, Monk RD: Calcium. Lancet 352:306–311, 1998.
Fouser L: Disorders of calcium, phosphorus, and magnesium. Pediatr Ann 24:38–46, 1995.

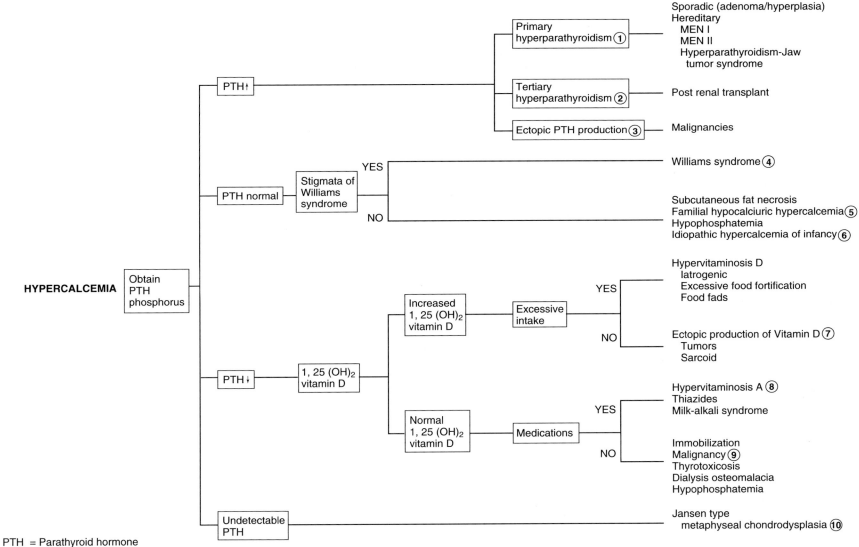

HYPERCALCEMIA — Obtain PTH phosphorus

PTH↑
- Primary hyperparathyroidism ①
  - Sporadic (adenoma/hyperplasia)
  - Hereditary
    - MEN I
    - MEN II
    - Hyperparathyroidism-Jaw tumor syndrome
- Tertiary hyperparathyroidism ②
  - Post renal transplant
- Ectopic PTH production ③
  - Malignancies

PTH normal — Stigmata of Williams syndrome
- YES → Williams syndrome ④
- NO → Subcutaneous fat necrosis / Familial hypocalciuric hypercalcemia ⑤ / Hypophosphatemia / Idiopathic hypercalcemia of infancy ⑥

PTH↓ — 1, 25 (OH)$_2$ vitamin D
- Increased 1, 25 (OH)$_2$ vitamin D — Excessive intake
  - YES → Hypervitaminosis D / Iatrogenic / Excessive food fortification / Food fads
  - NO → Ectopic production of Vitamin D ⑦ / Tumors / Sarcoid
- Normal 1, 25 (OH)$_2$ vitamin D — Medications
  - YES → Hypervitaminosis A ⑧ / Thiazides / Milk-alkali syndrome
  - NO → Immobilization / Malignancy ⑨ / Thyrotoxicosis / Dialysis osteomalacia / Hypophosphatemia

Undetectable PTH → Jansen type metaphyseal chondrodysplasia ⑩

PTH = Parathyroid hormone
MEN = Multiple endocrine neoplasia

Nelson chapters 44.10, 49, 543, 581, 712

INDEX

Note: Page numbers followed by the letter f refer to algorithm figures.